Orthodontic Treatment Protocols

by

Dr. Ivelina Koycheva

First edition
2020

https://StudyOrthodontics.com/

Editor: Velin Koychev;
Design: Stanislav Petkanov;

ISBN 978-619-91640-0-6

Content

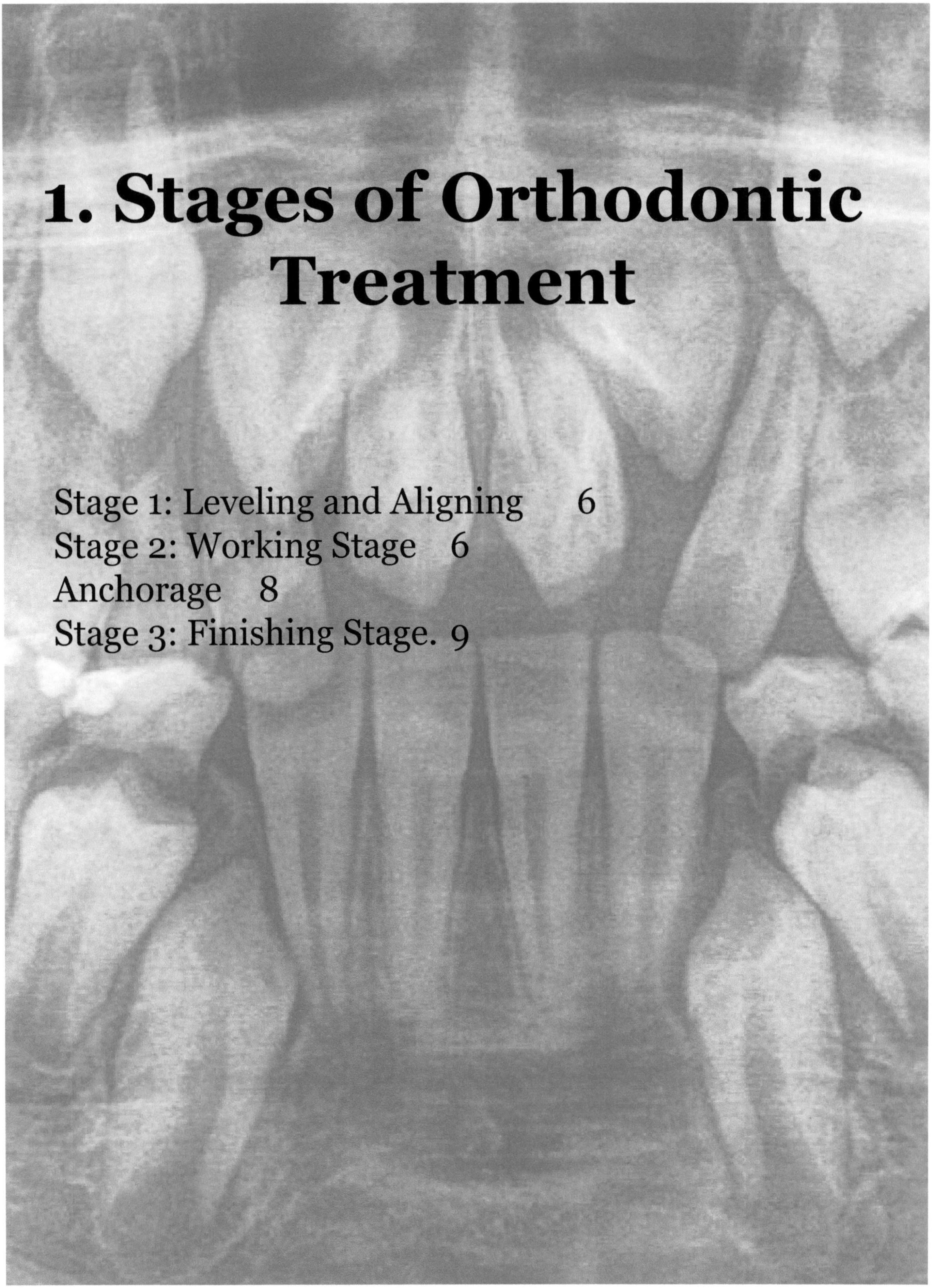

1. Stages of Orthodontic Treatment

Treatment with the Straight Wire Appliance can be divided into three stages:
Stage 1: Leveling and alignment;
Stage 2: Working stage;
Stage 3: Finishing stage.

Stage 1: Leveling and Aligning

- Leveling and aligning is a complex process in which all the crowns are moving at the same time and in different directions;
- All teeth should be engaged from the beginning to obtain maximum efficiency of tooth movement;
- Usually, at this stage, round small-diameter NiTi wires such as a 0.012-inch for severe crowding or a 0.014-inch for moderate to minimum crowding are preferred;
- These round wires can be in place for as long as 8 to 12 weeks;
- Next wire usually is a 0.018-inch NiTi for arch development and expansion;
    - It corrects most of the rotations left by the previously used round wires;
    - Provides more stiffness to start leveling the curve of Spee and therefore flatten the occlusal plane.
- Next wire in use is the rectangular 0.016 x 0.016-inch or 0.016x 0.022-inch NiTi which starts tipping and torque control, and continue arch development a flattening the curve of Spee;
- Next two wires are used for torque control - 0.017x 0.025 -inch and 0.019x 0.025-inch NiTi;
- Evaluate bracket placement and debond/rebond as necessary.

a b

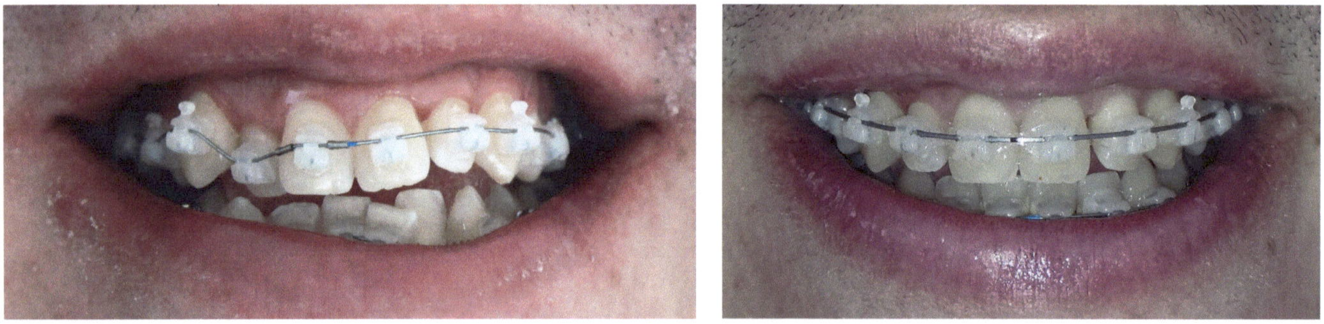

Figure 1.1 Levelling and aligning with small diameter round wires (a) and rectangular wires (b)

Stage 2: Working Stage

This stage of treatment is the one on which we will spend more time. At this stage, the maxillary and mandibular arches are coordinated, proper overbite and overjet are achieved, Class II or Class III are corrected, maxillary and mandibular midlines are aligned, extraction spaces are closed, and maxillary and mandibular occlusal planes are paralleled. Most of these corrections happen simultaneously.

- **Arch Coordination** (*Figure 1.2*)
    - The palatal cusps of the maxillary molars should intercuspate with the fossae and marginal ridges of mandibular molars;
    - The buccal cusp of the mandibular premolars should intercuspate with the marginal ridges of the maxillary premolars;
    - The mandibular canines and incisors should occlude with marginal ridges of the maxillary canines and incisors;
    - Overjet should be of 2 to 3 mm all around the arch from second molar to second molar;

- The maxillary archwire must be 2 to 3 mm wider than the mandibular archwire;
- The archwire coordination is done with stainless steel wire;
- The maxillary teeth should be upright and centered in the alveolar/basal bone and coordinated with the mandibular teeth, which should also be upright and centered in the alveolar/basal bone to obtain a proper intercuspation.

- **Overbite and Overjet Correction.**

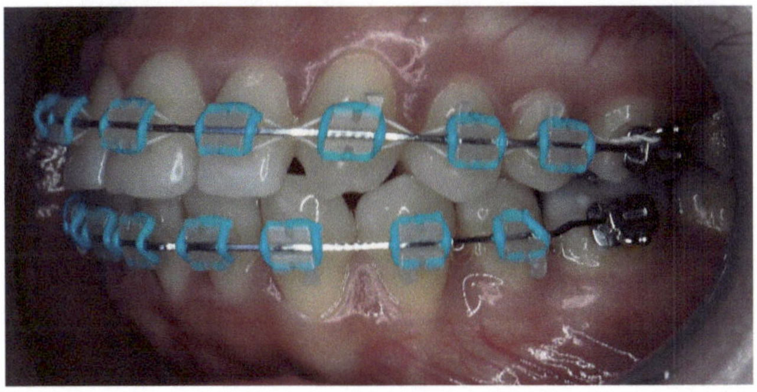

Figure 1.2 Arch coordination phase.

An optimal overbite/overjet relationship does not have to be a certain predetermined number of millimeters. More important is the functional relationship they have.

- Optimal overbite is usually around 4 mm and an optimal overjet is 2 to 3 mm;
- According to contemporary aesthetic trends and taking into account the aging process, for adolescents and young adults, maxillary incisors should have, at rest, an exposure of about 4 mm beyond the most inferior point of the upper lip known as upper stomion;
- The incisal edge of the lower incisors should be at the same level as the most inferior point of the upper lip.

- **Closing Extraction Spaces.** (*Figure 1.3*)

Usually, after leveling and aligning, the extraction spaces left are smaller than at the beginning of treatment because some of the space has been taken to unravel the initial crowding and to upright the maxillary and mandibular incisors.

- The maxillary and mandibular occlusal planes should be flat or almost flat;
- The six anterior teeth should be consolidated into one unit;
- Then we need to determine the anchorage requirement;
- The anchorage requirement can be minimum, medium, or maximum;
- Wires used at this stage are stainless steel and can be either 0.019 × 0.025 inch SS or 0.021 × 0.025 inch SS, depending on the anchorage situation.

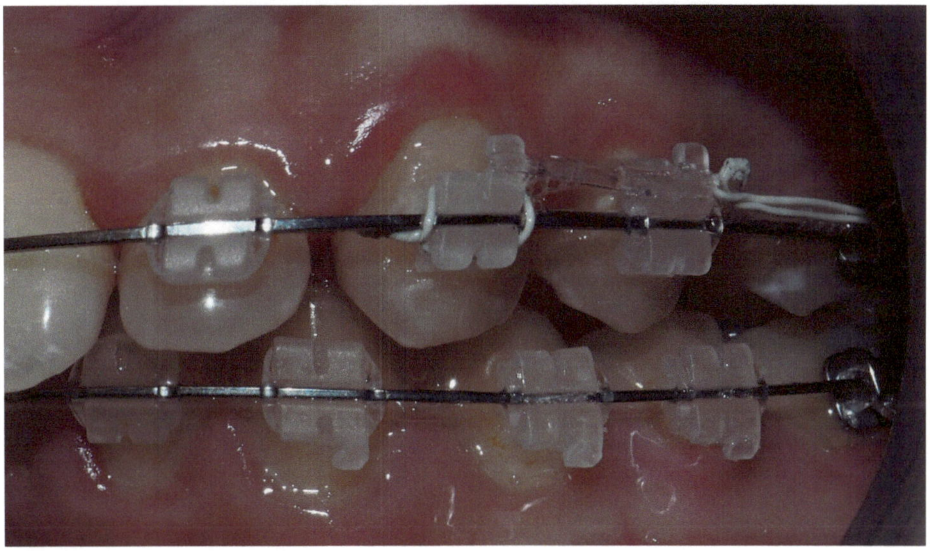

Figure 1.3 Closing extraction spaces with the use of retroligatures.

Anchorage

- **Minimum Anchorage.**

On a minimum anchorage situation, molars will be moved mesially to close the remaining extraction spaces. (*Figure 1.4*)

  - We use a 0.021 × 0.025 inch SS wire to express the buccal crown torque of the maxillary incisors and the mesial tip of the canines. In the mandible, this wire will express the mesial tip of the canine. This situation will increase the anchorage in the anterior part of the mouth because it would be more difficult to retract or even tip back the anterior teeth while moving the molars forward;
  - We can reduce the size of the wire in the posterior part, specifically the edges, in order to decrease the anchorage of the posterior teeth;
  - The force must be applied from the first molars;
  - After the first molar has been moved forward as desired, the second molar can be activated and moved forward, too. Often the second molars will travel forward as we move the first molars and then the space remaining between the first and second molars will be very small and easily closed with an elastomeric chain.

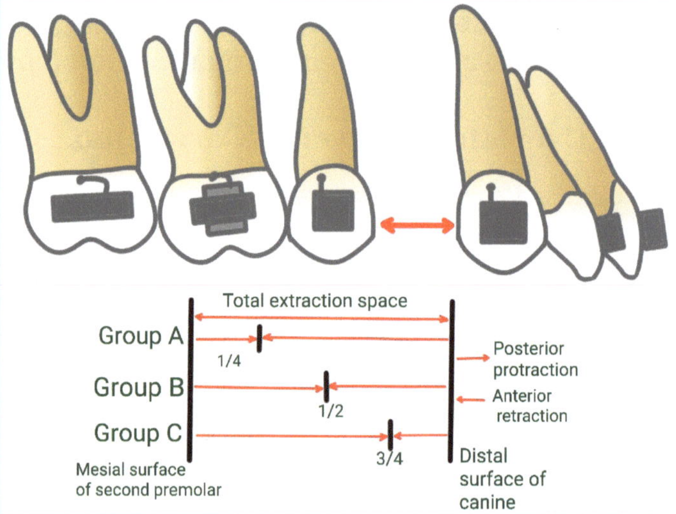

Figure 1.4 Types of anchorage

- **Moderate Anchorage.**

This is the most common anchorage situation we will encounter in our cases. Moderate anchorage means that the remaining spaces should be closed reciprocally.

  - For this situation, we use a 0.019 × 0.025 inch SS wire;
  - The activation is done from the first molar.

- **Maximum Anchorage.**

In a maximum anchorage situation, most of the remaining space left after leveling and aligning is closed due to the distal movement of the anterior teeth.

  - We use a 0.019 × 0.025 inch SS wire;
  - The force is activated from the second molars;
  - Auxiliaries to enhance posterior anchorage such as TADs, or extraoral force (headgear) can be used as needed.

- **Intermaxillary elastics.**

We use them, but it is important to understand how they are used to avoid problems. We do not use intermaxillary elastics in the following situations:

  - Round wires;
  - Initial leveling and aligning;

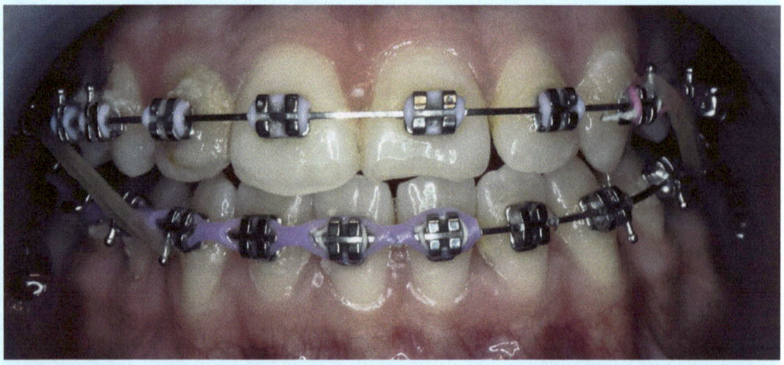

Figure 1.5 Use of intermaxillary elastics for anchorage during space closure. Class III elastics on patient right and class II elastics on patient left.

- Low-deflection wires;
- To a terminal tooth, the last tooth in the arch;
- In the anterior part of the mouth to close open bites;
- For an extended period of time.

We use intermaxillary elastics in the following situations:

- At the working and finishing stages *(Figure 1.5)*
- On square or rectangular stainless steel wires;
- On the buccal side of the mouth, short Class II or III and/or triangular verticals.

Stage 3: Finishing Stage.

At this stage, the goal is to place each tooth on its ideal position and flatten the occlusal plane, full bracket expression is desired.

- Larger wires such as a 0.021 × 0.025-inch stainless steel or a 0.022 × 0.028-inch stainless steel are required;
- We could use minor wire bends for repositioning;
- With a thin articular paper, all contacts must be checked.;
- Only tooth-tooth contacts should be allowed;
- All brackets, tubes, or bands' contacts must be removed to allow proper settling.
- Vertical triangular 3/16-inch elastics, either 6 oz or 8 oz, are used to achieve proper intercuspation.

a b

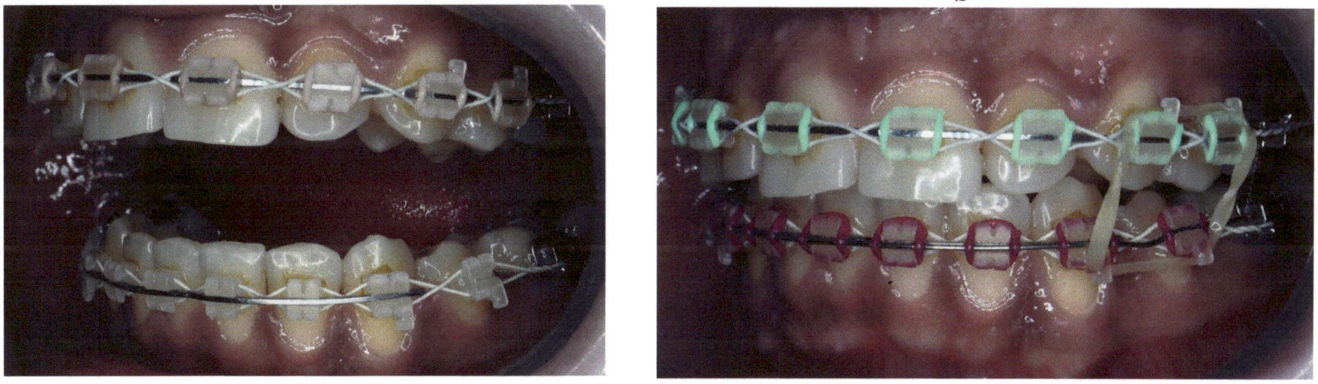

Figure 1.6 Finishing the orthodontic case. The main archwire is cut at the canine level (a). An additional small diameter round archwire is placed. Vertical elastics are used to help settling (b).

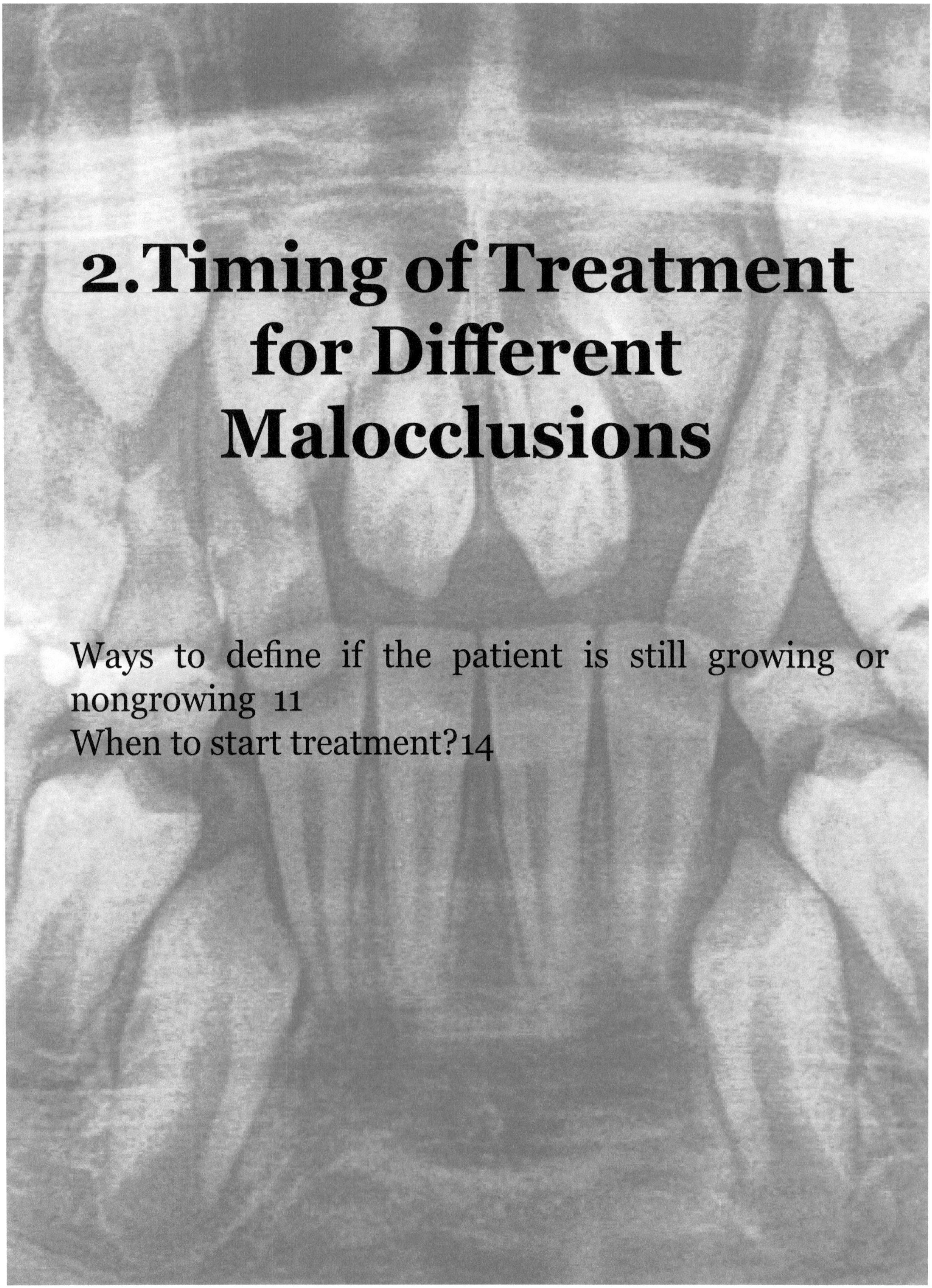

2.Timing of Treatment for Different Malocclusions

The timing of treatment is an important factor in planning and should be considered according to the malocclusion.

Ways to define if the patient is still growing or nongrowing

- Determining the skeletal maturational level of the patient;
- Chronological age;
- Dental age;
- Resent body growth described by the parents.

In some instances, it is desirable to treat the patient at the time when the patient is growing rapidly, as during the circumpubertal growth period, when functional jaw orthopedics has been shown to be particularly effective. In other circumstances, we would like to know if a patient has reached his or her growth potential, as in planning corrective jaw surgery or the placement of implants, so that substantial further growth is not anticipated or desired. We also would like to know if a patient is early in the growth process and would respond skeletally rather than dentally to forces placed against the maxillary sutural system (e.g., RME, facial mask therapy).

Use chronologic age as an indicator.

- It is one of the most inaccurate ways of determining a patient's maturational level;
- It is well known that females mature faster than males on average by at least a year.

Using the stage of dental eruption and development.

- It is more accurate than using chronologic age;
- It is expected to have the pubertal growth spurt by the time of the eruption of the second premolars or second molars;
- After the eruption of the second molars, growth potential is expected to be minimal.

The cervical vertebral maturation (CVM) method

This method has been available since the early 1970s.

- There are six stages of cervical maturation in all, as is shown diagrammatically in *Figure 2.1*

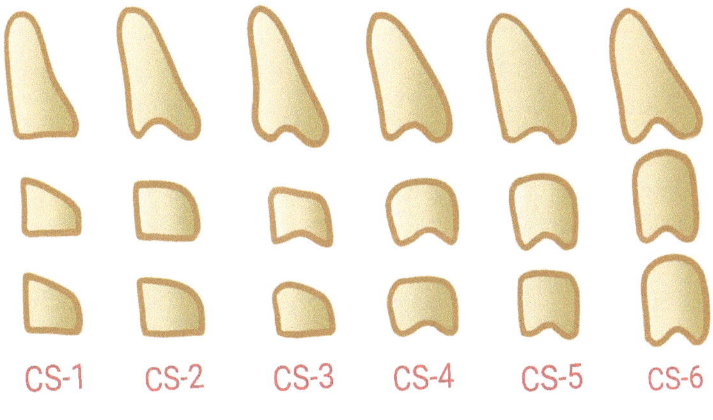

Figure 2.1 Cervical vertebral maturation (CVM)

- Using the lateral headfilm, only the bodies of the second, third, and fourth cervical vertebrae (C2, C3, and C4) are considered;
- Two morphologic characteristics are monitored;
- The presence or absence of a notch or indentation on the inferior border of each of the three vertebral bodies;
- The shape of the third and fourth cervical bodies, which vary from trapezoid to rectangular horizontal to square to rectangular vertical;
- The first three stages are differentiated by the presence or absence of the notch.

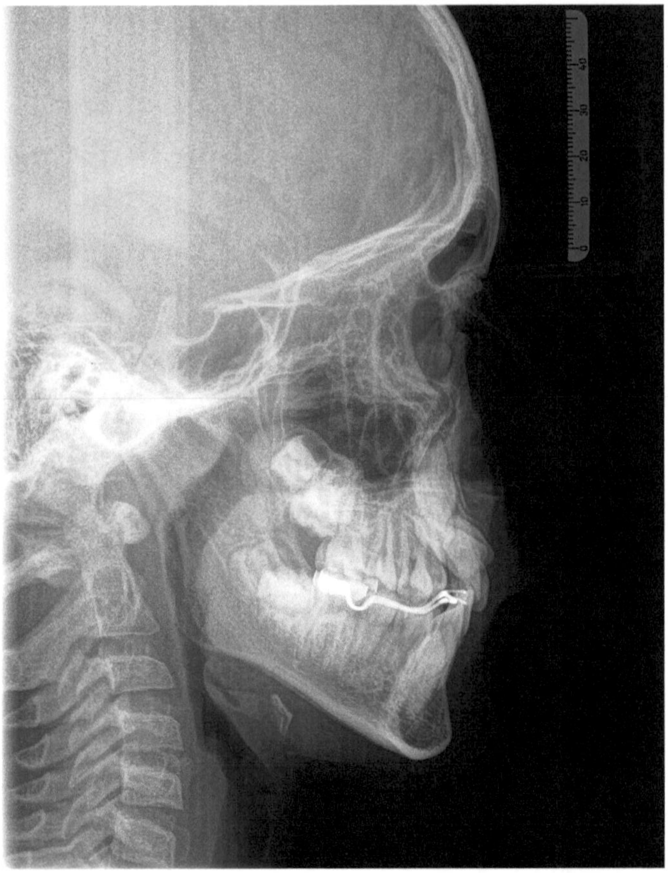

Figure 2.2

First cervical stage (CS-1), *Figure 2.2*

- The inferior borders of vertebral bodies 2 to 4 are flat (or sometimes slightly convex);
- The notch must be at least 1 mm in depth at the center in comparison with the anterior and posterior aspects of the inferior border of the body;
- The third and fourth cervical bodies are trapezoidal in morphology, assuming the shape of a wedge or "ski jump," with the posterior border of the vertebral body taller than the anterior border and the superior surface sloping forward and downward;
- This stage occurs from approximately the time of the eruption of the deciduous dentition until about 2 years before the peak in skeletal growth;
- The ideal age to intervene with facial mask (FM) therapy combined with RME is at CS-1.

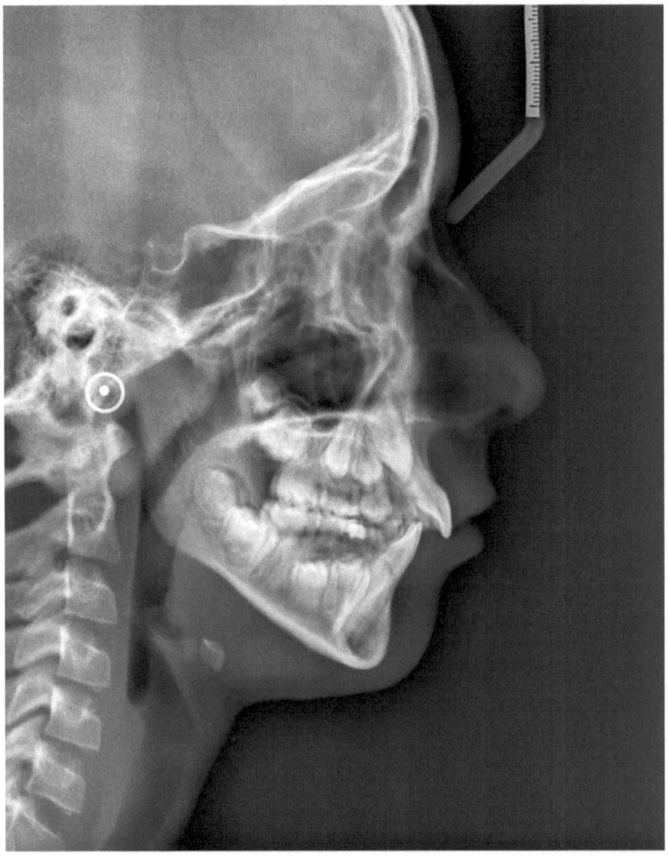

Figure 2.3

The second cervical stage (CS-2) *Figure 2.3*

- It is characterized by a notch present along the inferior border of the second cervical vertebra (odontoid process);
- The lower borders of the third and fourth vertebral bodies remain flat;
- Usually, both C3 and C4 retain a trapezoidal shape;
- CS-2 can be termed the "get-ready" stage because the peak interval will begin about 1 year after this stage is evident.

The third cervical stage (CS-3) *Figure 2.4*

- It is characterized by notching of the inferior borders of C2 and C3. C4 remains flat;
- At least one of C3 and C4 bodies still retains a trapezoidal shape while the other can assume a more rectangular horizontal shape;
- At this stage, the maximum craniofacial growth velocity is anticipated.

The fourth cervical stage (CS-4) *Figure 2.5*

- All three bodies have notches along their inferior bodies, so the more important factor is the shape of C3 and C4 ;
- At this stage, both vertebral bodies have a rectangular horizontal rather than a trapezoidal shape;
- During this stage continued craniofacial growth can be anticipated, but at a lesser rate than is seen at CS-3.

The fifth cervical stage (CS-5) *Figure 2.6*

- It can be differentiated from CS-4 based on the shapes of C3 and C4, with these bodies becoming square in shape;
- All three cervical bodies have notches;
- It is called the “marshmallow” stage;
- When this stage is reached, most substantial craniofacial growth has been achieved.

The sixed cervical stage (CS-6) *Figure 2.7*

- At least one of the third and fourth cervical bodies has assumed a rectangular vertical morphology;
- Anyone over the age of 20 years presumably would be at CS-6.

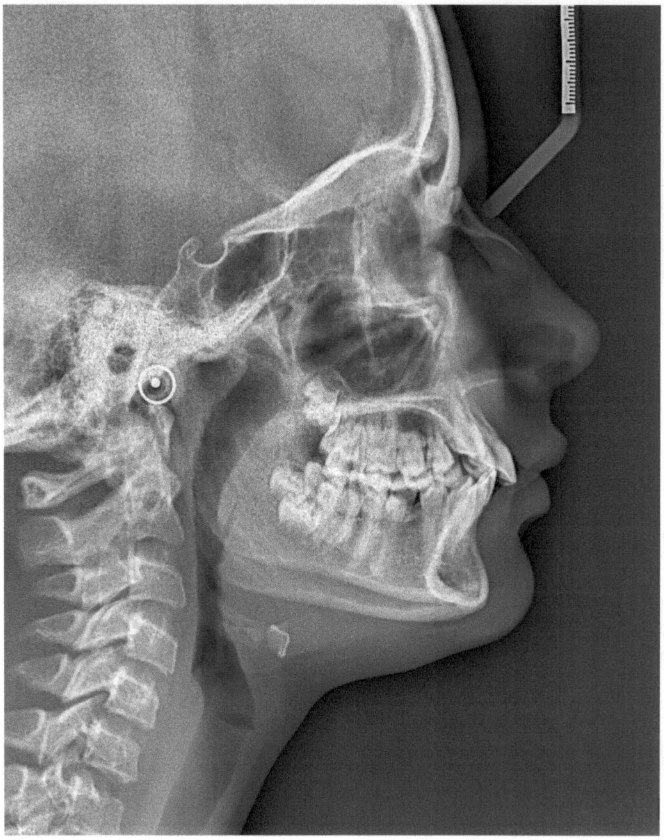

Figure 2.4

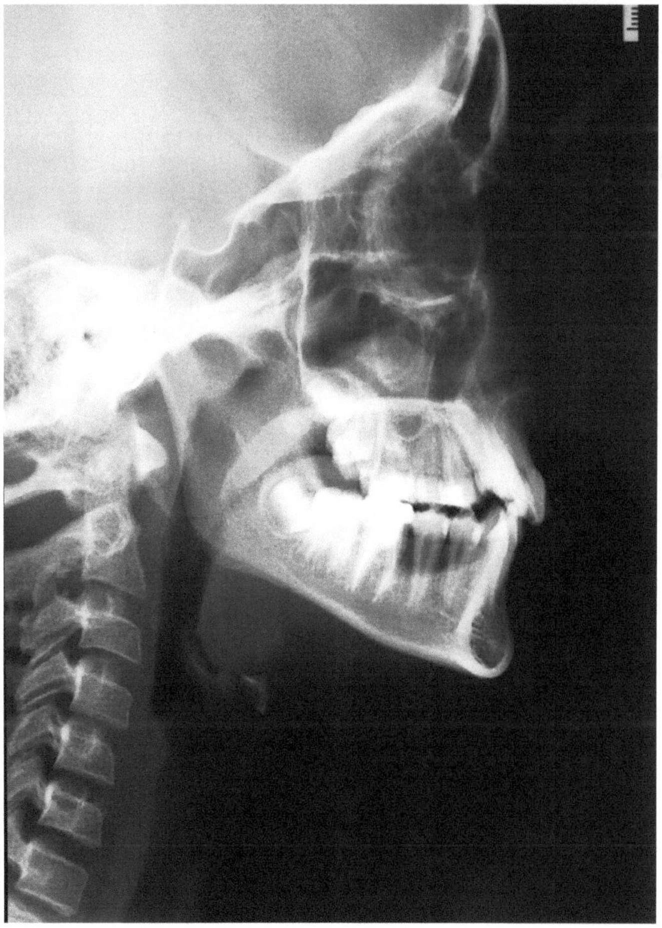

Figure 2.5

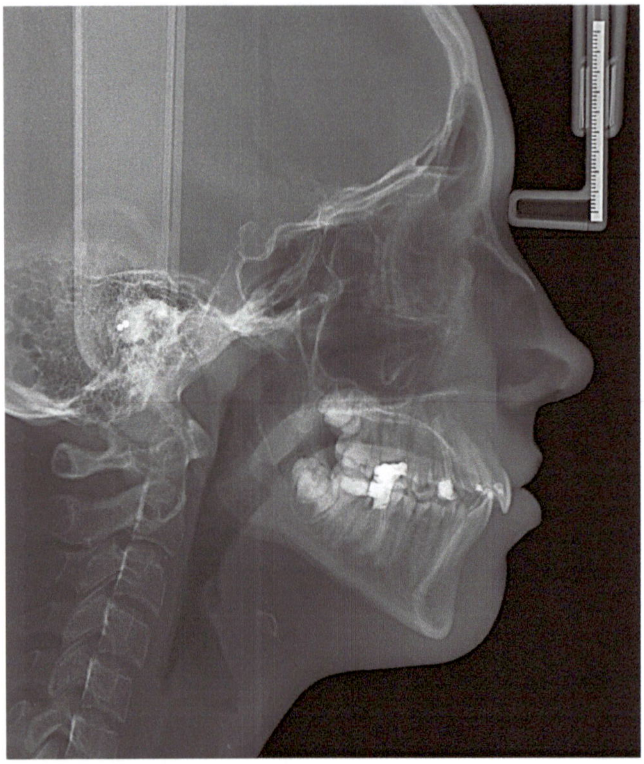

Figure 2.6

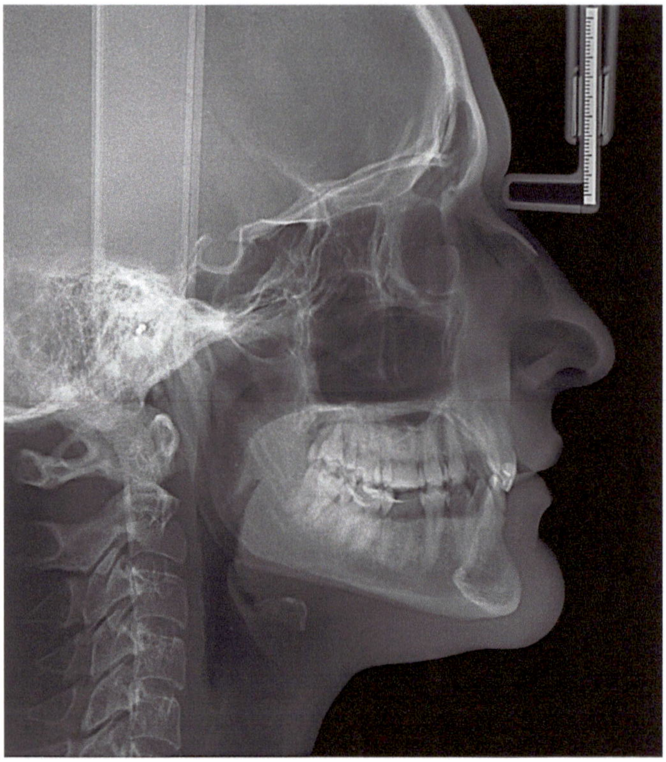

Figure 2.7

When to start treatment?

Early mixed dentition treatment

Many traits of malocclusion can manifest in the early mixed dentition and there is often a temptation to begin treatment at this stage.

Advantages of early treatment

- Maximize growth potential, compliance and orthopedic change in the young patient;
- Reduce the risk of trauma when maxillary incisors are prominent;
- Simplify any further treatment that may be required in the permanent dentition,
- Reduce the need for extractions;
- Establish a more stable result;
- Psychological benefit, promoting self-esteem by correcting potentially socially unacceptable malocclusions early.

Disadvantages associated with starting treatment too soon.

- The overall duration will be extended because almost inevitably the second phase of treatment will be required in the permanent dentition;
- Problems with compliance over the longer term;
- There is a growing body of evidence to suggest that the treatment result for growth modification will be the same whether carried out in the early mixed or permanent dentition, the only difference being the increased duration if started early (Harrison et al, 2007).

The appropriate time to start treatment

- When we aim growth modification, usually we start at late mixed dentition, just before the loss of the second deciduous molars;
- In the early permanent dentition is generally the best time to address problems of crowding;
- Class III cases associated with maxillary hypoplasia can benefit from interceptive treatment to move the maxilla forward with protraction headgear. This appears to be more effective if carried out in the early mixed dentition;
- Treatment to correct a class II skeletal base relationship is most effective during the adolescent growth spurt. In females, this will generally occur earlier than in males and is poorly correlated with dental age. Therefore, this type of treatment should often be started earlier in females than males;
- Certain malocclusions, especially increased overjet, can be a source of teasing and bullying, which can be very stressful. In these circumstances, early treatment may be indicated;
- An increased overjet increases the risk of dentoalveolar trauma, especially before the age of ten. Early treatment to reduce the overjet is indicated in those patients where little protection is provided by the lips, due to lip incompetence and marked maxillary protrusion;
- Early treatment of a posterior crossbite associated with displacement can prevent continuation into the permanent dentition.

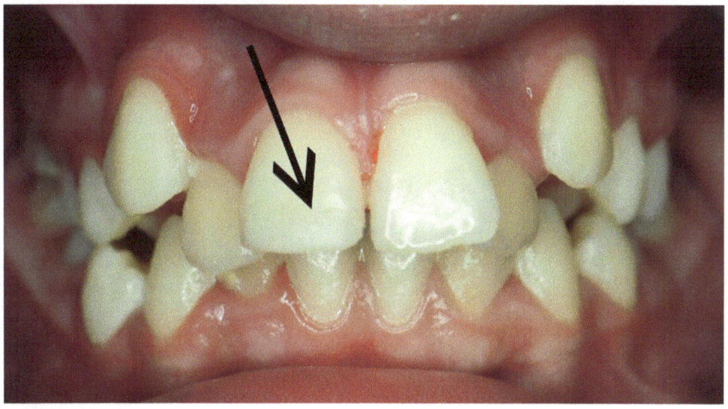

Figure 2.7

DECIDUOUS DENTITION 4-6 YEARS	EARLY MIXED 6-8 YEARS	LATE MIXED 8-11 YEARS	PERMANENT (GROWING)	PERMANENT (NON-GROWING)
Digital and pacifier habits	Posterior crossbite without functional shift			Surgical Class II
Space management	Severe crowding leading to serial extractions	Moderate to severe mandibular crowding		Surgical Class III
Posterior crossbite with functional shift	Single tooth anterior crossbite	Class II malocclusions		Camouflage treatment
	Class III malocclusions: facemask therapy			

Table 2.1 Appropriate time for treatment

Treatment of posterior crossbite without a functional shift

- It can be treated in the early mixed dentition or even closer to adolescence;
- The maxillary expansion involves the manipulation of the sutures within and surrounding the maxilla; This procedure should precede the ossification of these sutures, most likely before puberty.
- There is no evidence to suggest that expansion in the primary dentition is more stable than in the early-to-late transition dentition.

a *b*

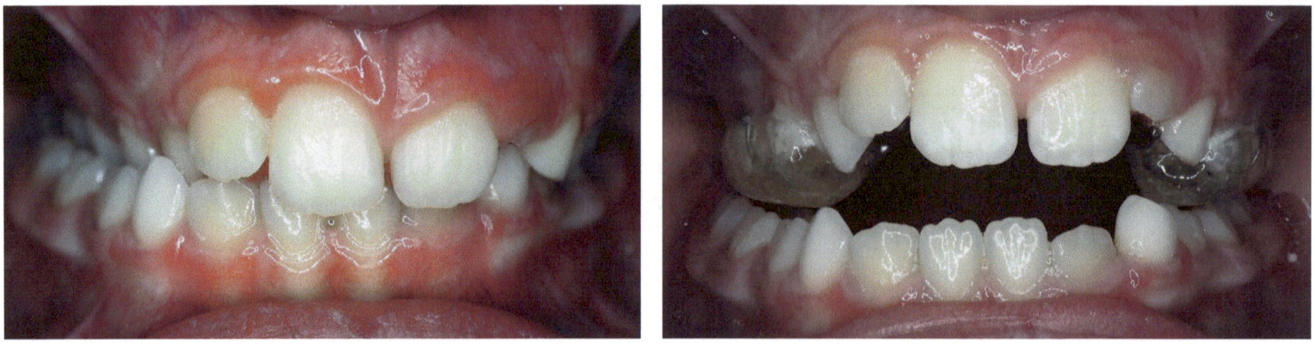

Figure 2.8 Asymmetric constriction of the upper jaw causing deviation of the lower jaw and crossbite on the right (a). Early treatment is done with a fixed expansion appliance (b)

The best time to treat crowding.

- With mild to moderate crowding is in the late mixed dentition, after the eruption of the first premolars;
- For the cases that need extractions, the timing of late mixed dentition is suitable because the first premolars have already erupted for extraction;
- Serial extraction is best done for a severely crowded malocclusion with a normal overbite.

The best time to treat open-bite malocclusion

- Various studies of dentoskeletal open bite treatments suggest that early functional therapy is able to seize the malocclusion to reduce the need for treatment during adolescence;
- This is especially true in the cases of open bite caused by oral habits.

a *b*

c

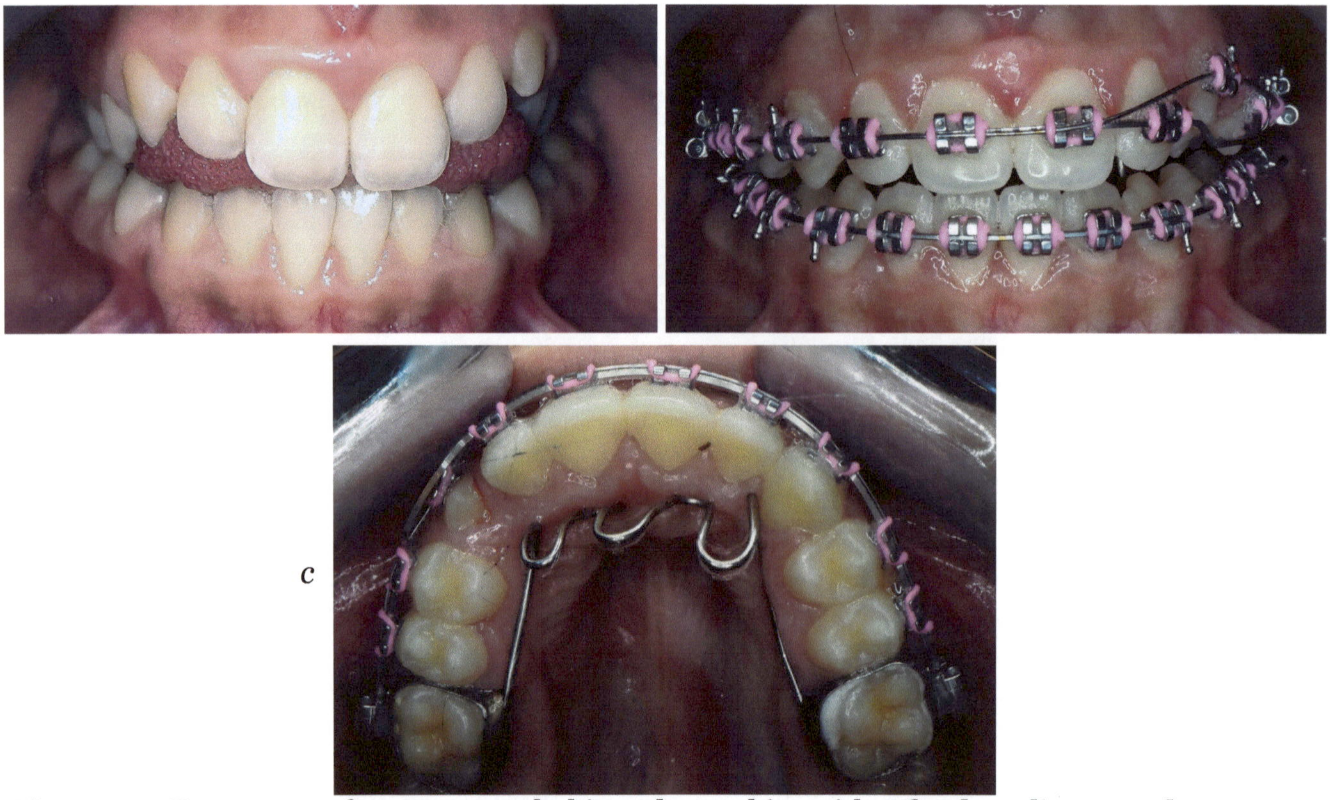

Figure 2.9 Treatment of tongue trust habit and open bite with a fixed appliance and tongue guard.

The best time to treat class II malocclusion

- There is a debate on whether to start early treatment with a functional appliance or to wait for treatment in the permanent dentition;
- Several studies suggest that starting early will accelerate growth temporarily but there is no evidence of stimulating more growth than the expected growth potential of the patient;
- Aside from the earlier improvement in self-esteem, it seems that early orthodontic treatment of Class II malocclusion does not offer an advantage over a later treatment.

Early treatment of Class III malocclusion

- Protraction facemask therapy, with or without maxillary expansion should be Initiated at the early mixed dentition stage;
- The application of prolonged force on the circummaxillary sutures may stimulate the formation of new bone, resulting in the forward and downward movement of the maxilla;
- Skeletal changes are primarily the result of anterior and vertical movement of the maxilla;
- The facemask and expansion therapy can also be a viable option for older children, although it is not as effective as it is in younger children and results in more dental rather than skeletal changes.

Appropriate time for orthognathic surgery

- The rule of thumb is to operate excesses late and deficiencies early;
- Mandibular prognathism cases should be treated after the cessation of mandibular growth. This is generally around 18 years of age males and 16 years for females;
- Early surgery on growing patients with mandibular prognathism will risk outgrowth of surgical correction and require retreatment;
- For patients with growth deficiencies, surgery can be considered earlier, but rarely before the adolescent growth spurt;
- Maxillary vertical excesses may be treated at age 14 or later since vertical growth is generally completed at this time.

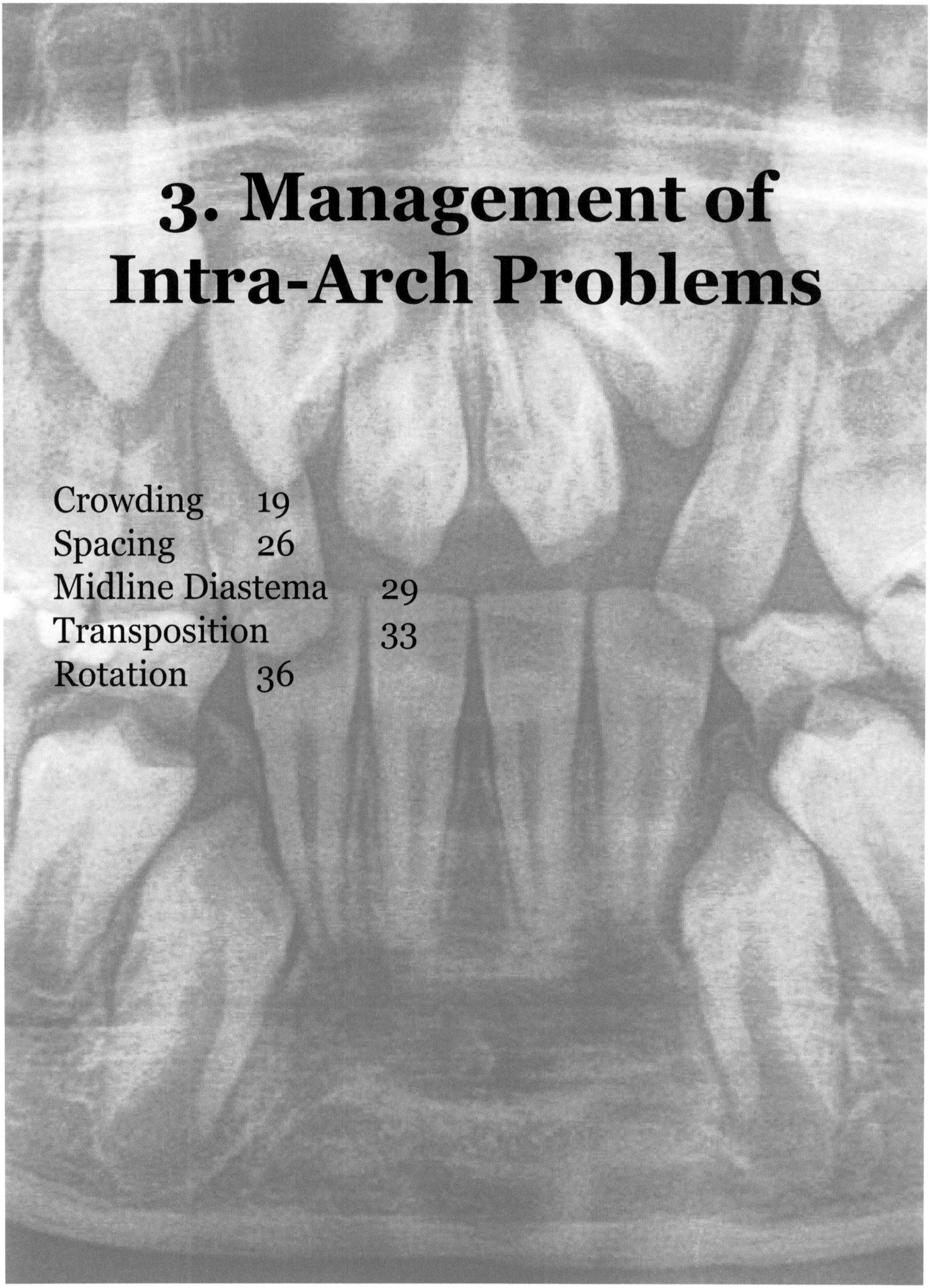

3. Management of Intra-Arch Problems

Intra-arch problems are crowding, spacing, or single tooth malposition.

Crowding

Crowding is a condition where there is malalignment of teeth caused by inadequate space (*Figure 3.1*).

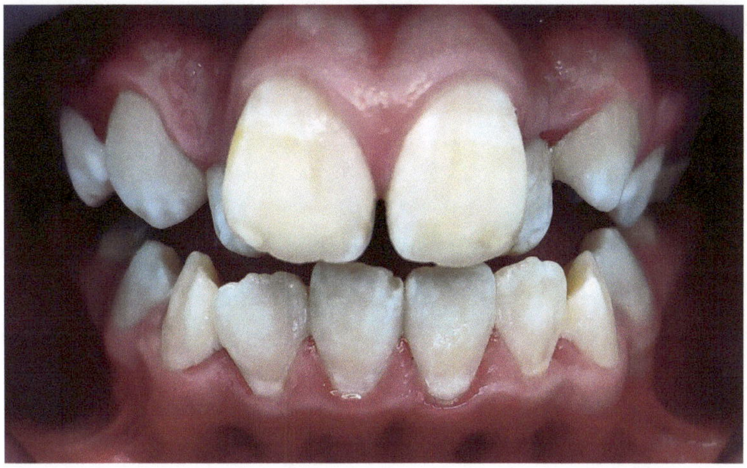

Figure 3.1 Patient with severe crowding of incisors

Etiology of Crowding

The etiology of crowding can be broadly classified into hereditary crowding and environmental crowding.

- Hereditary Crowding

Tooth size–arch length discrepancy is the reason for hereditary crowding. True hereditary crowding should be differentiated from environmental crowding. The signs of hereditary crowding are:

1. Protrusion of incisors without spacing;
2. Midline displacement of mandibular incisors with early exfoliation of deciduous canine or blocked lateral incisor on the affected side;
3. Ectopic eruption of first molars;
4. Impaction of teeth.

- Environmental Crowding can be due to:

1. Trauma;
2. Discrepancy in individual tooth size;
3. Absence of treatment of cavities and loss of arch length;
4. Abnormal or larger shape/size of the tooth (*Figure 3.2*);
5. Disturbed eruption path;
6. Rotation of teeth;
7. Transposition of a tooth;
8. Ankylosed primary tooth;
9. Premature loss of primary tooth;
10. Retained primary tooth;
11. Changed eruption sequence;

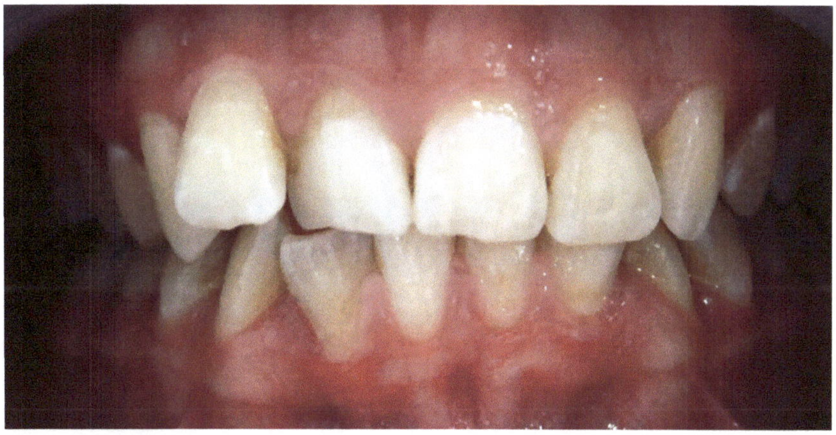

Figure 3.2 Large size of lateral incisor causing environmental crowding

Classification of Crowding

There are different methods of classification of crowding.

1. ***Hereditary crowding*** or ***Environmental crowding.***

2. ***Primary crowding:*** Determined genetically and is caused by disproportionately sized teeth and jaws.
Secondary crowding: Acquired crowding is caused by loss of arch length due to environmental cause.
Tertiary crowding: Also called late incisor crowding is due to late mandibular growth.

3. ***Simple crowding***: This is due to disharmony between the size of the teeth and the space available for them without skeletal, muscular, or functional occlusal problems.
Complex crowding. This is caused and associated with skeletal, muscular, and functional occlusal problems.

4. Crowding in mixed dentition

- First-degree crowding is a slight malalignment of the anterior teeth. No abnormality in the supporting zone (*Figure 3.3*)
- Second-degree crowding is a noticeable malalignment of anterior teeth. No abnormality in the supporting zone. (*Figure 3.4*)
- Third-degree crowding is a severe malalignment of all four incisors. (*Figure 3.5*)

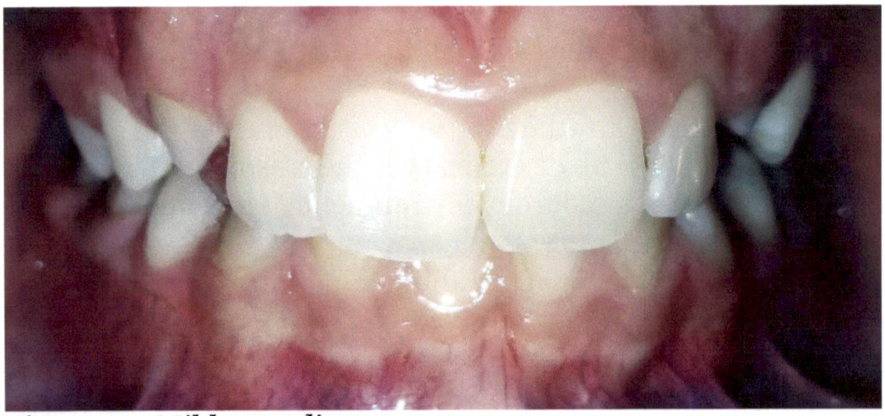

Figure 3.3 Mild crowding

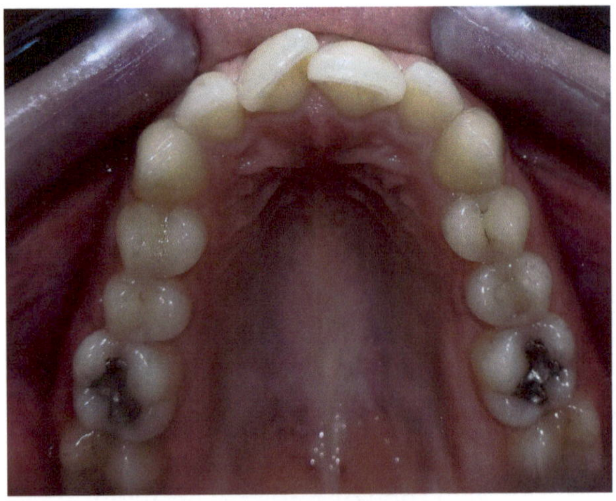

Figure 3.4 Moderate crowding

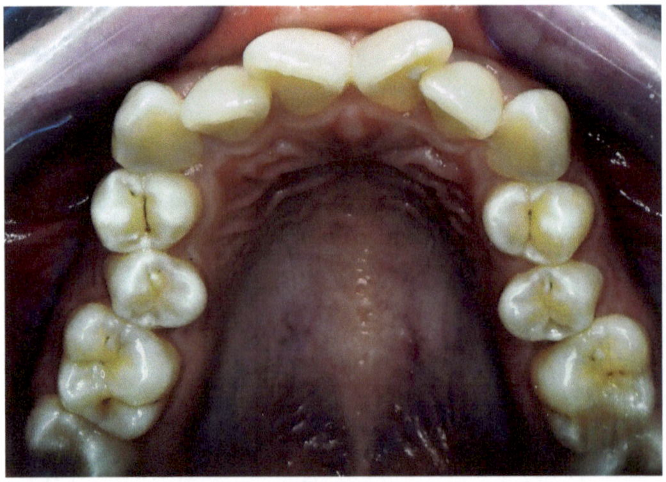

Figure 3.5 Severe crowding

Clinical Features of Class I Crowding

- Crowded mandibular incisor teeth;
- Premature exfoliation of deciduous canines on the crowded side due to a displacement of erupting tooth;
- Spreading out of maxillary permanent lateral incisor;
- Gingival recession on the labial surface of prominent mandibular incisors;
- Bulging of canines in the unerupted position;
- Reduced leeway space;
- Impaction of a second permanent molar, if no treatment is given. *Figure 3.6 (a)*

a *b*

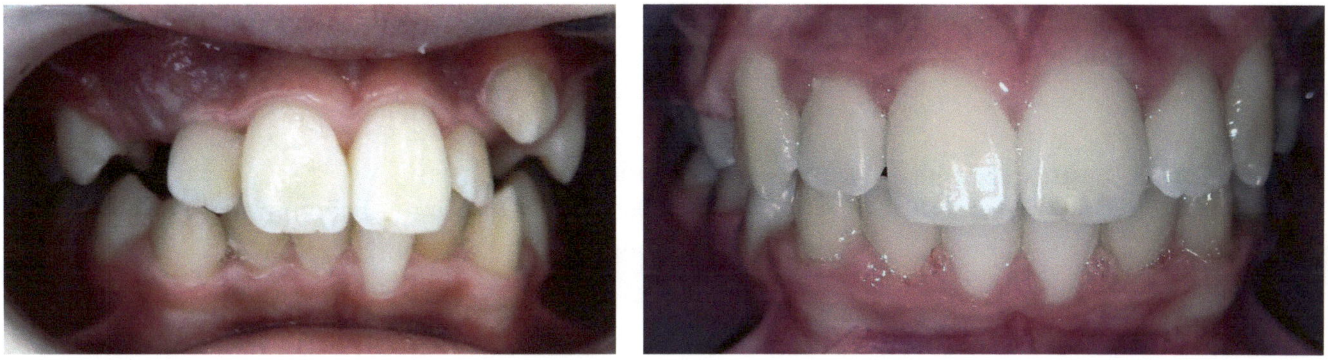

Figure 3.6 (a) Patient with crowded incisor teeth, spreading out of maxillary lateral incisor and prominent canine bulbs. (b) Treatment of the crowding was done with the expansion of the arches using a rapid maxillary expander. Lower arch perimeter slightly larges after upper arch expansion because of occlusal contacts.

Management of crowding in mixed dentition

- We should use mixed dentition model analysis like Moyers' analysis is carried out to find out the arch length discrepancy. Management of crowding in mixed dentition is shown in *Table 3.1*

Age [After Eruption of 21/12]	Timing	Treatment
Slight crowding: Slight changes in the position of anterior teeth	Wait and watch	No treatment
Moderate crowding: Lack of space by width of one lateral incisor	Can wait till (or) premolar eruption	Expansion Guidance of eruption
Pronounced crowding	Immediate treatment	Expansion Guidance of eruption Serial extraction Extraction and orthodontic treatment

Table 3.1 Management of crowding in mixed dentition

Management of Crowding in early permanent dentition

- Arch length analysis for permanent dentition like Carey's analysis should be carried out;
- Treatment can be either by non-extraction or extraction.

Non-extraction

- In cases with mild discrepancy, non-extraction method of treatment is used;
- Proximal reduction and treatment with either removable appliances or fixed appliance;
- Lip bumpers are useful in increasing the arch length;
- Arch expansion procedures also can be carried out to alleviate crowding;
- Molar distalization is another method to gain space in minor crowding correction depending on the type of the sagittal malocclusion. *Figure 3.6 (b)*

Extraction:

- Treatment planning should be aimed at the choice of extraction;
- After extraction, treatment is done with preferably fixed appliance mechanotherapy;
- If there is any unerupted tooth, it has to be brought into occlusion.

Management of crowding in adults

- Crowding can be classified as mild, moderate and severe;
- It could be associated with the upper or lower jaw or both;
- In case there are missing teeth at the beginning of treatment, the orthodontic plan should use the existing space whenever possible;
- If we have severely damaged teeth with poor prognosis, we should always consider extracting them instead of healthy premolars.

Treatment of mild, moderate and severe crowding

- In Class I cases if there is a different degree of crowding in the upper and lower jaw, we should perform Bolton analysis; *Figure 3.7*

a *b*

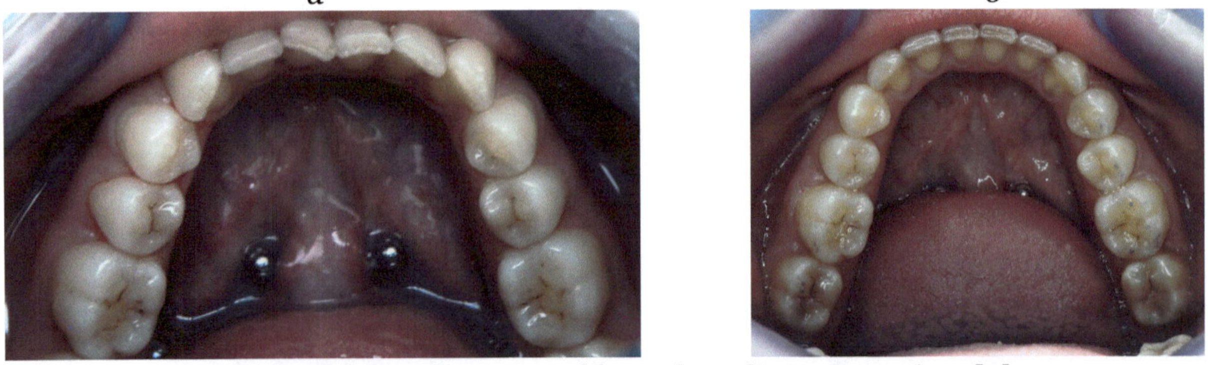

Figure 3.7 Treatment of mild crowding caused by Bolton discrepancy in adult.

- If we have Bolton discrepancy, we should perform interproximal enamel reduction;
- In class I cases with deep bite, after correcting the deep bite crowding should be resolved by leveling the curve of Spee and Wilson and alignment;
- In class II case treated with four premolar extractions, crowding should be resolved by using

the extraction space;

- In class II case treated with only upper premolar extractions, in the upper arch for alignment we use extraction spaces, in the lower arch we can use space from slight expansion or IER; (*Figure 3.8*)

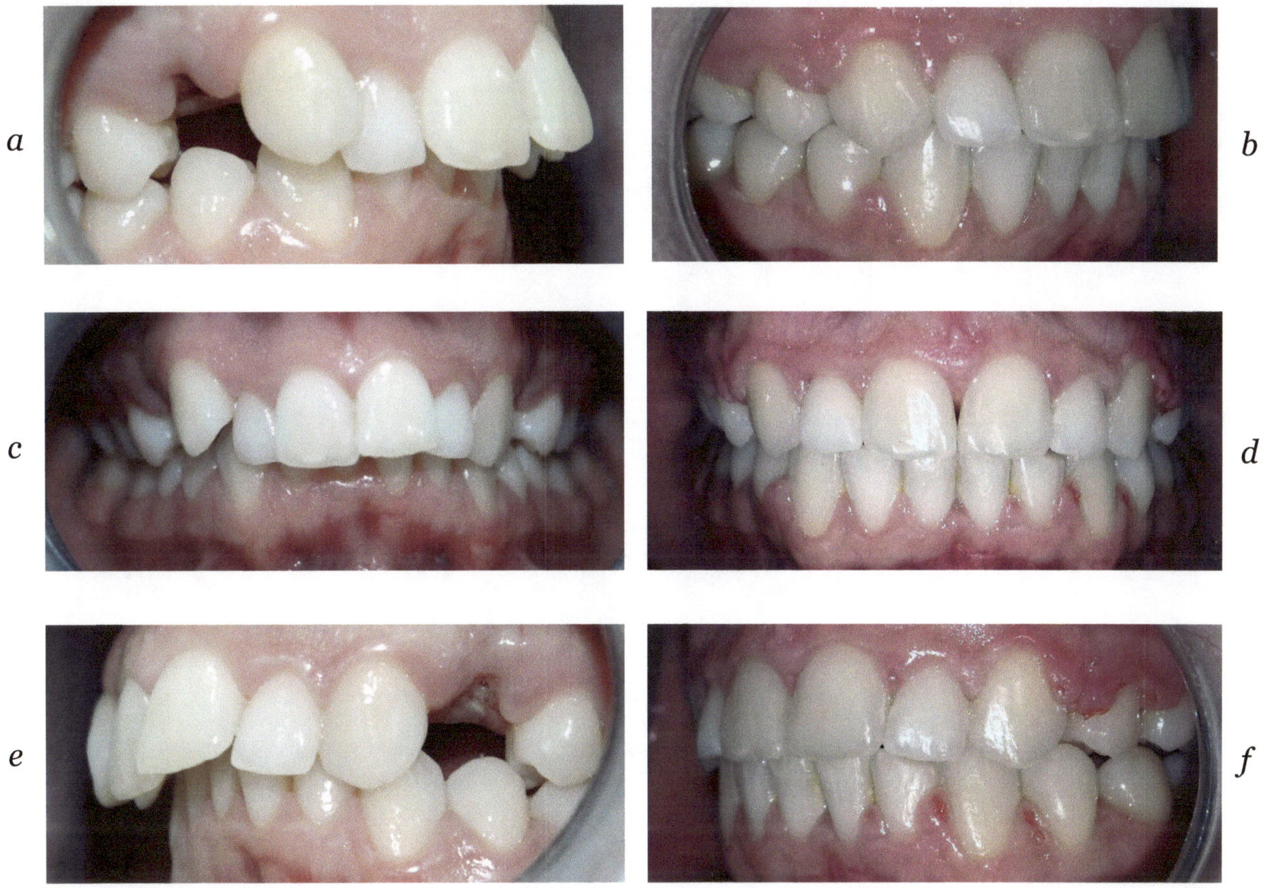

Figure 3.8 Class II treatment by upper premolar extractions. Before (a, c, e) and after treatment (b, d, f).

- In class III cases treated with four premolar extractions, we use extraction space for alignment; (*Figure 3.9*)
- In class III case treated only with two premolar extractions in the lower arch, upper arch crowding, if present, can be resolved with expansion, proclination of upper anteriors or with IER;
- In severe crowding situations in adults, the extraction of premolars is advocated.

Appliances and methods used for correction of crowding

- Expansion appliances – Quad helix, Rapid palatal expander, W- arch, transpalatal arch. You can find details of these appliances in the treatment of transversal malocclusions. (*Figure 3.10*)
- Distalization appliances – Pendulum appliance, Mini implants. Details about appliances are given in 'Management of Class II malocclusions'; *Figure 3.11*
- Interproximal enamel reduction.

Interproximal enamel reduction (IER) is a clinical procedure involving the reduction, anatomic recontouring, and protection of proximal enamel surfaces of permanent teeth in order to create space for orthodontic treatment. Anterior teeth are contoured during or after orthodontic treatment to create a balanced or harmonious appearance of teeth;

- It is recommended that careful stripping of the proximal surfaces of the anterior teeth is done when there was tooth-size discrepancy;

- Stripping is also carried out for the reshaping of enamel on some teeth, thus contributing to an improved finishing of orthodontic treatment and dental esthetics;
- Normalization of gingival contour and elimination of triangular spaces above the papilla;
- To provide space for correcting an exaggerated curve of Spee.

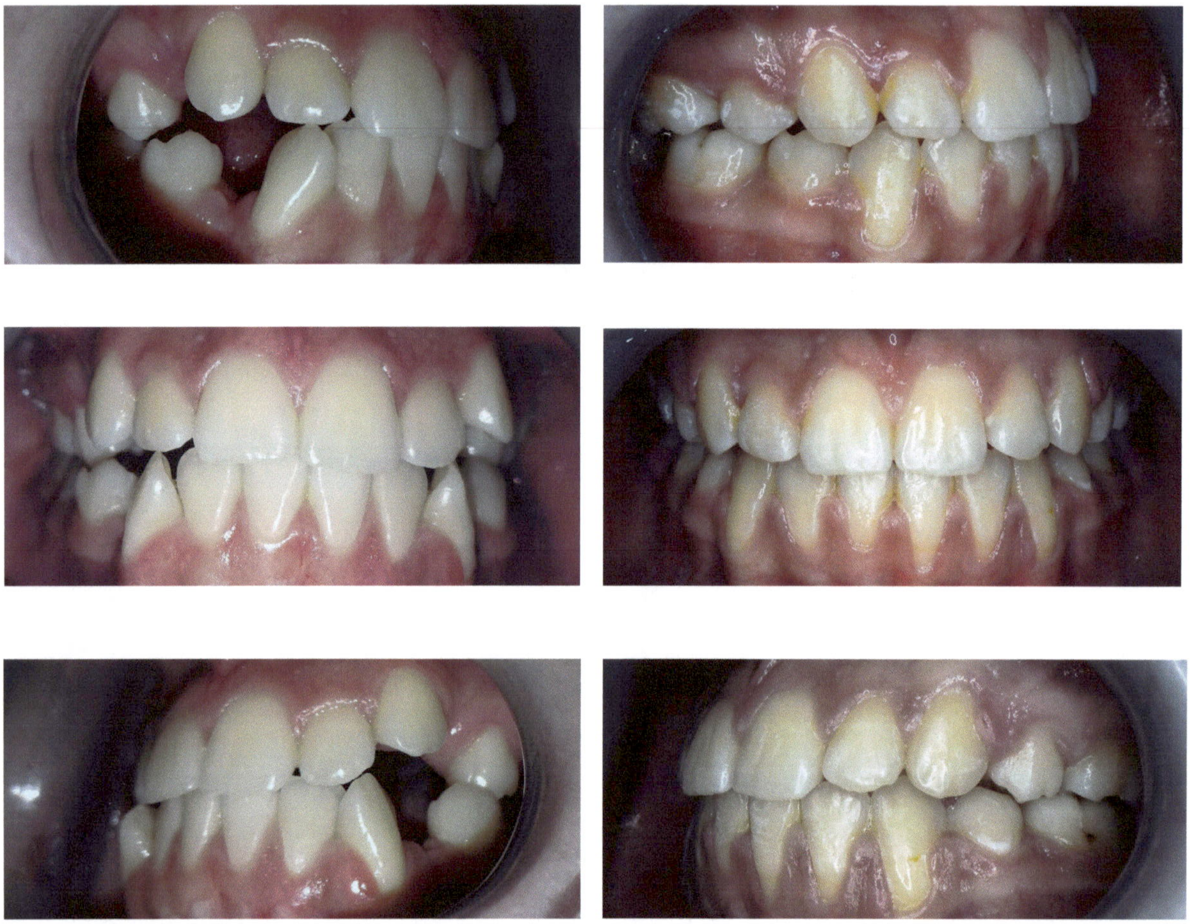

a *b* *c* *d* *e* *f*

Figure 3.9 Class III case treated with four premolar extractions. Before (a, c, e) and after treatment (b, d, f).

a *b*

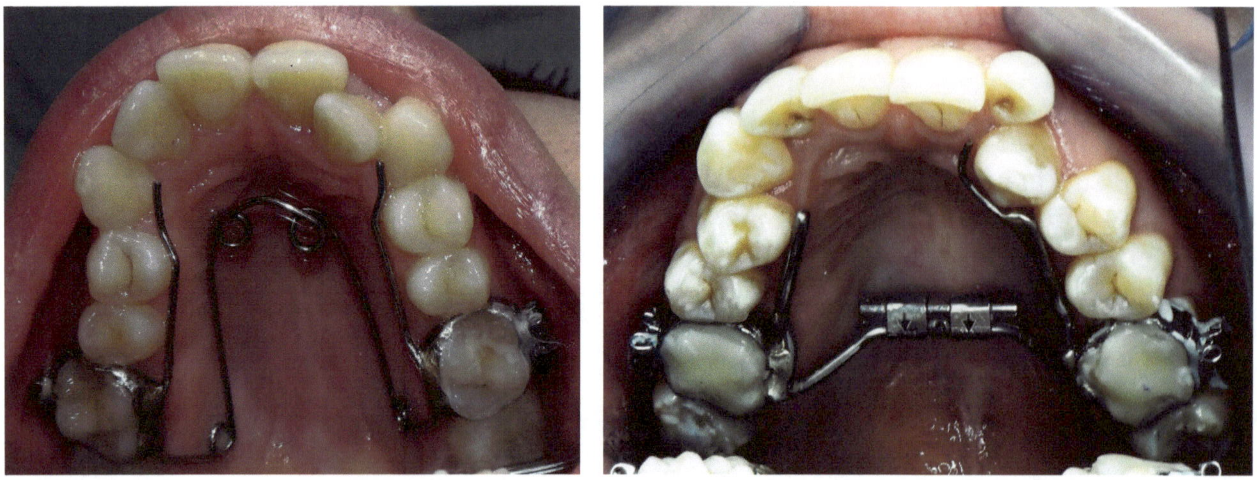

c 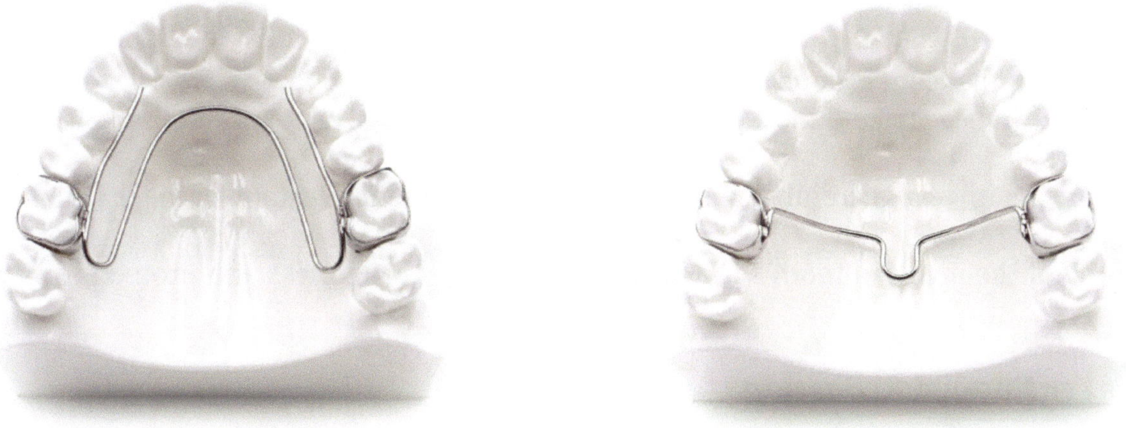 d

Figure 3.10 Expansion appliances - QuadHelix (a); Rapid-palatal (b); W-arch (c); Transpalatal-arch (d);

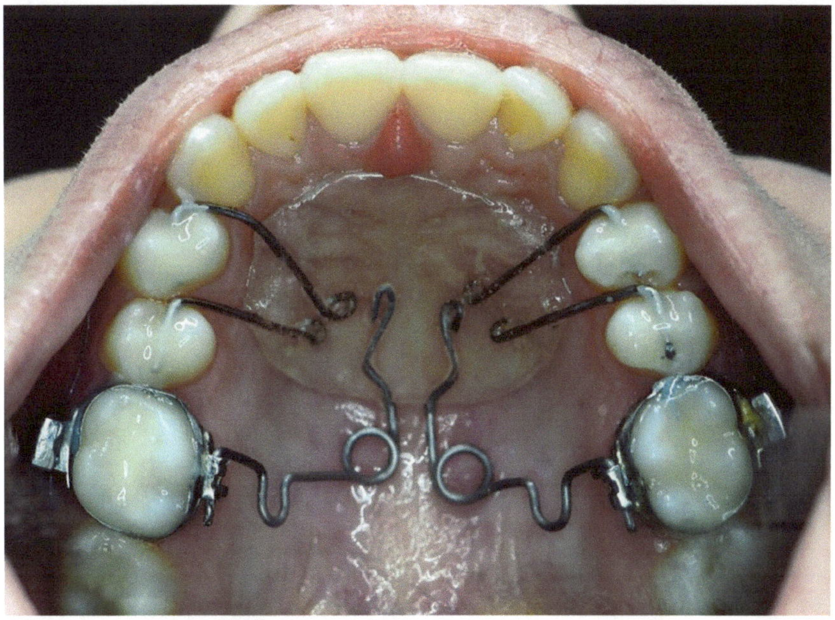

Figure 3.11 Pendulum appliance;

Camouflage of Class II and III malocclusions

- The use of mandibular stripping can be beneficial in camouflaging slight to moderate Class III conditions and overjet;
    - It is not recommended in severe crowding (more than 8 mm per arch);
- IER should not be used when there is active periodontal disease or lack of dental stability;
- IER should not be used when there is poor oral hygiene;
- Stripping should not be used in small and hypersensitive teeth;
- Stripping should not be carried out on 'square' teeth as teeth with straight proximal surfaces and wide bases produce broad contact surfaces, and could potentially cause food impaction and reduced interseptal bone;
- Interproximal reduction is composed of four stages: separation, reduction, recontouring, polishing, and protection

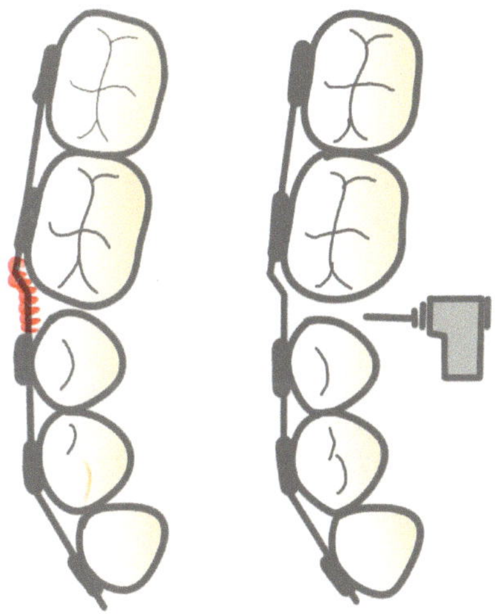

Figure 3.12 Stripping procedure

of the enamel (*Figure 3.12*).

- Separation of the teeth is done using separators;
- Reduction can be carried out by various methods using abrasive strips, diamond cutting disk or burs;
- Recontouring involves careful reshaping of the reduced teeth to establish the original contact contours;
- Polishing of the involved tooth surface to reduce enamel roughness and protecting by fluoridation.

Techniques for Enamel Reduction

- Manual Method This method consists of using metallic strips, impregnated with abrasive metal oxides, and numerous holding devices;
- Mechanical Method This technique greatly reduces working time. The tools for its use mainly consist of disks for handpiece or contra-angles, high-speed handpiece, and mechanical files for contra-angle heads with shuttle movement;
- Peck and Peck recommended the use of double-sided abrasive strips for gross reduction of less than 0.2 mm of enamel and safe-sided steel abrasive disks for reduction beyond 0.2 mm.

Retention after correction of crowding

- In the mixed dentition, we use removable orthodontic appliances as retainers so we do not interrupt the normal process of eruption of permanent teeth. After the establishment of permanent dentition, we can discontinue night ware of appliance;
- This appliance is also useful for correcting small rebounds;
- In the early permanent dentition after alignment, we can use permanent retention or removable splints – Essix or removable appliance. Retention should continue at least until 18 – 19 years of age after the late mandibular growth has stopped;
- In permanent dentition fixed retention is advisable.

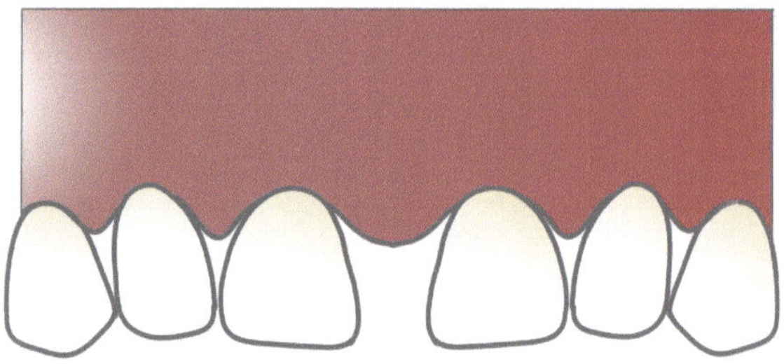

Figure 3.13 Spacing;

Spacing

Imperfections in the teeth alignment and distance, in which there is a gap between two teeth or many teeth describes spacing (*Figure 3.13*).

Classification of Spacing

- Localized spacing (*Figure 3.14*).
- It is a condition in which spacing is present in localized regions or areas;
- Generalized spacing (*Figure 3.15*)

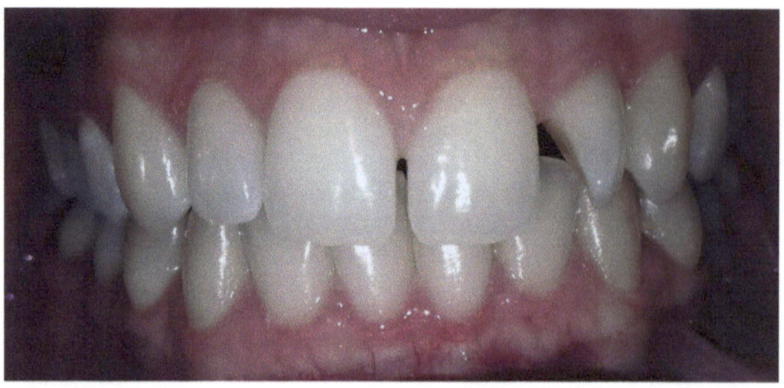

Figure 3.14 Localized spacing

a

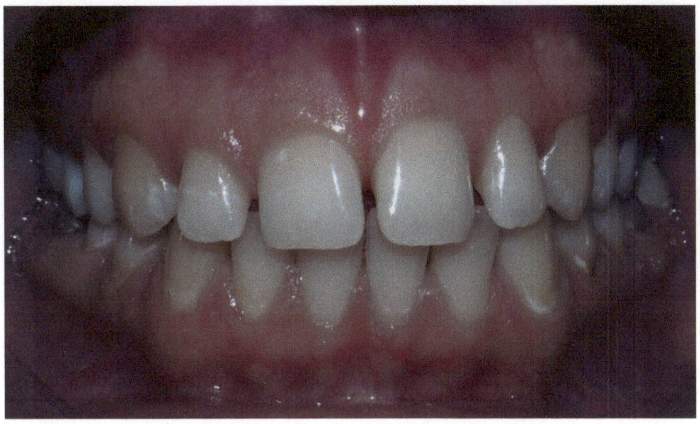

b

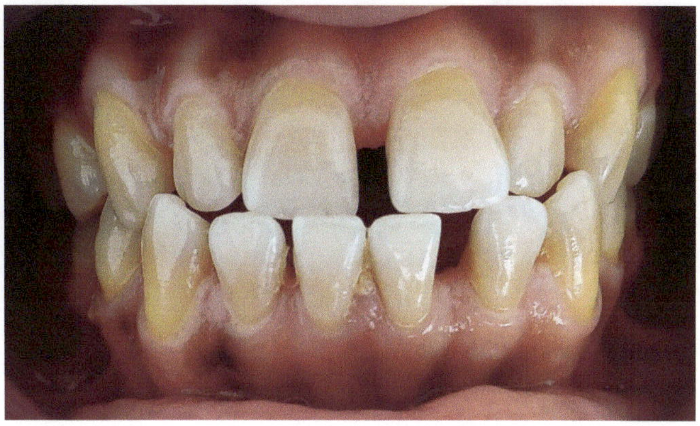

Figure 3.15 Generalized spacing (a,b).

Etiology of localized spacing includes:

- ***Missing teeth***: which can be
  - *Congenitally missing teeth.* This causes localized spacing but the problem may not be restricted to one particular spot;
  - *Unerupted teeth.* Impacted or unerupted tooth causes localized spacing. Assess whether the tooth can be brought into normal position;
- ***Premature loss of permanent teeth.*** In this situation, the decision has to be made whether to close the space or maintain the space and replace it with an implant or bridge.
- ***Prolonged retention of primary teeth*** results in:
  - Ectopic eruption of permanent successor;
  - When the primary tooth is exfoliated after the ectopic eruption of permanent successor space results;
- ***Sucking habits***: May cause localized spacing.

Etiology of generalized spacing (*Figure 3.16*)

The causes of generalized spacing are:

- ***Microdontia***

The presence of small teeth in the normal jaws will result in generalized spacing. Such conditions are best treated by, composite build-ups or consolidation of spaces and placement of bridges.

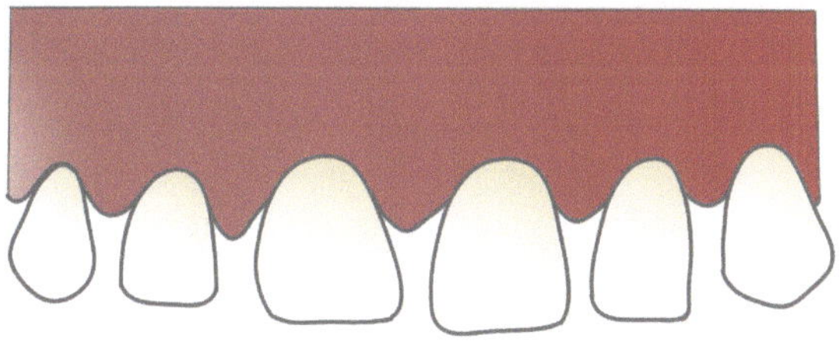

Figure 3.16 Generalized spacing.

- ***Macrognathia***

This also manifests in the same way as small teeth. But here the teeth sizes are normal, whereas the arch size is bigger (*Figure 3.17*).

- The best method of treatment is to protract the posterior teeth to close anterior spaces if the profile is acceptable;
- Other methods will be, composite build-ups or consolidation of spaces and placement of bridges.

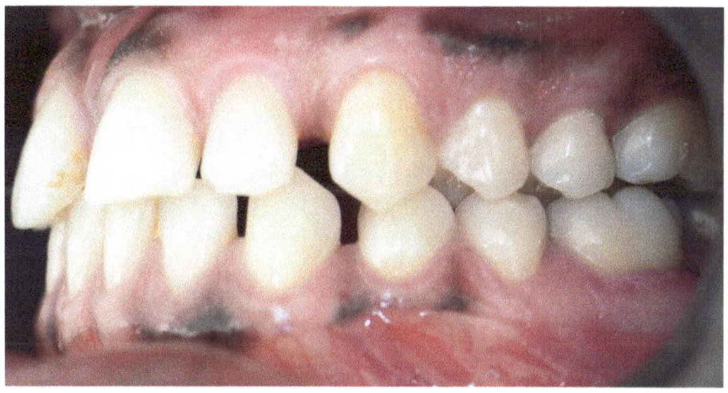

Figure 3.17 Macrognathia as a cause for spacing

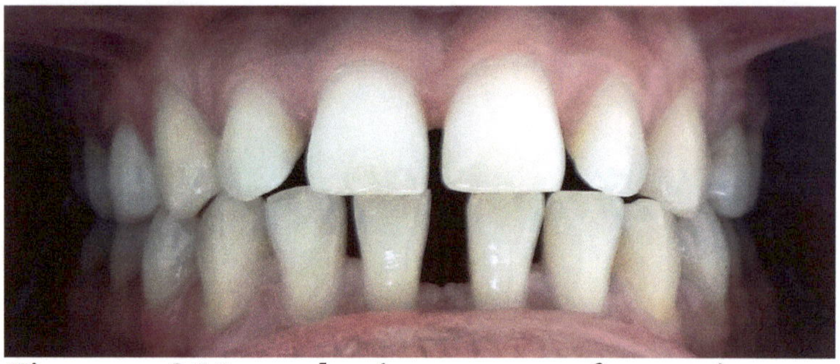

Figure 3.18 Macroglossia as a cause for spacing

- ***Macroglossia or an enormously large tongue*** causes generalized spacing (*Figure 3.18*).

In this case, the patient complains of generalized spacing increasing in the past few years. Ten years ago there were no spaces between the teeth. Since the cause is the enlargement of the tongue, after space closure the patient will need permanent retention.

- The lateral borders of the tongue show indentations;
- Treatment is not advisable unless the malocclusion is gross;
- If the malocclusion is gross, partial glossectomy or excision of a wedge of tissue from the tongue can be advised.

- ***Sucking habits*** may also cause generalized spacing;

- ***Abnormal tongue posture*** may also cause generalized spacing.

Clinical features of spacing

- There is a discrepancy between arch length and jaw size;
- Often we find proclination of the anterior segments;
- Rotations are rare but are found mostly in the premolar area;
- In the early mixed dentition, we have an ugly duckling stage before the eruption of permanent canines which is associated with midline diastema. This is a physiologic phase and the clinician should not attempt space closure.

Management of spacing can be done by orthodontic, or combined orthodontic and prosthodontic treatment.

Management in the mixed dentition

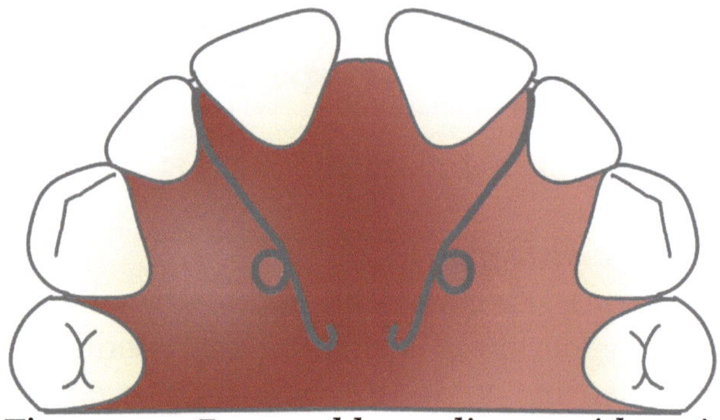

Figure 3.19 Removable appliance with springs.

- The orthodontist should be able to recognize the physiologic ugly duckling stage when spaces are temporarily seen in the dental arches;
- No treatment should be started before the eruption of the permanent canines unless incisor teeth have migrated to one side causing loss of space for an unerupted permanent tooth.

Orthodontic Management consists of:

- Elimination of the habits by habit breaking appliance;
- Localized spacing can be closed with removable appliances with springs (*Figure 3.19*);
- If there is proclination associated with spacing, Hawley's appliances are used for closing of spaces and retraction;
- Conditions, where spaces are to be closed by protraction of posterior teeth, can be achieved only by fixed appliance mechanotherapy.

Treatment in the early and adult permanent dentition

- All of the treatment methods used for mixed dentition can be used in the permanent dentition.
- Prosthodontic management
- Sometimes localized spaces are best treated by giving jacket crowns or composite build-ups.
- Combined orthodontic and prosthodontic management
  - If the space is excess or severe, then space is consolidated by using fixed appliance therapy;
  - In the consolidated space, either an implant is placed or a bridge is placed.

Appliances used for correction of spacing

- Removable appliance Hawley type with springs;
- Removable appliance with a modified anterior bow for hooking elastics (*Figure 3.20*);
- Aligner treatment can be used.

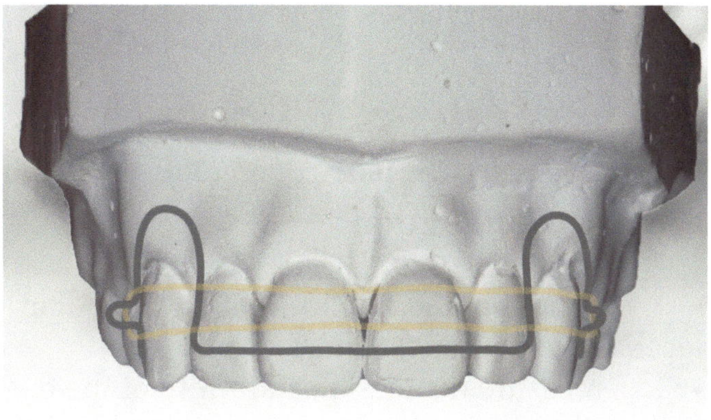

Figure 3.20

Fixed appliances

- Close spaces after alignment and leveling phase;
- Use elastic chain with rigid wire like 0.019 x 0.025-inch stainless steel for a 22-inch slot;
- Spaces can be closed with a combination of power chain and open coil spring on a rigid wire;

Retention

- Cases treated orthodontically usually require long-term retention;
- In most cases, fixed retention is chosen.

Midline Diastema

Median diastema is a form of localized spacing wherein there is a space present between two central incisors (*Figure 3.21*).

Classification

- Diastema with convergent long axes of central incisors;
- Diastema with divergent long axes of the central incisors.

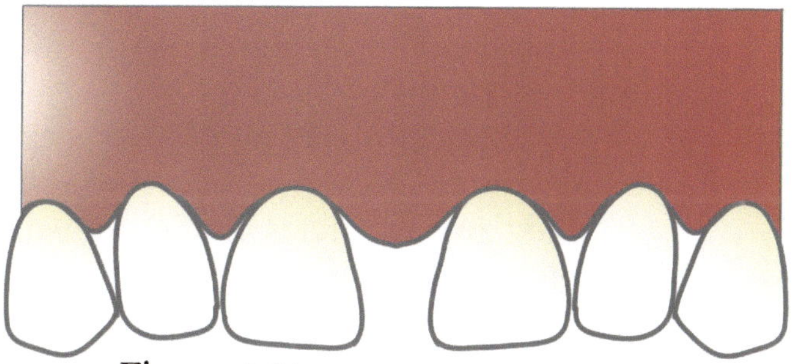

Figure 3.21

Etiology

The etiology of median diastema is depicted in *Table 3.2*.

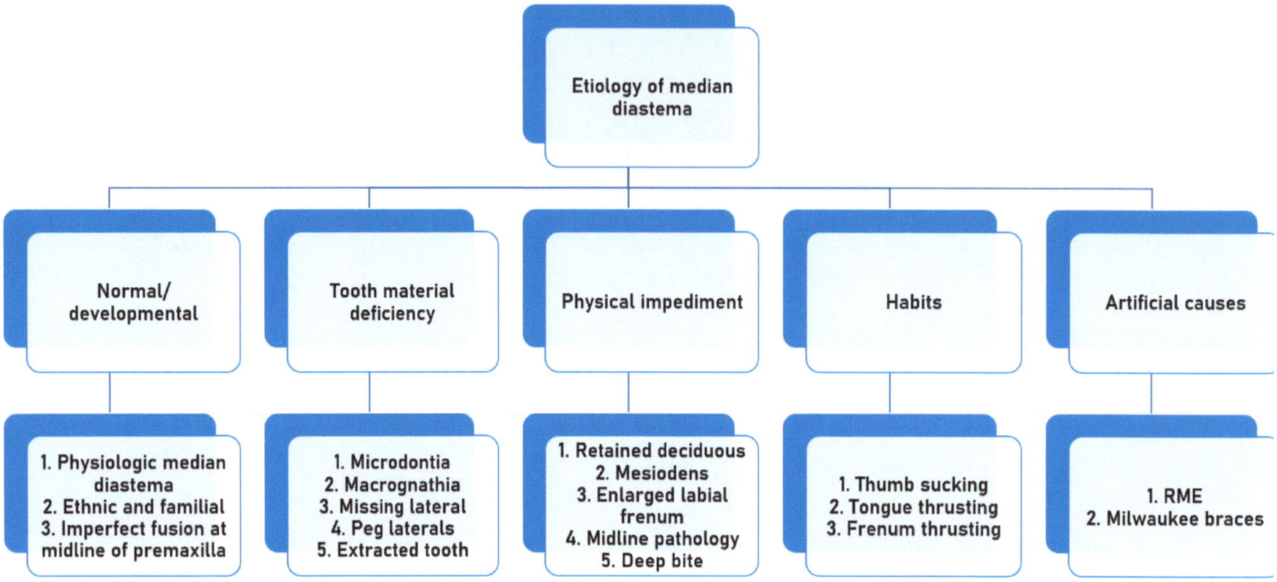

Table 3.2 Causes of Median Diastema

Clinical examination

- Examine and confirm whether median diastema is localized or part of generalized spacing;
- Measure the mesiodistal width of the teeth;
- Blanch test: Lift the upper lip and look for blanching of the soft tissues lingual to and between two central incisors. Presence of blanch indicates high frenal attachment as the cause of midline diastema;
- Assess the depth of the overbite;
- Look for any malicious oral habits;
- On a periapical radiograph, there may be a V-shaped notching present between the central incisors.

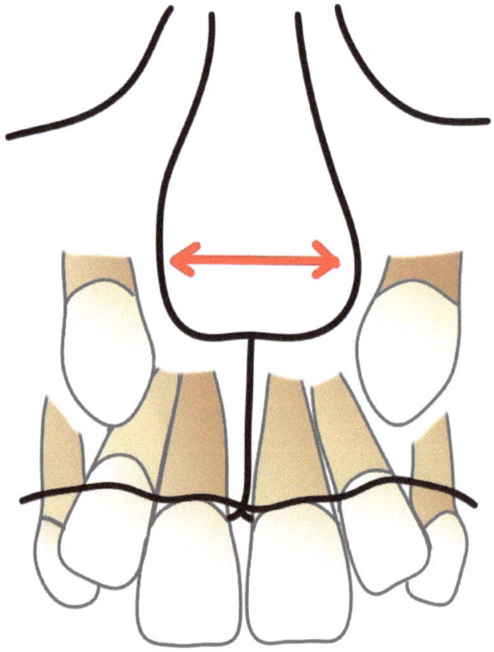

Figure 3.22 Ugly duckling stage

Management

- We need to keep in mind that During Physiologic median diastema or ugly duckling stage spacing between central incisors is part of normal growth (*Figure 3.22*).
  - This space becomes smaller as the lateral incisor erupts into the arch.
  - The appearance of the permanent canine brings about total closure of the median diastema.
  - This condition requires no treatment.
- Ethnic and familial:
  - A certain group of peoples, especially African populations, exhibit median diastema as an ethnic norm.
  - Median diastema is seen in some families also *(Figure 3.23)*.
- Imperfect fusion at the midline:
  - Median diastema occurs due to imperfect fusion at the midline of the premaxilla;
  - A V-shaped or W-shaped osseous septum may be associated with this condition;
  - Treatment consists of excision of included interdental tissue between the incisors;
  - A flap is raised interdentally and fissure bur inserted into the cleft;

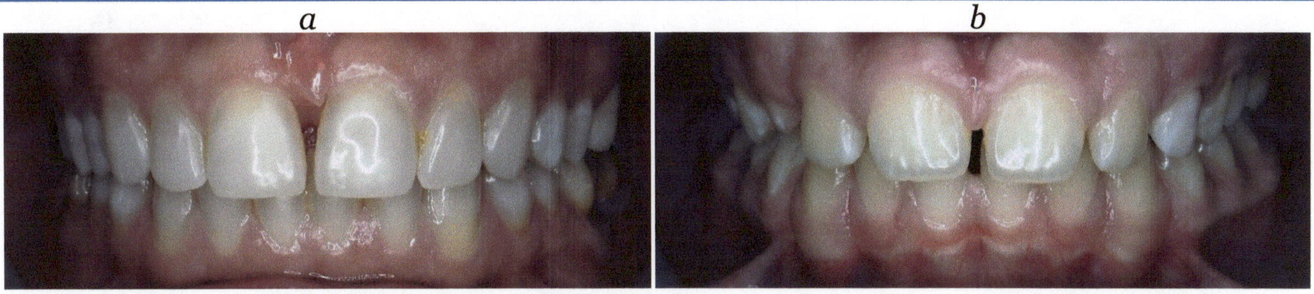

Figure 3.23 You can see on these two photos a mother on the left (a) and daughter on the right (b). The cause of the median diastema in both cases is Bolton anterior discrepancy. The proposed treatment in the mother case is aesthetic build up. In the younger patient, we are waiting for the upper canines to erupt and close some of the spaces. After orthodontic space closure, there would also be an aesthetic build up.

- With the bur, the included tissues are removed and flap sutured;
- An orthodontic appliance for the closure of median diastema is given during the healing process.
- Small teeth/microdontia and macrognathia. Such conditions can be treated either by orthodontic methods or by mean of or composite build-up;
- When there are missing teeth or extracted teeth space can be consolidated and replaced with implant or bridge;
- Peg shaped lateral incisor can also be the cause for spacing. After median diastema closure with an orthodontic appliance, the peg-shaped lateral incisors are reshaped either by crowns or composite build-up;
- Retained deciduous teeth: This will cause an ectopic eruption of the tooth and median diastema;
- The retained deciduous tooth has to be extracted at the earliest and allow for spontaneous closure of median diastema;
- Mesiodens: If there is a mesiodens diagnosed, it should be extracted and space closed.
- Enlarged frenum: If we notice abnormal frenulum tissue, frenectomy should be done after bringing the incisors together. Scar tissue formed will help in retention;
- Midline pathology: Midline pathology, like cysts, has to be treated first and then closure attempted;
- If the cause of spacing is a deep bite, along with the closure of space, bite opening is done to achieve stable results;
- Elimination of habits: Median diastema due to pernicious habits requires simultaneous discontinuation of the habit.

Management in the mixed and early permanent dentition

Orthodontic management for median diastema can be divided into four main categories:

- Closure by mesial tipping movements:
- Appliances used are:
- Removable appliance with two finger springs for mesial movement of central incisors (*Figure 3.24*);
- Removable appliance with a split labial bow (*Figure 3.25*);
- Closure by bodily movement: This can be achieved with the use of fixed orthodontic appliance (*Figure 3.26*);
- If we start treatment in the mixed dentition, we use the 2x 4 bracket system which consists of four brackets on the permanent incisors and molar tubes on the first molars.

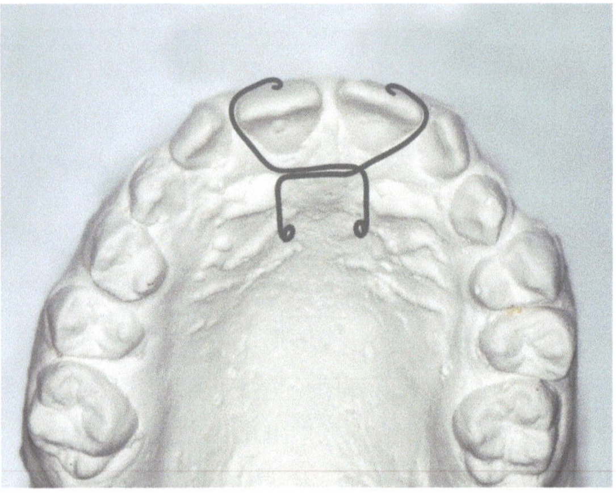

Figure 3.24

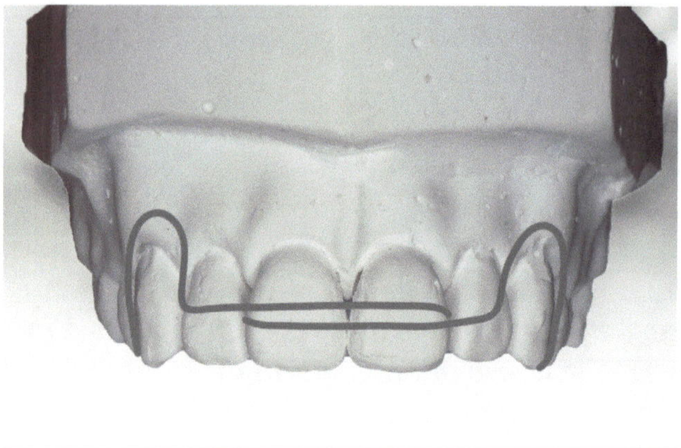

Figure 3.25

- Closure by reduction of overjet:
  - In the case of patients, with increased overjet, reduction of overjet will close the median diastema;
  - The maxillary labial segment that exhibits median diastema is drawn into smaller perimeter when the overjet is reduced;
  - This causes spontaneous closure of diastema along with overjet reduction;
  - Removable Hawley's appliance can be used for this purpose;
  - Fixed appliances also are used.

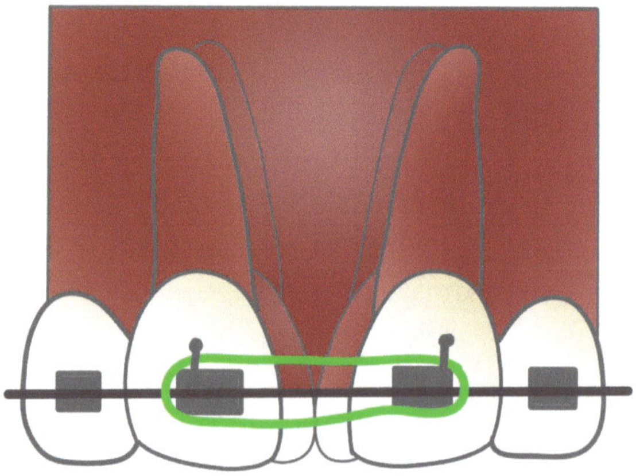

Figure 3.26

- Full orthodontic treatment:
  - When median diastema exists with other types of malocclusion, closure of median diastema is carried out along with other correction;
  - This is best achieved by fixed appliance mechanotherapy.

Management in adults

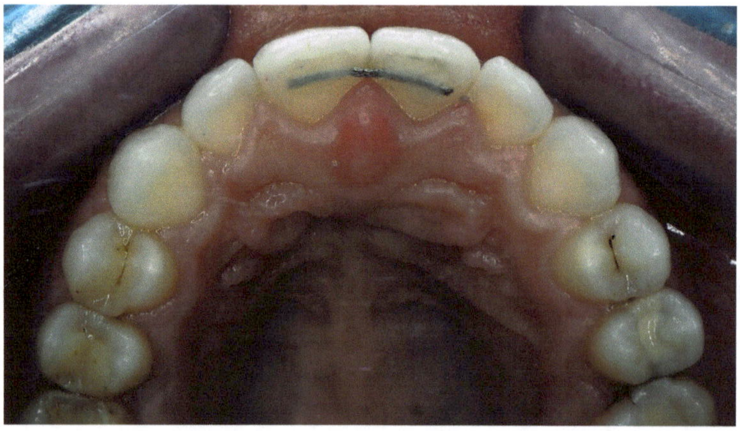

Figure 3.27 Fixed retainer for upper central incisors

Other methods of treatment include:
1. Restorative management: Very small median diastema is closed using composites.
2. Prosthetic management: If the diastema is big, closure by light-cure composite will increase the mesiodistal width of the tooth to an unesthetic level. In these cases, if the arch is well aligned, closure by implant or bridge is suggested.
3. Surgical management: Surgery is done in some cases where there is a median diastema in otherwise normal occlusion.

Retention

- Fixed retention is advised between the two central incisors (*Figure 3.27*);
- We could use a fixed retainer only or a combination of fixed and removable Essix appliance.

Transposition

A transposed tooth is that which is:
- Changed in positional location to an adjacent tooth, or
- Erupting into a position normally occupied by a nonadjacent tooth (*Figure 3.28*).

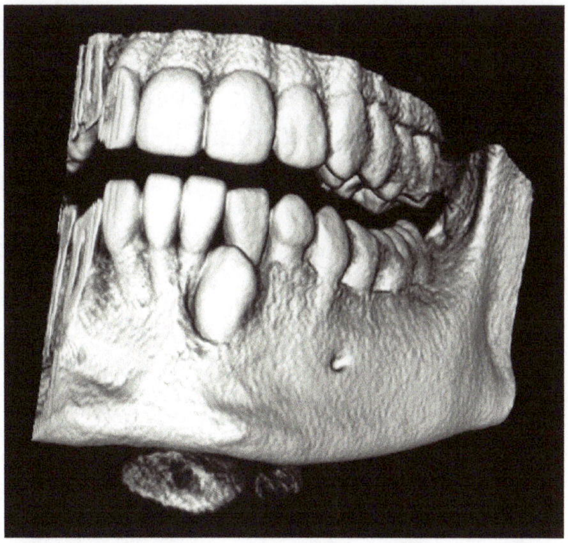

Figure 3.28 Transposition of lower canine and lateral incisor.

Classification

Classification can be done on three levels:
- First level is the jaw of occurrence;
- Second level is the transposed tooth;
- Third level is the site of transposition.

For example, MxCP1 means transposition of maxillary canine to first premolar position.

- Incomplete transposition displays only crown misplacement;
- Complete transposition involves the whole tooth.

Epidemiology

Peck and Peck (1995) have quoted the most common transposition in decreasing order of occurrence as follows:
- Maxillary canine with first premolar;
- Maxillary canine with lateral incisor;
- Maxillary canine with first molar;
- Maxillary lateral with central incisor;
- Maxillary canine with central incisor.

There is no definite evidence of sexual differences in the transposition of canines.

Etiology

- Retained primary canines are the best documented etiologic factor;
- Roots of primary tooth deflect the permanent tooth;
- Trauma in primary dentition;
- Unknown: etiology is still unclear.

Clinical features

- Transposition is detected most often because of the absence of eruption of the teeth involved;
- During the clinical examination, we find delayed eruption of teeth on one side compared to the other;
- On palpation we would feel the bulge of the teeth;
- Radiographic examination confirms the diagnosis;
- A three-dimensional examination is often necessary to establish a treatment plan.

Management

The management depends on the diagnosis and time of treatment;

- Early recognition might help to change the eruptive path;
- Leaving the transposed teeth is a sensible alternative sometimes, followed by occlusal equilibration;
- If associated with crowding, extraction, and treatment with fixed appliance.

Management in the mixed dentition

- Early diagnosis of a developing transposition is extremely important and has a great influence on prognosis;
- This may usually be performed by a radiographic examination when the patient is between 6 and 8 years of age;
- When the alteration is detected early, interceptive procedures including extraction of deciduous teeth and placement of eruption guides for the permanent teeth may be performed, thus preventing complete development of the anomaly.

Management in the early and adult permanent dentition

Treatment options include alignment of the trans-posed teeth in their transposed state, extraction of one of them, or complete correction of the transposition.

- The ideal approach will be to completely correct the transposition of the teeth but most of the times it may not be possible;
- Factors to be considered when transpositions are being corrected;
- Positions of root apices;
- Facial esthetics;
- Malocclusion;
- Age of the patient;
- Motivation and expectations of the patient;
- The risk to the teeth and adjacent tissues and treatment time must be discussed with the patient before correction;
- Alignment in the transposed position will involve reshaping the crown morphology and periodontal gingival recontouring procedure. On the other hand, when transposition is detected at a later stage, orthodontic treatment planning and intervention must be addressed.

Transpositions in the maxillary arch - treatment options

- In incomplete transposition, where the crowns are transposed but the root apices are in their relatively normal positions, uprighting and rotating the involved teeth is the procedure most often required to place them in their normal alignment, provided enough space is available in the arch (*Figure 3.29*).

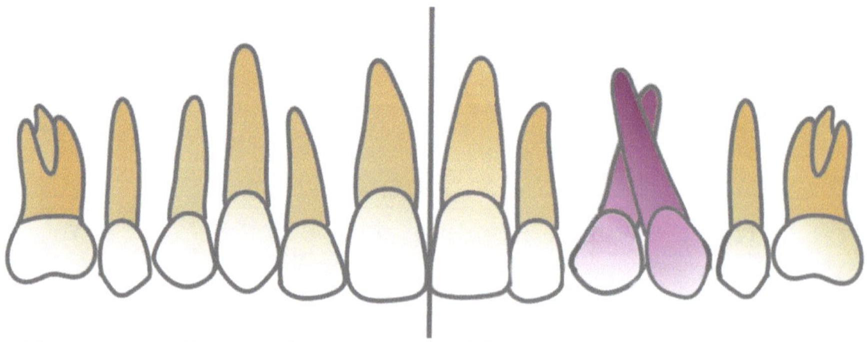

Figure 3.29 Incomplete transposition

- Upper canine premolar transposition in adult patients allows consideration of several treatment options, with or without extraction of the premolar;
- When there is a severe arch length deficiency, treatment with premolar extraction is considered as one of the alternatives. The transposed tooth is then moved to its natural position;
- If the mandibular canine and lateral incisor have already erupted in their transposed position, correction to their normal position should usually not be attempted;

When a transposition is complete, with root apices in their transposed positions, repositioning the teeth to their normal relationship in the arch is complex and may be damaging to the teeth or supporting structures; Alignment of these teeth in their transposed position is often an acceptable compromise (*Figure 3.30*);

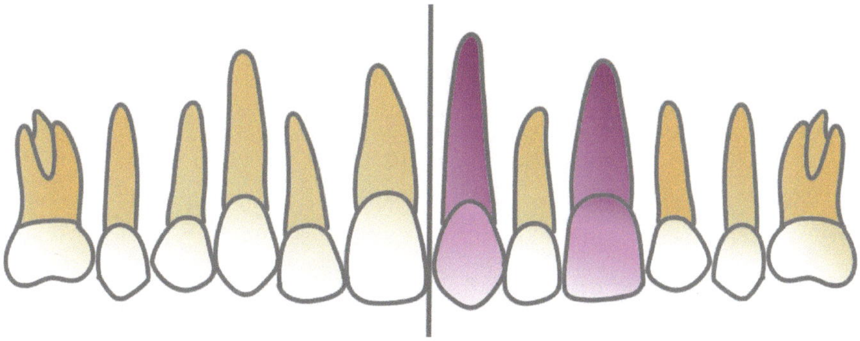

Figure 3.30 Complete transposition

- If one of the transposed or adjacent teeth is severely affected by caries or trauma, extraction of that tooth (usually the first premolar) should be considered;
- When sufficient space cannot be gained to align transposed teeth, extraction of the tooth should be considered;
- More complex treatment options include the attempt to move transposed teeth to their normal positions in the maxillary arch in selected cases;
- To avoid root interference or resorption during treatment, and to prevent bony loss at the cortical plate of the labially positioned canine, the transposed tooth (premolar or lateral incisor) should first be moved palatally, enough to allow for a free movement of the canine to its normal place;
- Afterward, the other transposed unit can be moved labially, back to its normal position in the arch;
- Attempts to correct transposed teeth in the mandible are often unsuccessful periodontically because of the limited amount of bone in the anterior mandible (*Figure 3.31*).

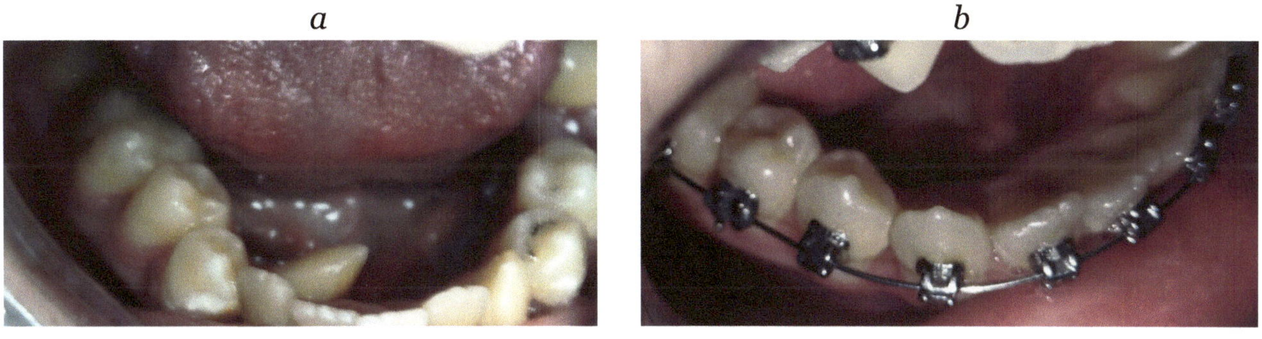

Figure 3.31 Successful treatment of incomplete mandibular transposition.

Retention

- We should consider permanent retention for at least 6 months after alignment so the intercrestal periodontic fibers would reorganize;
- After that period we can transfer to removable retainers

Rotation

Rotation is malposition due to abnormal turning of a tooth to its long axis (*Figure 3.32*).
Rotation can be defined as the spinning of the tooth around its long axis.

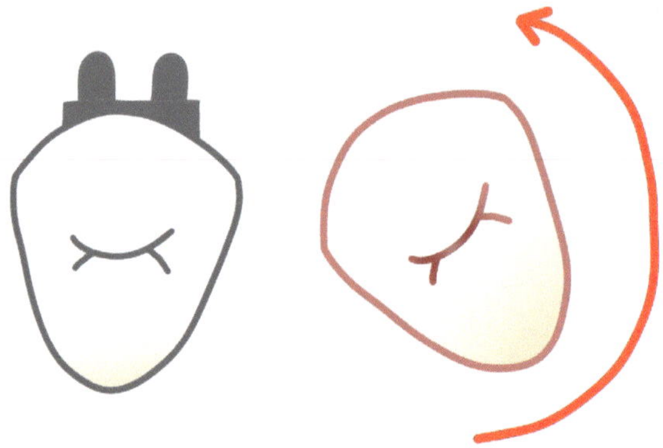

Figure 3.32

Clasification

1. Centric rotation—only rotation around the long axis.
2. Eccentric rotation—rotation with tipping of the tooth also.

- Derotation can be achieved by applying a couple;
- The forces get neutralized and only moment exists which causes rotation;
- The force required for rotation correction is 35–60 grams;
- There is a greater tendency for the rotation to relapse after correction;
- Rotation can be achieved by two ways: by using a couple forces, by using a single force and a stop (*Figure 3.33*).

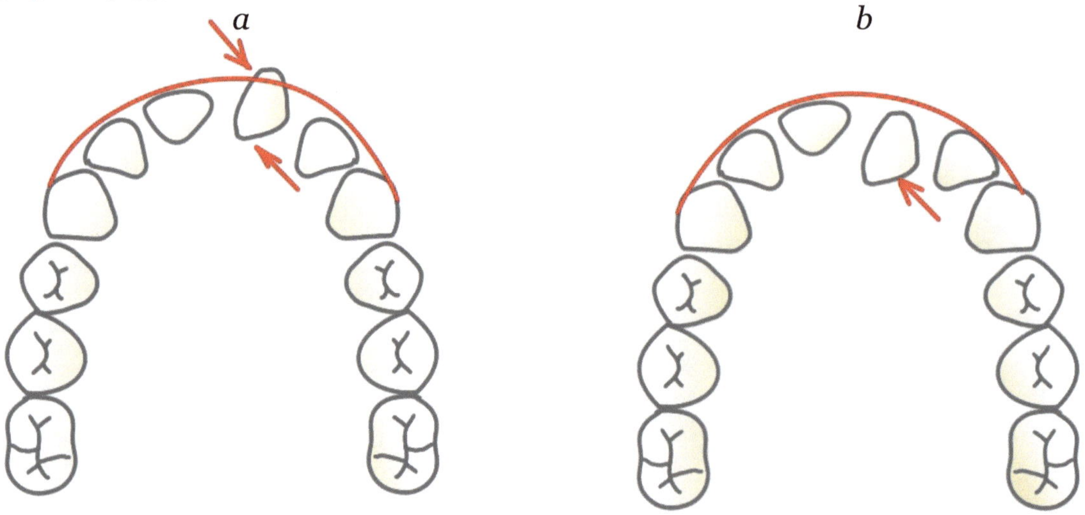

Figure 3.33 Methods of rotation (a) use of couple for correction, and (b) use of single force and stop

Etiology

Most often we find rotations in crowded dentitions. Reasons for crowding are:

- Discrepancy between tooth material and arch size;
- Bolton discrepancy;
- Supernumerary tooth;
- Persisting oral habit;
- Constriction of the arch;

- Crossbite;
- Retroclination of teeth.

Management of rotations in the mixed dentition

- We can use a removable appliance with springs creating a couple of forces (*Figure 3.34*);
- 2 x 4 bracket bonding is the best appliance to correct rotations in the mixed dentition.

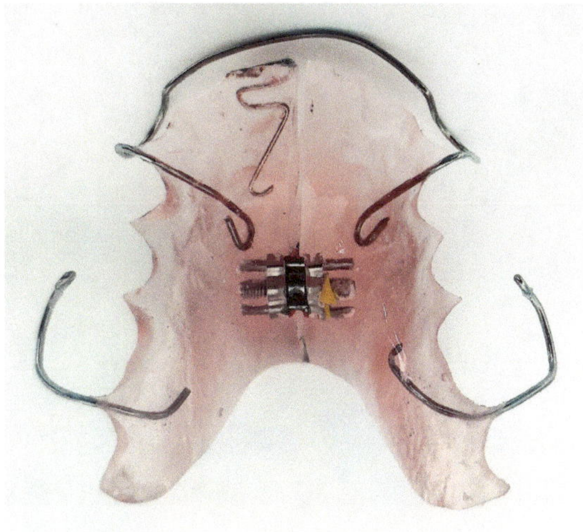

Figure 3.34 Removable appliance with springs for derotation

Management in the early and adult permanent dentition

- In the permanent dentition is best to use a fixed appliance;
- Bonding the bracket on the rotated tooth slightly closer to the rotated side (*Figure 3.35).*
- The second proposed treatment includes an auxiliary rotational wedge. The wedge is put on the distal two wings of the bracket and archwire is ligated to the mesial wings;

a *b*

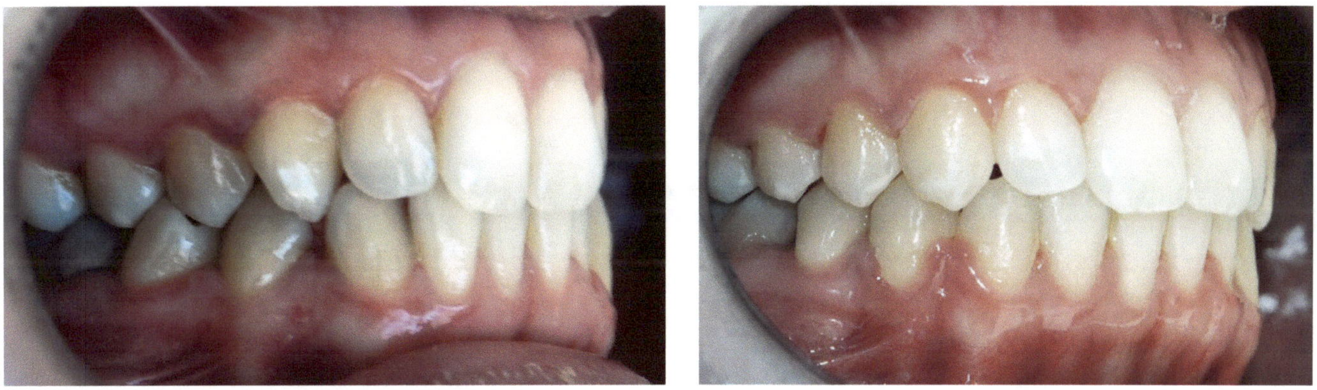

Figure 3.35 In this case, we have upper right canine rotated mediopalatally at 90 degrees. We would bond the bracket slightly more mesial in this situation.

- The second proposed treatment includes an auxiliary rotational wedge. The wedge is put on the distal two wings of the bracket and archwire is ligated to the mesial wings;
- The third method to derotate a tooth is to use the rotation side effect of the open coil spring. The spring would be put between the brackets of the tooth to be rotated and the next tooth. Wire ligature is put on the bracket of the anchor tooth to minimize unwanted rotation and the elastic ligature is ligated on the tooth to be derotated. A side effect is space opening between these two teeth which can be corrected later (*Figure 3.36*).
- Another method for derotation is the use of an additional palatal button on the tooth to be rotated and use couple of forces in opposite directions (*Figure 3.37*).

a

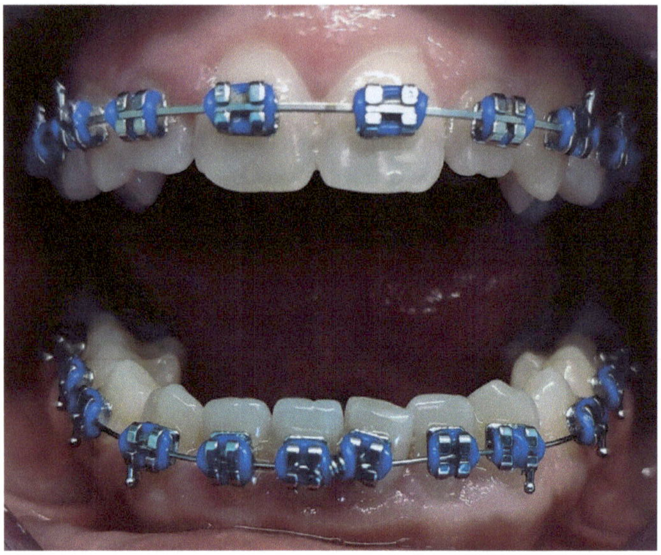

b

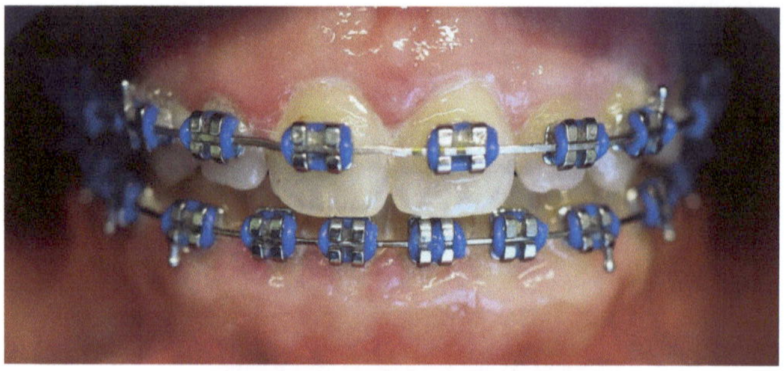

c

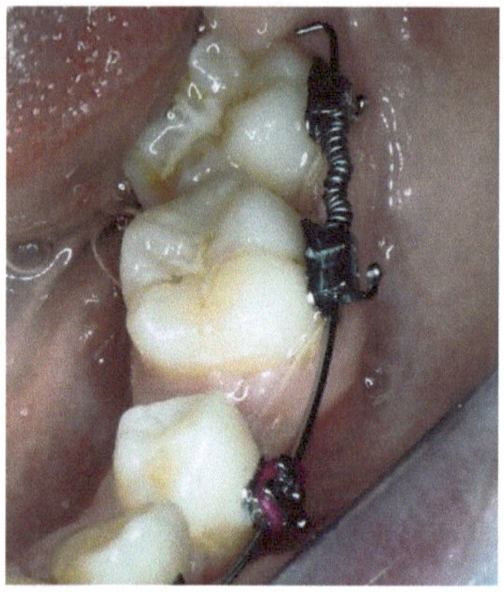

Figure 3.36 Derotation by the use of open coil spring

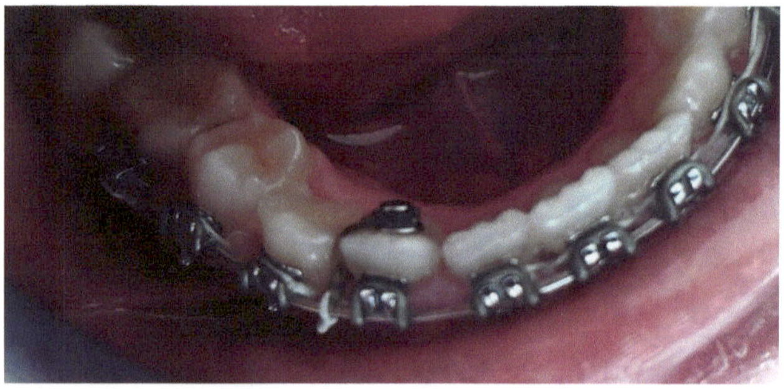

Figure 3.37 Derotation with couple of forces.

Retention

- Rotations tend to rebound easily so permanent retention is advised;
- Roth advocates overcorrection of rotated teeth to compensate for rebound;
- A combination of fixed retainer for the first year and removable retainer later is a good alternative.

4. Management of Developmental Problems

Management of oral habits

Abnormal functions such as mouth breathing, tongue thrust swallowing, low tongue position at rest, unilateral chewing, and abnormal postures of perioral musculature can cause malocclusion.
Research has shown that many deformities caused by muscle dysfunction during the primary or mixed dentition are not self-corrected and become worse in older age.

Non-Nutritive Sucking

Non-nutritive sucking has been defined as sucking on an object (digit or pacifier) not related to the ingestion of nutrients.

Etiology

- Still unknown;
- The psychoanalytic schools regard the habit as a symptom of some emotional disturbance;
- Behaviorists view the habit as a simple learned act with no underlying neurosis;
- Inadequate sucking activity. Digit sucking has also been related to inadequate sucking activity, based on the findings that children who did not suck their fingers were nursed longer.

Thumb or Finger Sucking

Thumb or finger sucking is one of the most common types of non-nutritive oral habit present in children.

- Reported prevalence rates in the first year vary from 50% to 70% and decrease thereafter;
- Persistence beyond the age of 5 is considered a chronic non-nutritive habit that needs some type of intervention.

Clinical findings

- Depend on the duration, frequency, and intensity of the force;
- According to Proffit, sufficient time must be more than a threshold duration, which is 6 hours or more per day. Therefore, if the habit has a shorter duration, little or no effect is seen.

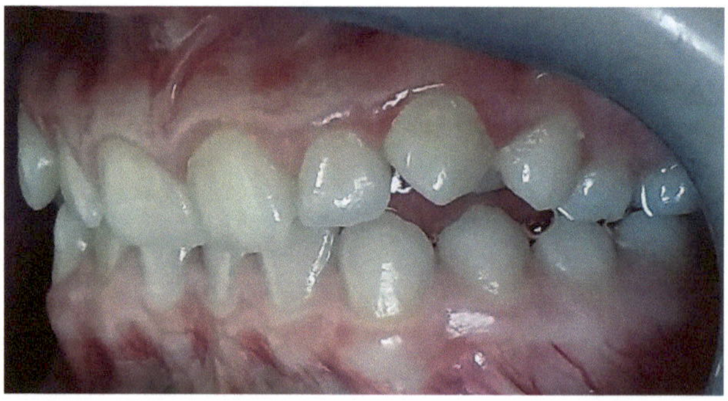

Figure 4.1 Posterior open bite caused by finger sucking

Clinical Features

When the object is positioned in the anterior part of the dentition we can observe:

- Maxillary incisor flaring, retroclination and crowding of the mandibular incisors, or both (maxillary incisor protrusion and mandibular incisor retrusion;
- Anterior open bite due to anterior undereruption, posterior overeruption, or a combintion of both;

• Posterior crossbite.

Dental effects

- Increased overjet due to incisor flaring;
- Anterior open bite;
- Interdental spacing;
- Posterior crossbite;
- Mandibular incisor crowding;
- Lingual tipping of mandibular incisors;
- Undereruption of maxillary incisors;
- Overeruption of posterior teeth;
- Class II molar relationships;
- Narrow (V-shaped) anterior maxillary arch.

a *b*

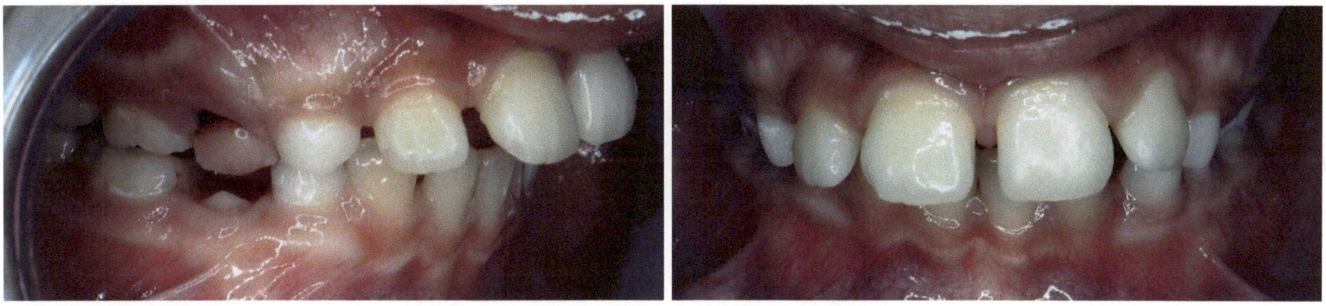

Figure 4.2 Effects of finger sucking habit to the dentition (a b)

Skeletal effects

- Counterclockwise maxillary rotation;
- Clockwise mandibular rotation;
- Increased mandibular plane steepness;
- Increased Class II relationship (forward positioning of point A);
- Increased anterior facial height maxilla, bilateral crossbite, and Class II malocclusion.

Management

Age of intervention

- Sucking habits during the primary dentition years usually have little if any long-term effect and usually stop around 4 to 5 years of age;
- Intervention is recommended after 4 or 5 years of age but should be considered earlier if a high-intensity and long duration are involved and there is severe damage to occlusion or to the jaw, such as clockwise rotation of the mandible and antegonial notching.

Treatment Approaches

1. Psychoanalytic methods: remainder therapy, reward therapy;
2. Behavioral modification techniques;
3. Use of orthodontic appliances;
4. Combination method.

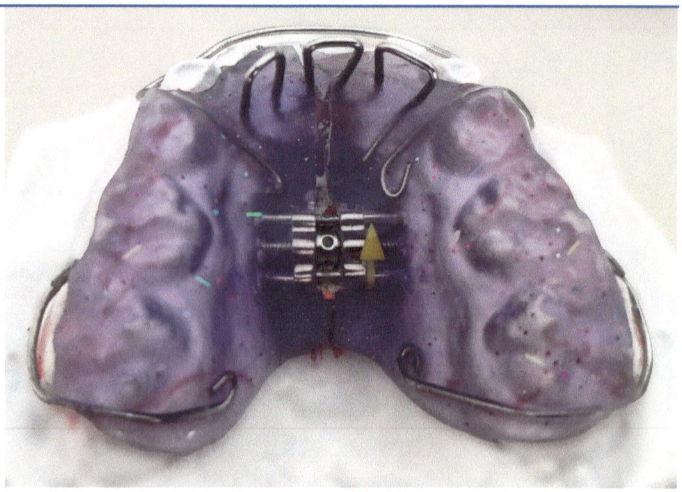

Figure 4.3 Removable habit breaker

Use of orthodontic appliances

- Habit-discouraging appliances usually have positive effects within 2 to 3 months, but they
- should be left in place for at least 6 months to make sure the habit is completely controlled;
- Depending on the patient's cooperation, the kind of habit, and the type of deformity, several kinds of removable, fixed, or semi removable appliances can be used.

Removable habit breakers

- Simple Hawley appliance with a piece of wire embedded in the acrylic resin portion behind the incisors; it can be a useful reminder device and has the advantage of allowing the patient to remove it for eating and maintaining good hygiene (*Figure 4.3*).
- The disadvantages of this type of appliance are that patient compliance is a major factor and the appliance can be easily misplaced or lost.

Fixed habit breakers

- They do not rely on patient compliance;
- A palatal archwire soldered to the bands forms the base of the appliance, to which a crib or some loop is soldered to the anterior portion of the arch, behind the incisors (*Figure 4.4*).
- Bluegrass appliance can be used during the primary or mixed dentition.
- The Bluegrass consists of a six-sided roller that is slipped over a 0.045-inch stainless steel wire soldered to molar bands;
- The child is instructed to turn the roller with his or her tongue instead of sucking the digit (*Figure 4.5*).

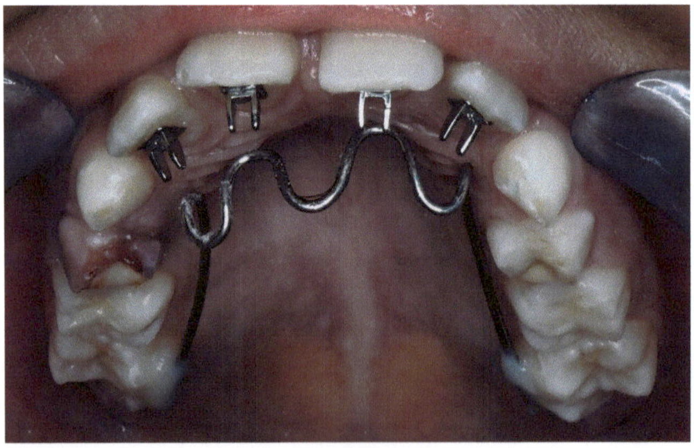

Figure 4.4 Fixed habit breaker

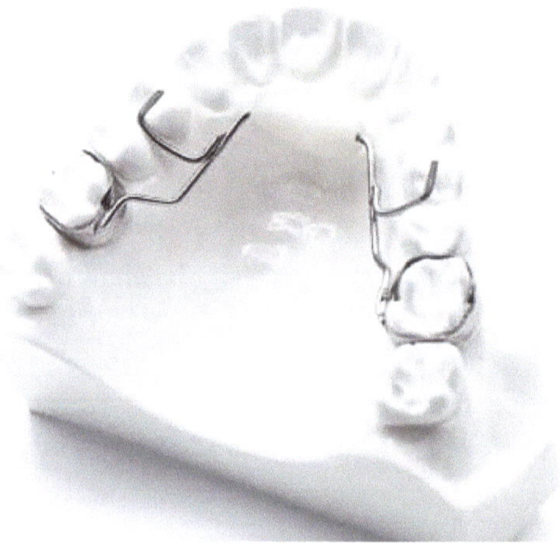

Figure 4.5 Bluegrass habit breaker

Palatal bar

- It is constructed of two molar bands and 0.036-inch stainless steel wire to serve as the base of the appliance;

- A shield or crib made of 0.030-inch wire is adapted to the deepest anterior part of the palate, separating the thumb or finger from the soft tissue;
- A short vertical extension in the front serves as a reminder (*Figure 4.6*).

Quad helix (*Figure 4.7*)

- It is applied during the primary or mixed dentition for transverse expansion of the maxillary arch;
- A combination of the quad helix and habit controller soldered to the anterior part of the helix can be useful in patients who have thumb-sucking habits and also need palatal expansion;
- The quad helix alone, without a habit controller, also can prevent thumb sucking.
- It is a combination of tongue guard and transpalatal arch with some modifications;
- This appliance is constructed of two maxillary molar bands and two pieces of 0.036-inch stainless steel wire;
- One wire serves as a transpalatal arch with an omega loop of 10- to 12-mm diameter toward the distal side. This arch should be soldered to molar bands so that it is separated by at least 1 mm from the palate to facilitate maxillary molar intrusion without impinging on the palate;
- The second wire is used to form a tongue guard wide enough to cover the incisor gap. It should be long enough to stay below the level of the mandibular incisal edge at occlusion.

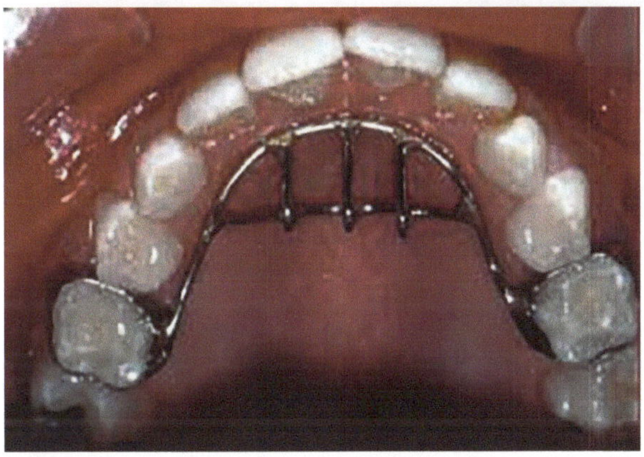

Figure 4.6 Palatal bar appliance

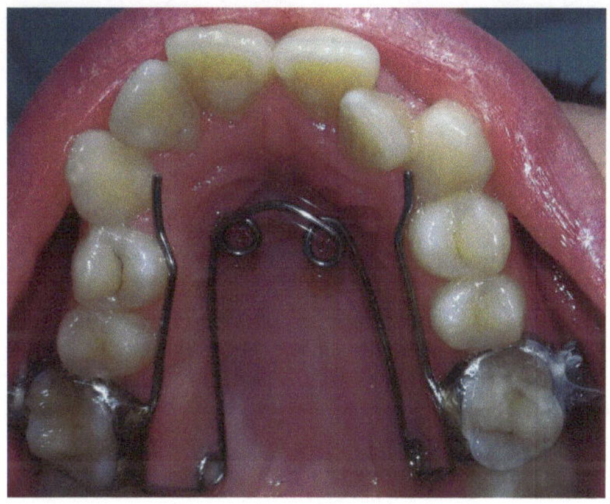

Figure 4.7 Quad helix appliance

Pacifier Habits

Sucking is a powerful reflex in infants in their early days of life.
The American Academy of Family Physicians (AAFP) recommends weaning children from pacifiers between 6 months and 12 months of age to prevent otitis media.

Clinical effects

- Flaring and spacing of upper anterior teeth;
- Retroclination and rotation of anterior lower teeth;
- Anterior open bite;
- Thong trust developed because of anterior open bite;
- Extrusion of posterior teeth;
- Elongation of the lower third of the face;
- Posterior crossbite;
- Speech problems;
- Incising of food problems.

Management of pacifier sucking habit

- Discontinuation of the use of pacifier;
- Careful observation of the child because of the risk of exchanging pacifier for finger sucking;
- The transverse occlusal relationship should be evaluated between 2 and 3 years of age, particularly in children who suck pacifiers;

Tongue Thrust

Clinically, tongue thrust is defined as a forward placement of the tip of the tongue between the anterior teeth during swallowing. The constant pressure of the tongue may force the teeth out of alignment. This myofunctional disorder of the tongue in the oral cavity has been referred to as deviate swallow, infantile swallow, abnormal swallow, reverse swallow, and immature swallow (*Figure 4.9*).

a *b*

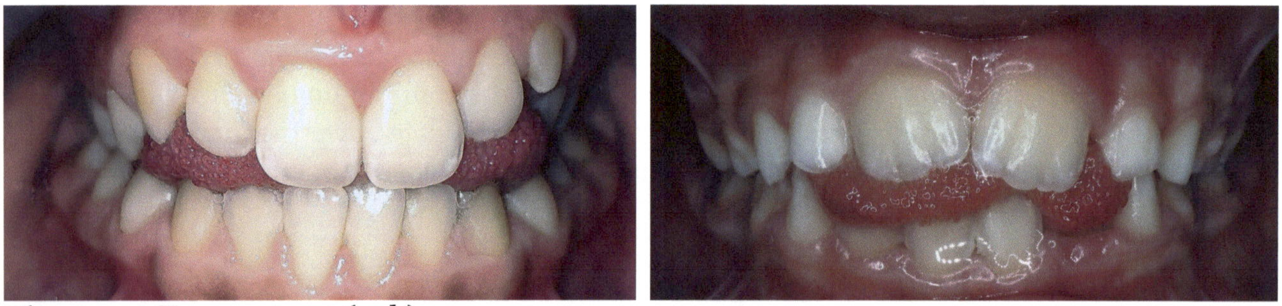

Figure 4.9 Tongue trust (a, b)

- Tongue thrust can develop following finger sucking or because of other factors leading to tongue protrusion during swallowing;
- It can be present without any visible muscle contraction and can be self-corrected or reduced by age.

Classification

- Moyers divided classified abnormal swallowing into three types: the simple tongue-thrust swallow, the complex tongue-thrust swallow, and retained infantile swallow.

1. Simple tongue thrust
   - Simple tongue thrust is usually associated with a history of digit sucking that has led to open bite;
   - The sucking habit may no longer be practiced, but the tongue must thrust forward into the open bite area to maintain an anterior seal with the lips during swallowing.
2. Complex tongue thrust
   - It is a more complicated type of swallowing pattern associated with chronic nasorespiratory issues such as mouth breathing, tonsillitis, or pharyngitis;
   - When the tonsil is inflamed and enlarged, the root of the tongue exerts a force on the tonsil and causes pain. To avoid this force and resulting pain, the mandible will drop reflexively, separating the maxillary and mandibular teeth, enlarging the freeway space, and providing more room for the tongue to move forward.
3. Retained infantile swallow
   - It is an abnormal swallowing pattern in which the infantile swallow remains and the transition to an adult swallowing behavior has not occurred.

Etiology

The following have been proposed as local or general causes for these types of abnormal swallowing:

- Hereditary factors, such as a large tongue;
- Vertical skeletal problems such as a steep mandible or wide gonial angle;
- Thumb or another finger sucking;
- Short lingual frenum;
- Mouth breathing, which might be due to many factors that cause nasal obstruction, such as allergies, nasal congestion, deviated conchae, or large adenoid;
- Certain artificial nipples used in bottle feeding;
- Sore throat, enlarged tonsils, or adenoids that cause difficulty in swallowing;
- Premature loss of primary teeth and abnormal tongue adaptation;
- Muscular, neurologic, or other physiologic abnormalities, such as loss of muscle coordination.

Types of tongue thrust

Anterior tongue thrust (Figure 4.10)

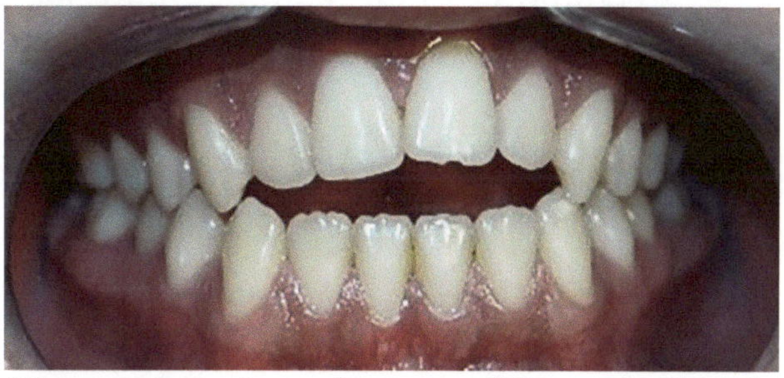

Figure 4.10 Anterior open bite associated with anterior tongue thrust

- The resulting occlusal problem is anterior open bite;
- Sometimes anterior tongue thrust is accompanied by macroglossia;
- Anterior tongue thrust combined with strong mentalis muscle dysfunction exaggerates maxillary incisor protrusion, mandibular incisor retroclination, and crowding and consequently causes severe overjet;

Lateral tongue thrust

- It can cause unilateral or bilateral open bite;
- The anterior bite is usually closed;
- The posterior teeth may be open on one or both sides, from the first premolar to the distalmost molars;
- Lateral tongue thrust usually develops following undereruption of primary molars due to ankylosis;
- Early detection and extraction of ankylosed primary molars can prevent these abnormalities.

Bilateral tongue thrust

- It can develop following primary molar ankylosis on both sides;
- Macroglossia can cause the tongue to rest over occlusal surfaces;
- Another possible cause is a bilateral failure of eruption.

Clinical Features

- Open bite;
- Dental protrusion;

- Spacing;
- In patients with narrow maxillary arches who have a persistent tongue thrust, the maxillary expansion will accommodate the tongue and produce better treatment results.
- Orthodontic treatment will relapse if the force of the tongue is not controlled;
- Speech problems are also a consequence of tongue dysfunction and affected occlusion. The /s/ sounds are most affected, and lisping can result;
- Lateral lisping can occur in patients with lateral open bite caused by lateral tongue thrust during swallowing.

Examination of a child to determine the presence or absence of tongue dysfunction
The following may indicate the presence of tongue dysfunction:

- Initial cause of open bite, such as thumb and finger sucking, prolonged use of pacifiers, and bottle feeding;
- Mouth breathing resulting from a history of allergies or enlarged tonsils or adenoids;
- Open mouth posture (lip incompetence);
- Tightening of facial and lip muscles (grimace or pursing of lips) during swallowing;
- Speech difficulty during sounds such as /s/ and /z/;
- Skeletal malformation of genetic origin.

Management

Two methods for treatment of tongue thrust have been proposed:

- *Mechanotherapy with an orthodontic device*
  - Mechanotherapy in tongue thrust patients can be accomplished with either a removable or a fixed appliance;
  - The part of the appliance that controls the abnormal pressure from the tongue (tongue crib or tongue guard) must be designed in such a way that it covers the entire anterior tooth gap but does not interfere with the bite during chewing;
  - Palatal expansion of the narrow palate and correction of mouth breathing would facilitate the correction of tongue dysfunction.
- *Oral habit training*
  - Oral habit training is an exercise technique taught by a qualified speech therapist who tries to reeducate the muscles associated with swallowing by changing the swallowing pattern;
  - In cases of severe tongue thrust, proper myofunctional therapy might be advised in addition to mechanotherapy;
  - Good results can be achieved when the patient is instructed to complete daily exercises and use the fixed tongue guard;
  - Example exercise: The appliance is inserted, and the child is instructed to close the teeth, put the tip of the tongue behind the tongue crib, and swallow while trying to hold the tongue tip so that it does not touch the crib. This exercise should be repeated several times during the day.

Lip sucking or lip interposition habit

This habit is usually secondary to a finger or thumb habit or to an atypical deglutition pattern, because this type of patient has a great overjet, and consequently, the lower lip is placed behind the upper incisors maintaining or aggravating the condition.

Clinical features *(Figure 4.11)*

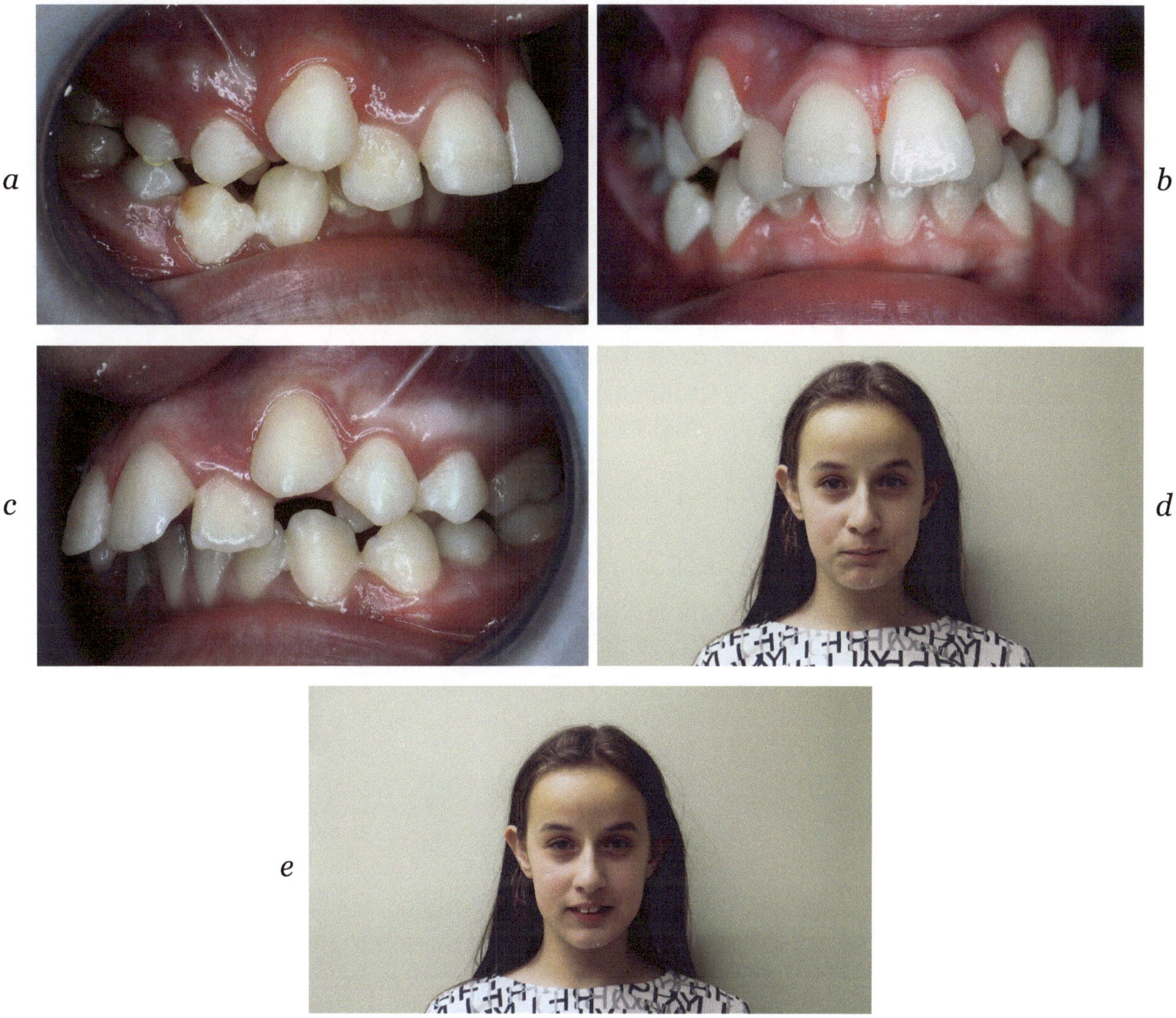

Figure 4.11 Dental features of lip interposition habit (a,b,c,d,e)

- Upper dentoalveolar protrusion;
- Lower incisor retroclination;
- Hypotonic upper lip;
- Hypertonic lower lip;
- Lip incompetence;
- Hypertrophy of the mentalis muscle;
- The excessive pressure of the lower lip impedes the correct development of the lower dental arch;
- Deep bite;
- Generally, the lower incisors occlude on the palatine mucosa;
- Mandibular retrognatia.

Management

- Elimination of the habit;
- Correction of the protruding upper incisor teeth;
- Reduction of the overjet.

Appliances used for management

The lip bumper

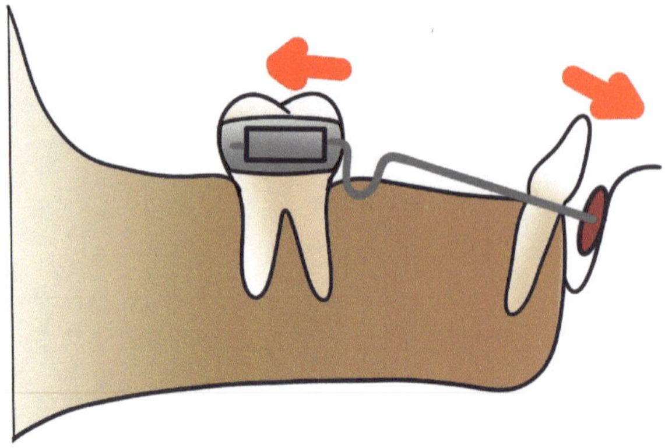

Figure 4.12 Lip bumper appliance

- It is a fixed and passive appliance that has one or two acrylic shields on the anterior sector that separate the lower lip from the anterior teeth, not allowing the lip between the buccal aspects of the lower incisors and the palatine aspects of the upper incisors (Figure 4.12);
- This appliance will have a favorable influence on the development of the lower dental arch, because it will separate the lip from the anteroinferior teeth, producing spontaneous lower arch expansion.

The 2 x 4 technique

- Placing brackets on the anterior sector and with the action of upper retrusion arches or lower protrusion arches; according to the cephalometric requirements of the case, we can correct the overjet by reducing the space needed for the interposition of the lower lip.

Mouth Breathing

Normal respiration requires adequate airway space through the nasal and nasopharyngeal areas. If the structures within this passage, such as the adenoids, tonsils, or nasal turbinate, are enlarged pathologically or anatomically, nasal respiration is precluded; the result can be an adaptation to oral respiration.
The adenoid facial type is characterized as:

- Long, narrow face with an anterior open bite (*Figure 4. 13*);
- Dental protrusion;
- Incompetent lip;
- Narrow maxillary arch;
- Deep palate.

a

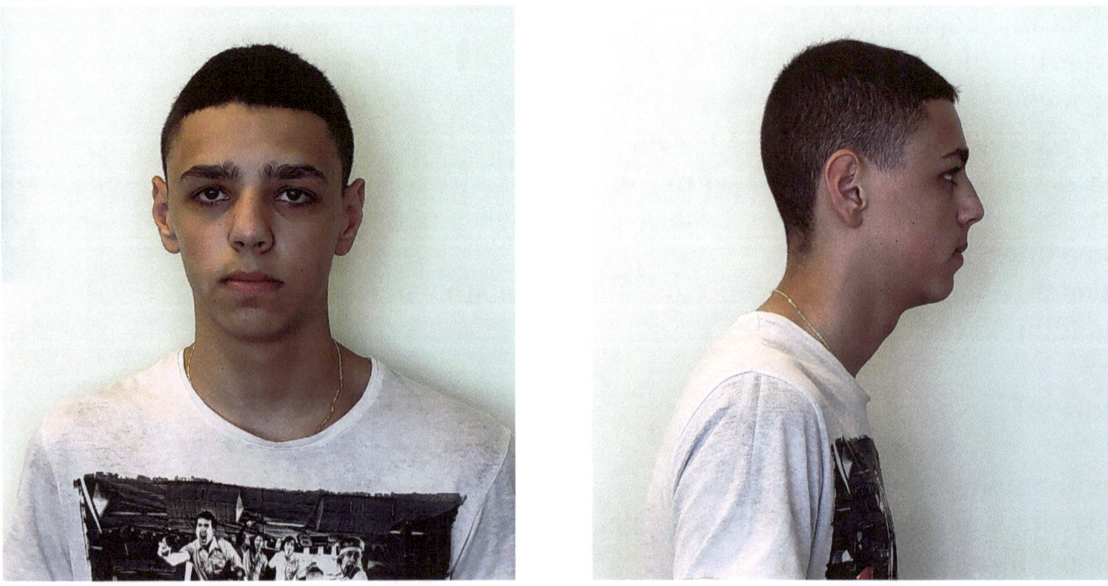

b

c d e

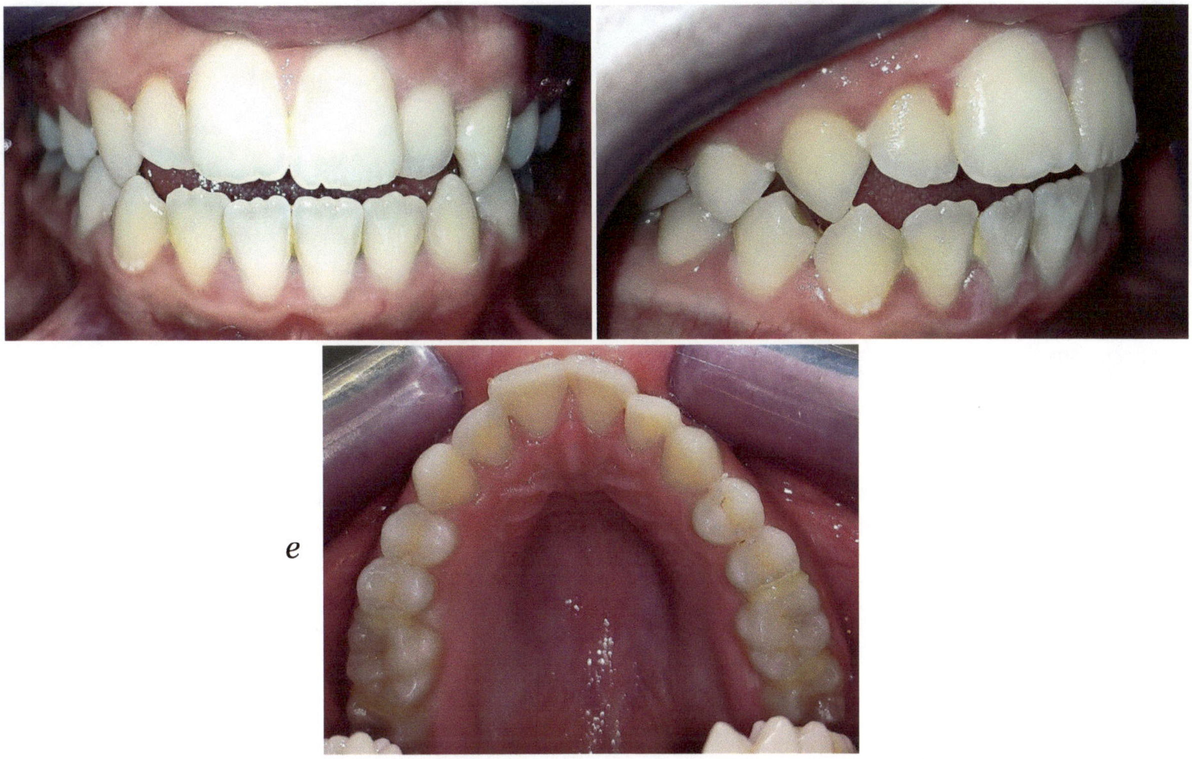

Figure 4. 13 Adenoid facial type patient (a,b) Intraoral features (c,d,e)

Effects on occlusion and dentoskeletal structures

- Maxillary retrusion;
- Maxillary deficiency;
- Counterclockwise rotation of the palate;
- Deeper palatal height;
- Retroclined mandibular incisors;
- Increased total anterior facial height and lower facial height;
- Larger gonial angle;
- Greater sella-nasion plane, palatal plane, and occlusal plane to mandibular plane angles.

a b

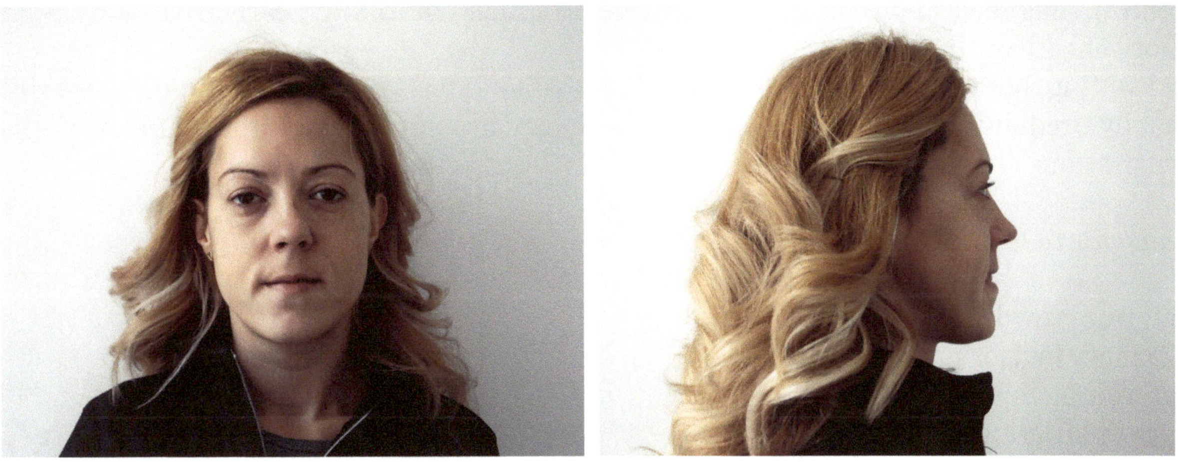

c

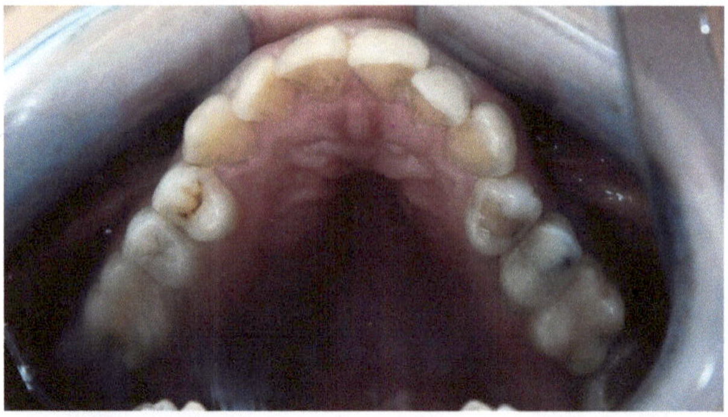

d

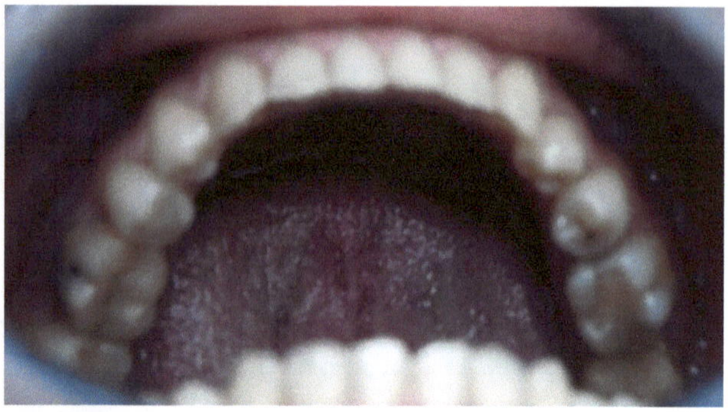

e

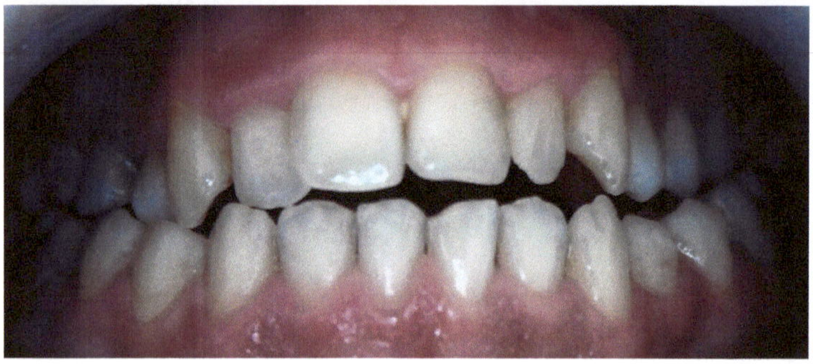

Figure 4.14 Typical characteristics of patients with mouth breathing caused by nasal obstruction: narrow, dolichocephalic face; convex profile; tapering, narrow maxillary dentition; and anterior crowding.

Etiology

- Allergies. Allergies cause swelling of the mucous membranes that line the nose. Even mild swelling can affect lung oxygenation by closing off the sinus openings;
- Inflammation and enlargement of tonsils and adenoids;
- Congenital malformations that cause structural deformities can also block nasal airways. These include deviated or enlarged conchae and deviated septum;
- Trauma such as a broken nose can distort the anatomy of the nose and cause a blockage.

Clinical Features

General body growth and posture.

- The sleep cycle is disrupted, growth hormone production is interfered with, and general body growth (size and weight) and even school performance are affected;
- Obstructive sleep apnea syndrome (OSAS) is a severe sleep disorder of early childhood, and any delay in diagnosis and treatment may cause prolonged morbidity; early treatment is simpler and more effective;
- Bedwetting, poor-quality sleep, and obesity are other effects on these children. These children are usually tired during the day, and their performance in school is poor; they often exhibit anger and frustration.

Dentofacial characteristics

- Anterior crowding;
- Maxillary incisor proclination;
- Anterior open bite;
- Narrow anterior maxilla;
- Narrow maxillary arch and bilateral posterior crossbite;
- Overeruption of molars;

- Dry lips;
- Bad breath and periodontal disease, caused by the shift in the bacterial flora in the mouth;
- Dark circles under the eyes

Skeletal changes

- Clockwise rotation of the growing mandible;
- Increased anterior facial height;
- Increased lower anterior vertical face height;
- Long, narrow face;
- Retrognathia of the mandible;
- Antegonial notching;
- Increased mandibular steepness;
- Maxillary constriction, deep palate, and posterior crossbite;
- Downward rotation of the posterior palate;
- Maxillary deficiency;
- Narrowed nasal airway passage and decreased intranasal capacity.

Clinical examination

Early detection and diagnosis of mouth breathing is an important part of children's dental examination.

Evaluation for mouth breathing consists of four steps:

1. The patient and parent should be questioned regarding the child's general health, the possibility of any allergy, the type of breathing during the day and while sleeping, the presence of daytime sleepiness, the presence of snoring, and the child's activities and school performance;
2. The child's general growth and posture, such as height and weight as compared with a normal growth chart, should be assessed. The child's posture should be observed while he or she walks, sits, is weighed, and is measured for height. The child's shoulders should be watched for the presence of any asymmetry, and the natural head posture, which can be altered in mouth breathers, should be noted;
3. Dentoskeletal characteristics of mouth breathers can be checked by extraoral and intraoral examination. Incompetent lips, forward position of the tongue, increased overjet, maxillary anterior crowding and tapering arch, posterior crossbite or crossbite tendency, and deep and narrow palate are visual signs of mouth breathing;
4. Direct examination for evaluation of the child's breathing can be performed in the clinic while the patient is seated straight and relaxed on a dental chair:

- First the patient's breathing is observed indirectly without informing the child;
- Then the patient is asked to take a deep breath without closing the lips, while the examiner watches the patient's lip position and alar muscle reflex carefully;
- The child is asked to close the lips and take a deep breath. Nose breathers dilate the external nares on inspiration by controlling alar muscles;
- Other kinds of direct examination can be done, such as holding a cold dental mirror in front of the nose for a little while.

Differential diagnosis for lip incompetence

Lip incompetence can be a sign of mouth breathing. Other factors can cause lip separation during the rest position; these must be differentiated during the patient's examination:

- Short lips;
- Hypotonic lips;
- Increased lower facial height;
- Severe dental protrusion.

Management

Orthodontic appliances

- Rapid palatal expansion results in significant changes in children's breathing patterns (*Figure 4.15*);
- This type of treatment corrects transverse occlusal disharmony and functional problems and provides more space for teeth;
- It increases nasal airway capacity as an immediate result of rapid skeletal expansion;
- The expansion provides room for the tongue to rest and function normally in the palate.

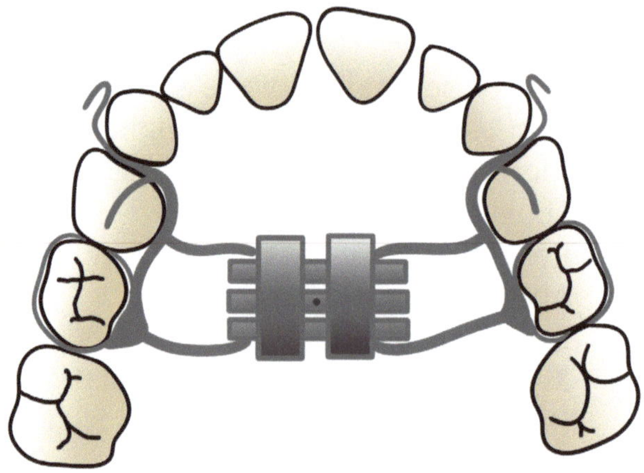

Figure 4.15 Rapid palatal expander

Suggestions for breaking this habit

- Use of a piece of surgical tape to keep the mouth closed;
- Use of an oral screen with a thin piece of rubber behind and between the lips to block airflow.

Muscle Exercises

- Lip exercises will strengthen the seal of the lips and obstruct the mouth to force breathing through the nose. For example, the patient can be instructed to hold a sheet of paper between the lips and try to breathe through the nose for a period of time, a few times a day, to improve lip seal;
- Another exercise involves the use of a button with a piece of string tied to it. The patient should hold the button behind the lips and stretch the string while the lips are resisting; this exercise can improve lip seal and tonicity;
- Hypotonicity of the upper lip. The child is advised to extend the upper lip as much as possible, curving the vermilion border under and behind maxillary incisors. When a child has a short upper lip, the exercise should be done 15–30 minutes per day for a duration of 4–5 months.

Muscle Exercise	Procedure	Indications
Pterygoid muscle Exercise	Consists of: • Bringing the mandible forward so that the mandibular incisor teeth are held anterior to the maxillary incisors, provided that the maxillary incisors are in normal position. • Then the patient is instructed to relax the muscles and allow the mandible to recede to the point where the dental arches are in their relatively correct mesiodistal relationship.	• In the treatment of distocclusion, as the weakness of this muscle can be responsible for this type of malocclusion.

Muscle Exercise	Procedure	Indications
Masseter-temporal muscles exercises	• Consists of the contraction and relaxation of the masseter group of muscles with the mandible in normal position. The patient places the tip of the forefinger over the muscle near the angles of the mandible to feel the contracting and relaxing movement. • This exercise should not be performed if the patient is unable to place the mandible in its correct position.	• Correction of infraocclusion. • In correction of Distocclusion
Tongue exercise	• The patient is instructed to position the tip of the tongue against the mucous membrane directly behind the mandibular incisors, and with each contraction of the masseter-temporal group of muscles to press the tongue against the anterior section; at the same time, by widening the tongue to force it against the lateral sides of the alveolar process.	• It is an adjunct to the masseter-temporal exercise. • Trains the tongue to remain in its proper position. • Has tendency to prevent the narrowing of the mandibular arch, facilitating the early removal of retainers.
Orbicularis oris and facial muscle exercise	• Orbicularis oris exercise is best performed with the aid of an exerciser design so that it is difficult to keep it within the oral orifice unless the orbicularis oris muscle is contracted properly. The exerciser is made of two curved bars of acrylic or stainless steel, and united near their centers by a joint to which handle at right angle is attached. There are notches at one end of the bars, to which elastic bands are attached so that there is a resistance to approximate the free ends of the bars. The free ends are shaped to engage the angle of the mouth. This exercise is continued with one elastic band during the first week or two, and contractions are increased daily until they reach 50-60 a day. • General tonic exercise: Influences not only the orbicularis oris, but also the muscles that work with the orbicularis oris. It consists in taking a generous mouthful of warm saline solution, at a temperature that is bearable to the mucous membrane of the mouth, and with the teeth held firmly in occlusion the solution is forced through the interproximal spaces into the buccal cavity and then back into the lingual space. The exercise is usually performed morning and night. The patient is directed to continue each exercise until the muscles are slightly fatigued.	• Increases the tonicity of muscle. • Oral hygiene is also improved.
Mentalis muscle exercise	• The exercise to develop the upper lip: o Grasp the chin firmly between the thumb and index finger with the lips relaxed. o Hold the lower lip down. o Close the lips. o Relax and repeat from 10 to 50 times at a specified time, as before meals. • The exercise for the pronunciation of the letter "P": o The sound should be made forcibly. o It should be made before a mirror. o The patient should be instructed how to make the sound. o Whether the mentalis shows excessive muscular activity at the beginning of the sound must be noted. o Two exercise periods of 5 or 10 min each must be observed daily. • Whistling: Is an exceptionally fine exercise for the orbicularis oris, mentalis and the associated muscle. The muscular activity is much more vigorous and powerful than that used in making the sound "P". The higher the note, the greater the muscular activity.	• Development of the orbicularis oris and the associated muscles. • The exercises should be started as soon as the protrusion has been reduced to the extent that it is possible for the patient to close the lips without stretching them.

Table 4.1 Muscle Exercises

Speech and Malocclusion

The majority of the sound is developed by the tongue and anterior teeth, and a causal relationship between speech defects and malocclusion has long been assumed to exist. One example is a lisping sound associated with malocclusion of the anterior teeth. Some other teeth irregularities that can be suspected to cause speech disorders are narrow, high palates; incisal irregularities; and spaced or absent teeth. Anteroposterior arch malrelationships (Angle Class II and Class III malocclusions) are also commonly listed as the malocclusions chiefly associated with defective speech.

Effects on occlusion

- The majority of children with speech defects protrude the tongue tip between the incisors during speech and swallowing;
- There can be anterior open bite;
- Increased overjet;
- Upper anterior protrusion.

Management

- It is done by a speech specialist;
- Orthodontic correction of existing malocclusion may be needed alongside with speech therapy;
- Some spontaneous correction of speech sound articulation occurs during the eruption of some permanent teeth at the first phase of mixed dentition.

Bruxism

- Bruxism is defined as the grinding of teeth resulting from a nonfunctional rhythmic contraction of the masseter, temporalis, and internal pterygoid muscles. Bruxism usually occurs while the patient is sleeping;
- Tooth grinding is a subconscious action that is characterized by a noticeable sound; it is silent during the daytime;
- Bruxism is a destructive habit that may result in structural damage, tooth wear, temporomandibular dysfunction (TMD), facial pain, muscle pain and tenderness, muscle spasms, headache, stiffness of the neck, and periodontal problems.

Incidence

- According to Peterson and Schneider,3 the prevalence of bruxism in children is very high, ranging from 5.1% to 96%.

Etiology

- The exact cause of bruxism is unknown;
- Most explanations center on local, systemic, and psychologic factors;
- The local theory suggests that bruxism is a reaction to an occlusal interference of opposing teeth, high restoration, or some irritating dental condition during function or at rest;
- Systemic factors in relation to bruxism include intestinal parasites, nutritional deficiencies, allergies, or endocrine disorders. Nervous disorders, psychologic dysfunction, emotional illness,

anxiety, frustration, stress, and asthma are other proposed factors.

Effects on the dentition are

- Tooth wear;
- Thermal hypersensitivity;
- Tooth hypermobility;
- Injury to the periodontal ligament and periodontium;
- Hypercementosis;
- Fractured cusps;
- Pulpitis, and pulpal necrosis.

Management in the mixed dentition

- Treatment can include occlusal adjustment of the dentition;
- Use of interocclusal appliances;
- Behavior modification;
- Pharmaceuticals;
- A soft or hard occlusal bite plate is a useful orthodontic appliance. Vinyl bite guards are fabricated to cover the occlusal surfaces of all teeth and can be worn at night to prevent continuing abrasion (*Figure 4.16*);
- Application of a simple Hawley appliance with an anterior bite plate is one method of choice, which is not only easy for children to wear but also prevents occlusal wear;
- It opens the posterior bite;
- Promotes posterior tooth eruption and alveolar growth;
- Reduces the deep bite and enhances lower facial height during the early and middle mixed dentition.

a

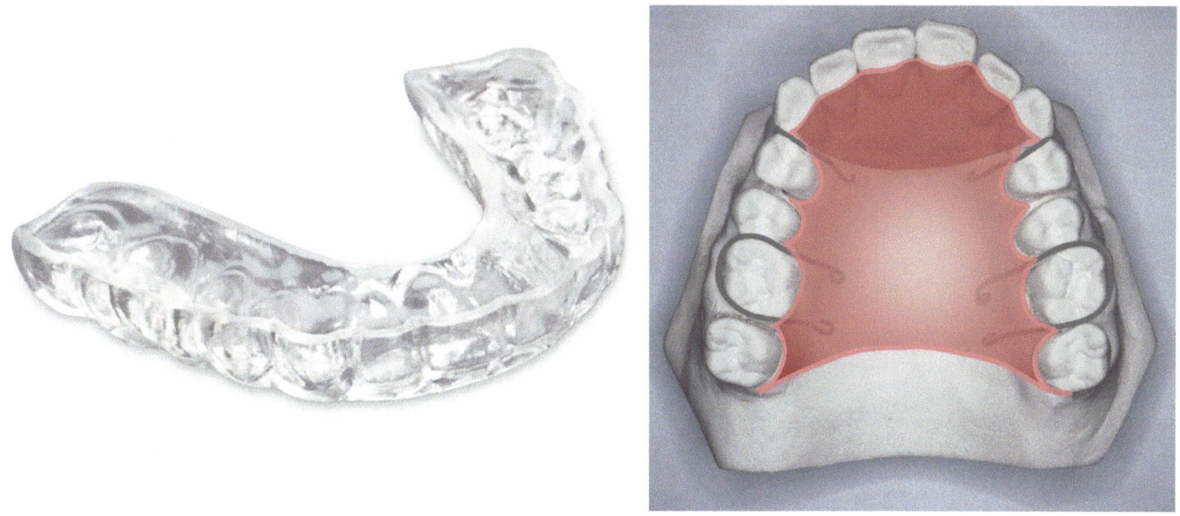

b

Figure 4.16 Appliances used for bruxism. Acrylic guard (a), removable Hawley appliance (b);

Management of Hypodontia

Tooth agenesis (hypodontia) is the most common craniofacial malformation; it can occur as an isolated condition (non-syndromic) or in association with other developmental anomalies (syndromic).

- It can result in abnormal spacing, tipping of adjacent teeth, abnormal tooth relationships, and disturbed intercuspation and interdigitation;

- Inclined teeth can result in occlusal trauma to the affected teeth, areas of stagnation susceptible to caries, periodontal problems, bone loss, and mandibular shift;
- Missing anterior teeth can disturb physiologic functions such as speech and mastication and can seriously impair the patient's esthetics (*Figure 4.17*).

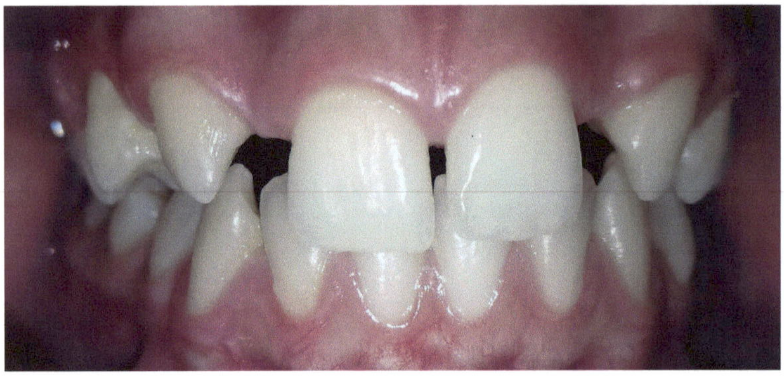

Figure 4.17 Patient with agenesis of upper lateral incisors

Classification

- Hypodontia is a general term used for the congenital absence of teeth. This anomaly can appear as an absence of a single tooth, agenesis of several teeth, or even complete tooth agenesis in patients with ectodermal dysplasia syndrome;
- Oligodontia or partial hypodontia is a term that has been used to describe the absence of multiple teeth (*Figure 4.18*);
- Anodontia (total hypodontia), or absence of all teeth, is a very rare anomaly that has occurred in some patients with ectodermal dysplasia.
- Anodontia (total hypodontia), or absence of all teeth, is a very rare anomaly that has occurred in some patients with ectodermal dysplasia.

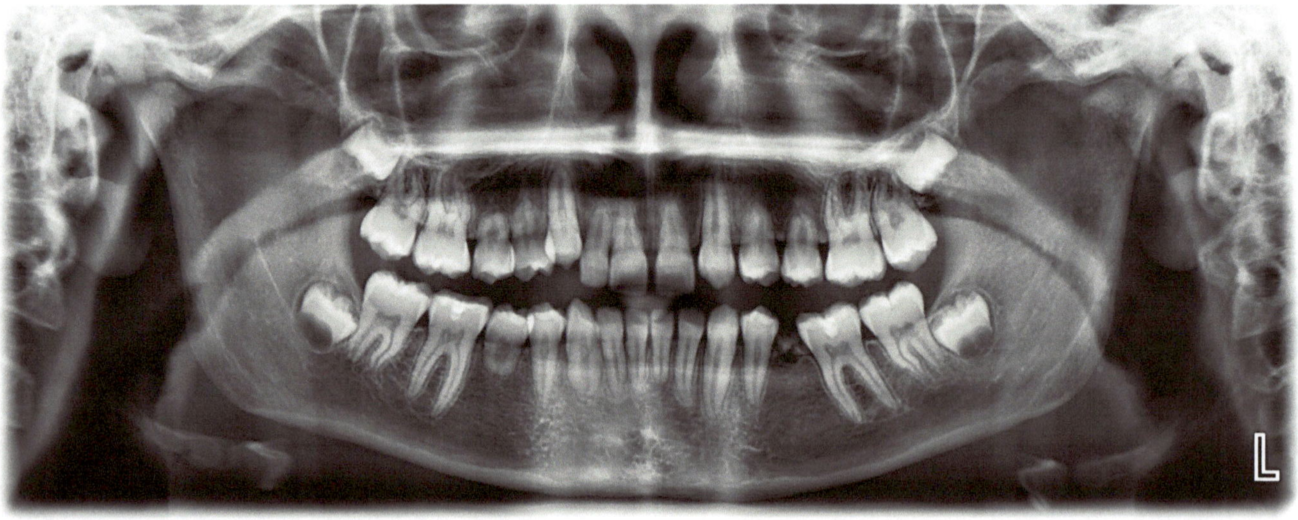

Figure 4.18 Patient with multiple missing teeth

Prevalence

- Excluding third molars, the incidence of other missing teeth has been reported to be between 1.6% and 9.6%;
- The teeth most frequently absent are the maxillary lateral incisors and mandibular second premolars and mandibular third molars (*Figure 4.19*).

a

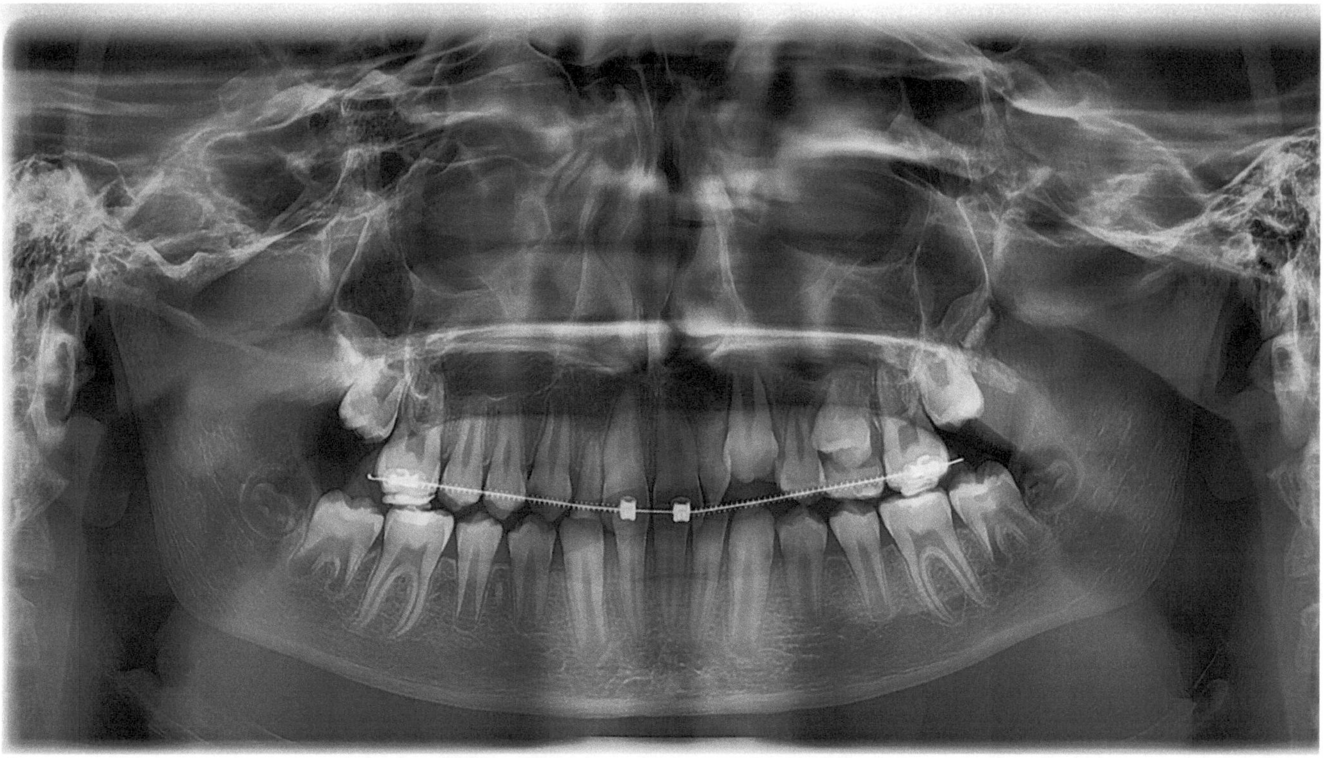

b

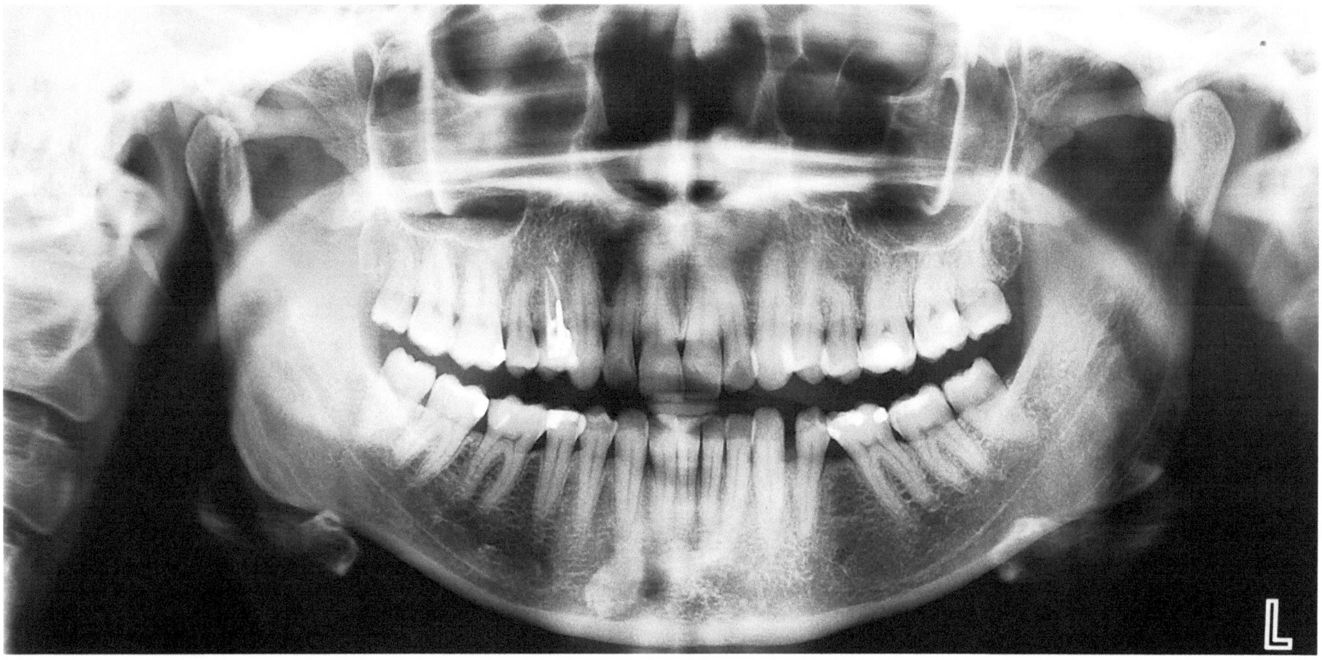

Figure 4.19 Patient with agenesis of upper lateral incisor and lower central incisor (a); Patient with agenesis of lower second premolar (b);

Etiology

Different etiologic factors have been proposed for this anomaly:

- Genetic factors;
- Environmental factors:
  - Allergy;
  - Facial trauma;
  - Maternal medications during pregnancy;

- Endocrine disturbances;
- Maternal health during pregnancy;
- Maternal rubella (German measles) during pregnancy;
- Evolutionary dental changes;
- Localized inflammation and infection during the initial stage of tooth formation;
- Systemic conditions (rickets, syphilis);
- Dysplastic syndromes (ectodermal dysplasia) and abnormalities of the ectodermal structures;
- Chemotherapy and irradiation.

Effects of hypodontia on occlusion

Depending on the number of missing teeth and the area where the teeth are missing, the following anomalies may result from hypodontia:

- Spacing;
- Midline shifting;
- Tipping of adjacent teeth;
- Tooth displacement;
- Overeruption of teeth in the opposing arch;
- Canine impaction;
- Premature contacts, occlusal trauma, crossbite;
- Mandibular shift;
- Abnormal path of growth;
- Soft tissue retrusion;
- Increasing numbers of missing teeth also resulted in a decrease in the mandibular plane angle and a reduction in the anterior lower facial height.

Clinical features of Hypodontia

- Overretained primary teeth;
- Incomplete eruption and ankylosis of primary teeth;
- Abnormal spacing and tipping of adjacent teeth;
- Midline shift;
- Microdontia;
- Asymmetric exfoliation of the primary dentition;
- Evidence of hypodontia in other members of the family.

Management

Treatment options

Generally, there are four treatment options for the management of missing teeth:

1. Moving the adjacent tooth to close the space created by the missing tooth, such as canine substitution for a lateral incisor;
2. Opening and aligning space for a conventional prosthesis or an implant-supported replacement;
3. Retaining the primary tooth;
4. Autotransplantation.

To determine the appropriate treatment option, the clinician must consider factors that can vary for each patient:

- The type of malocclusion;
- Anterior tooth relationships;
- The patient's profile;
- Space requirements;
- Condition of the adjacent teeth;
- The patient's desires.

Management of missing lateral incisors

General Factors	Space closure	Space opening
Facial profile	Convex or straight	Straight, Concave
Shape of the canine	Normal shape and color, not too large in comparison with central incisor	Large size, Darker color, high gingival margin
Type of malocclusion	Class I, Class II malocclusions, absence of posterior crossbite. Normodivergent or Hyperdivergent with an anterior open bite or open bite tendency	Class I, Class III malocclusion, anterior or posterior crossbite. Normodivergent or Hypodivergent with a deep bite.
Space available in the upper arch	Less than 8 mm	More than 8 mm
Wisdom teeth	Not erupted in a good position	Absent or extracted
Age	Adolescent patient	Adult patient
Patient`s wish		

Table 4.2 Decision between space opening and space closure

Space closure by canine substitution

Indications

- Class I crowded mandibular dentition requiring mandibular extraction;
- Class II division 1 malocclusion with severe overjet and good mandibular dentition;
- Canine with proper form, size, and color;
- Normal or moderate overbite;
- Concomitant missing maxillary lateral incisor and missing mandibular incisor;
- Patient's profile - balanced and relatively straight one or slightly convex;
- Lip line. Patients who show excessive gingiva on smiling because of an excess of vertical alveolar size or short upper lip are not good candidates for canine substitution *(Figure 4.20)*.
- Contouring and reshaping the canine crown may lead to dentin exposure, which requires restorative intervention *(Figure 4.21)*.

a *b*

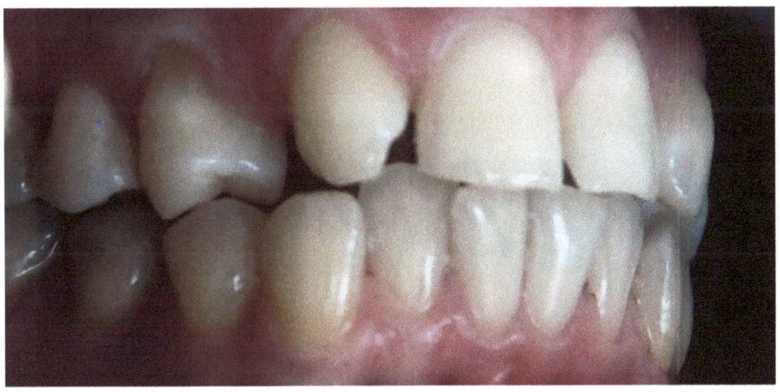

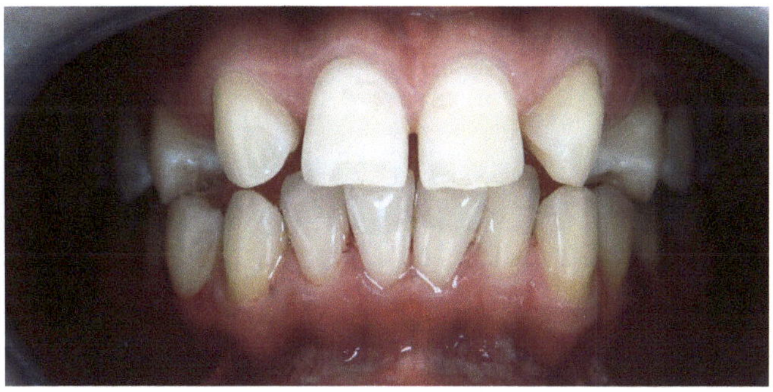

c d e f g h

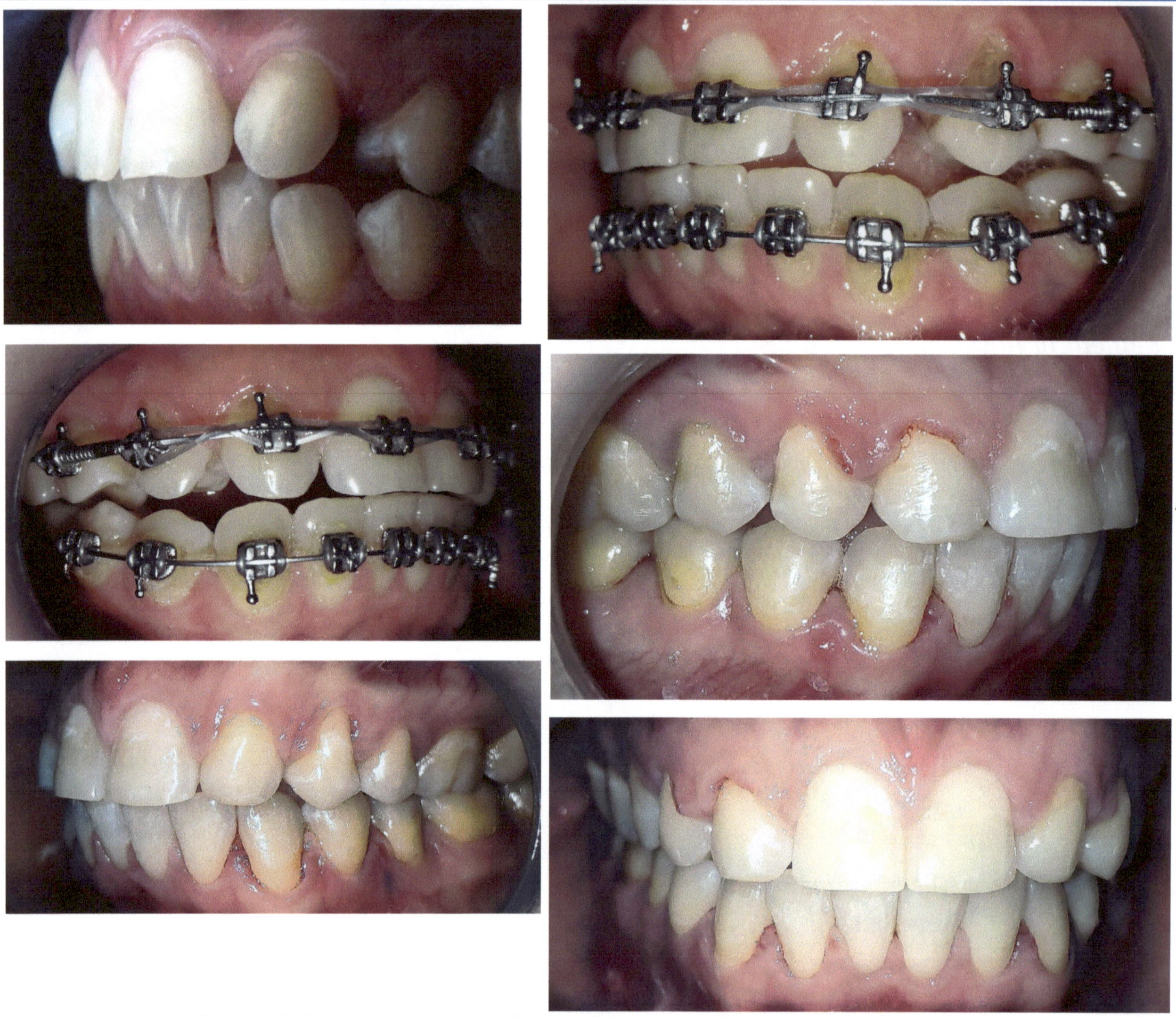

Figure 4.20 Patient with missing upper lateral incisors before (a,b,c) and after treatment (f,g,h). Closing of the spaces was done with a combination of elastic chain and open coil spring (d,e). Anchorage has been obtained with class III elastics.

Space creation and alignment for a prosthesis

Another option for management of hypodontia is an alignment of adjacent teeth in the region and preparation of the occlusion for prosthetic replacement or implants (*Figure 4.22*).

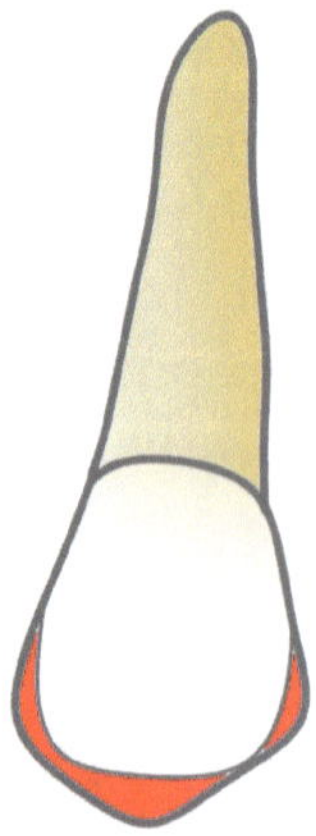

Figure 4.21 Reshaping of the canine tooth.

Indications

- Class I malocclusion, minimum overjet, and good mandibular dentition;
- Maxillary deficiency with normal mandibular dentition;
- Severe deep bite.

Treatment approaches

Prosthetic replacement options

- Fiber-reinforced composite resin fixed partial denture;
- Removable partial denture;
- Single-tooth implant.

a b c d
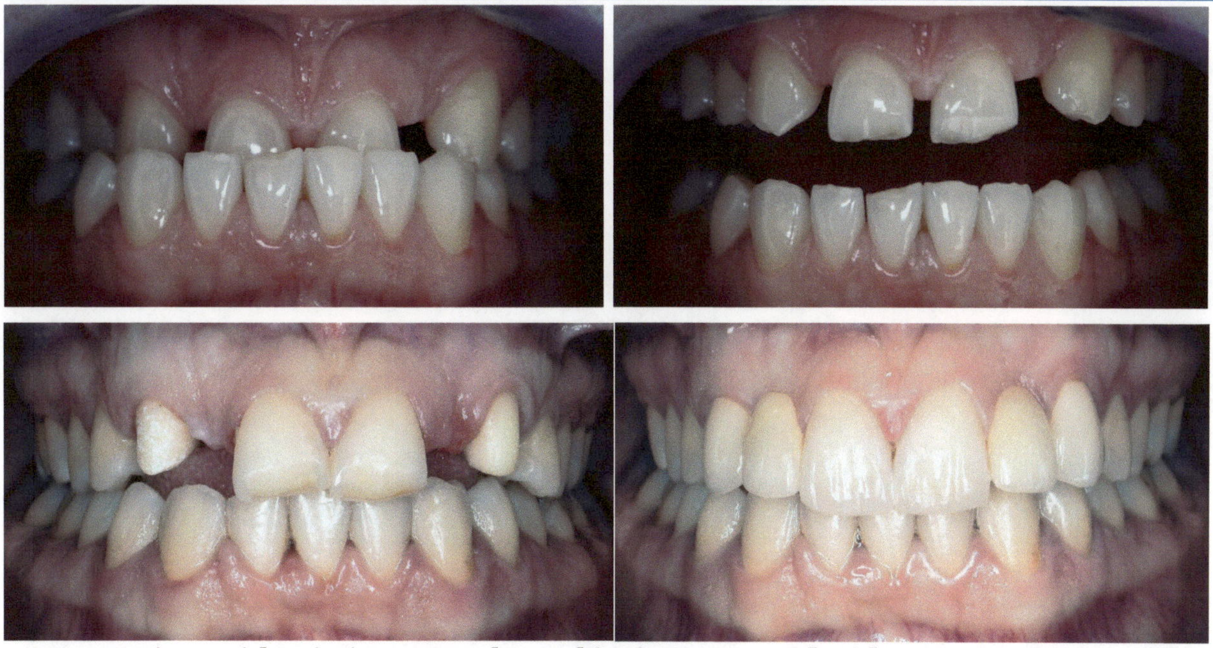

Figure 4.22 Patient with missing upper lateral incisors, treated with space opening and prosthetic restoration (a,b). The treatment plan included extraction of a lower incisor, correcting the reverse overbite, and space opening. After the debonding of brackets (c), the patient was sent to the restorative team (d).

Autotransplantation

- Autotransplantation is surgical repositioning of a tooth from one site to another within the same individual. The new location may be a fresh extraction socket or an artificially prepared socket in an edentulous alveolar ridge;
- Evidence for the successful transplantation of premolars and molars to the incisor region has also been presented.

Management of Missing Mandibular Second Premolars

The second premolar is one of the most common congenitally absent teeth. Its absence can cause serious problems for occlusion and represents a complicated treatment situation.

- There are two general strategies for management of congenitally missing second premolars:

1. Space opening for future restorations;
2. Space closure so that natural teeth touch each other

Treatment options for congenitally missing premolars:

- Retaining the primary molar;
- We must consider the age of the patient, the occlusal status, the condition of the infraoccluded tooth, including the degree of infraocclusion and root resorption, and adjacent alveolar bone levels (*Figure 4.23*);
- If the primary tooth is in normal condition and in a normal relationship to the adjacent and opposing teeth (excluding the aforementioned abnormal condition) but the succedaneous tooth is missing, it can be preserved as long as it remains naturally;
- Alveolar bone can also stay intact for a future implant or prosthetic replacement. In cases of infraocclusion of primary molars;
- Building the occlusal surface with composite is recommended.

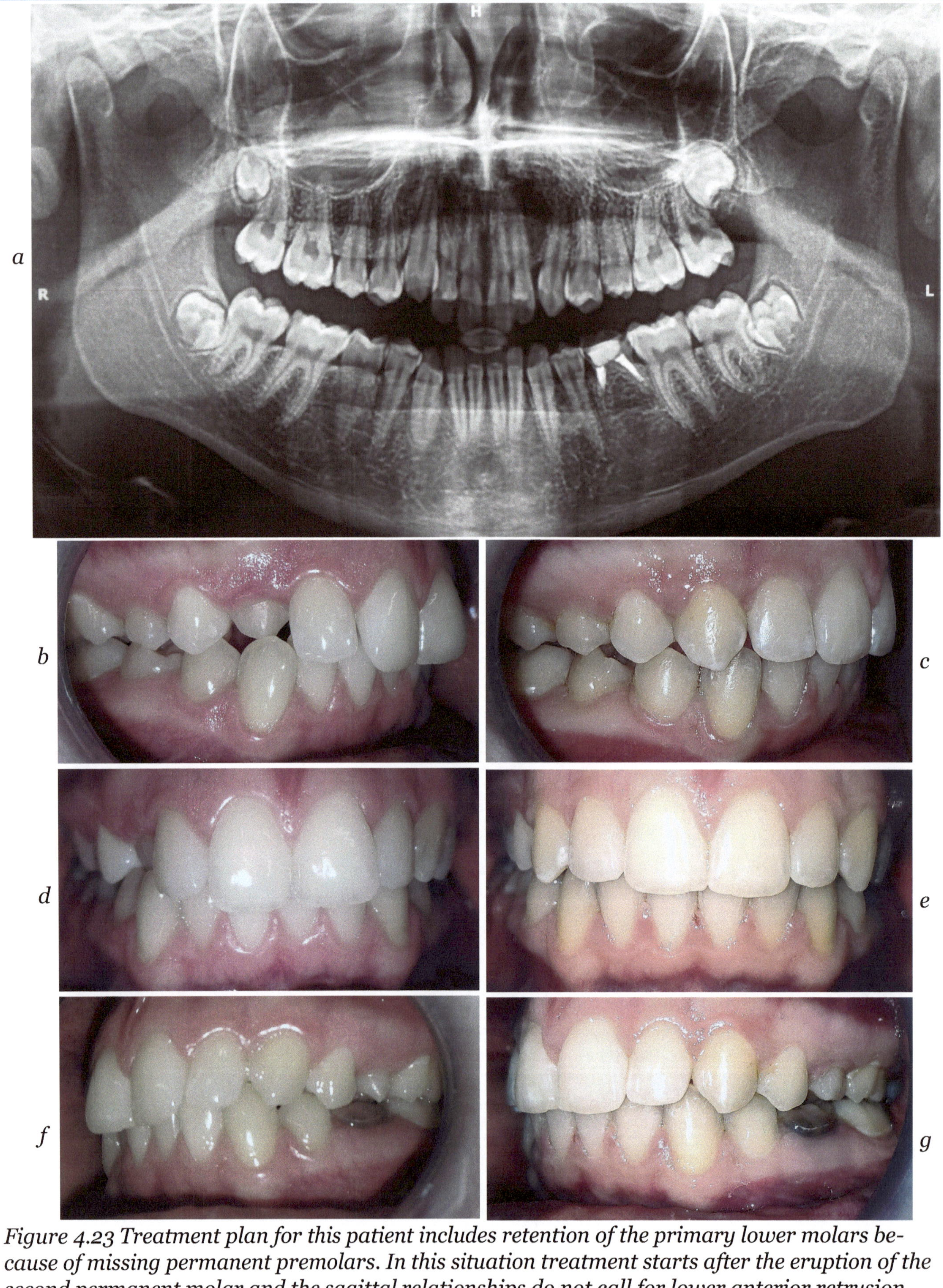

Figure 4.23 Treatment plan for this patient includes retention of the primary lower molars because of missing permanent premolars. In this situation treatment starts after the eruption of the second permanent molar and the sagittal relationships do not call for lower anterior retrusion.

- Closing the space left by the missing tooth

There are two different orthodontic treatment approaches to closing the premolar space:

- Gradual slicing of the distal surface of the primary second molar to allow the permanent first molars to drift slowly, thus facilitating future orthodontic treatment;
- Extraction of the primary second molar to allow the permanent first molar to drift mesially followed by immediate orthodontic uprighting and closure of residual space.
- Placing a tooth-supported restoration or a single-tooth implant
  - This option is usually applied in the permanent dentition;
  - Preparation of the occlusion may include uprighting of teeth, root paralleling, correction of rotations, leveling, and, in cases of overeruption, an intrusion of the opposing teeth.
- Autotransplantation

Orthodontic management of supernumerary teeth

Supernumerary teeth are defined as teeth formed in excess of the normal dental complement in a normal primary or permanent dentition. This phenomenon, also known as hyperdontia, is a disorder of odontogenesis that develops at the stage of initiation during teeth formation (*Figure 4.24*).

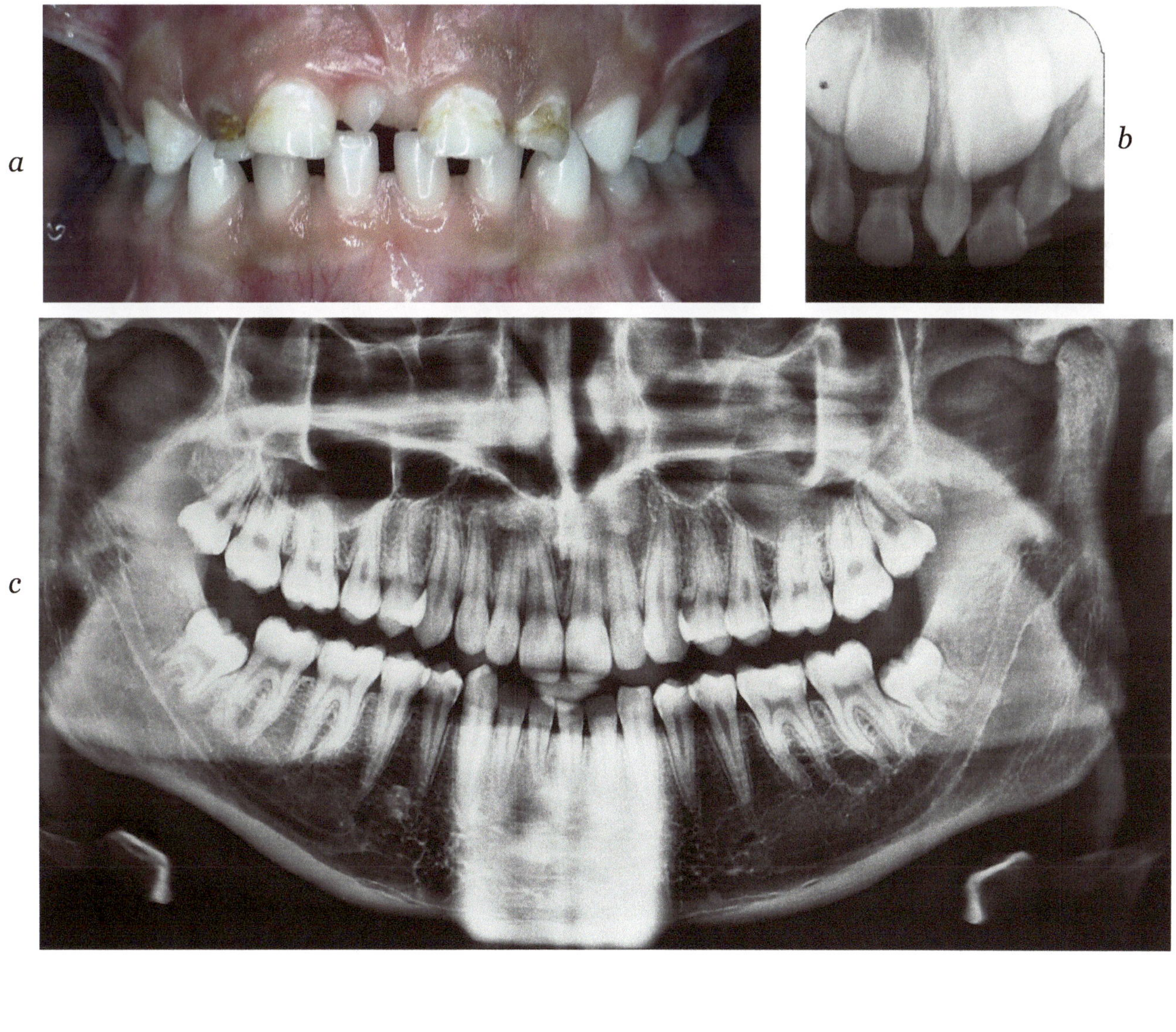

d

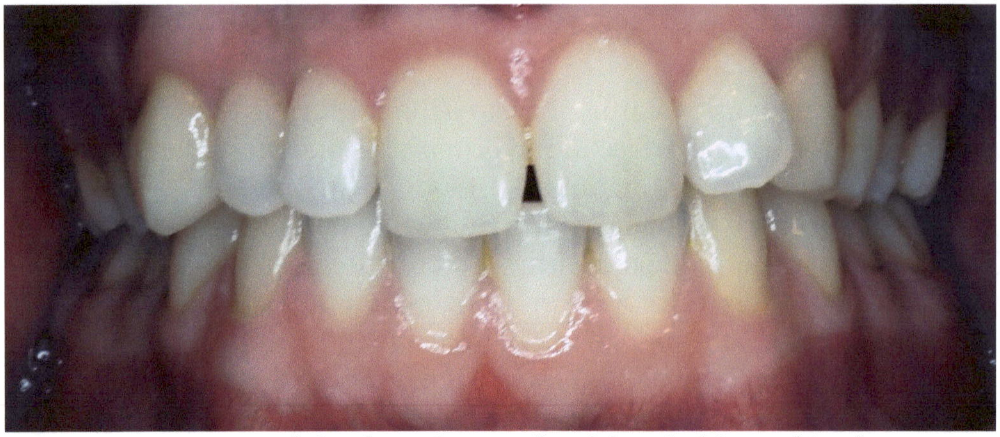

Figure 4.24 Supernumerary tooth in the primary dentition (a,b); and in the permanent dentition (c,d)

Prevalence

- Supernumerary teeth are relatively common in the general population;
- They can affect both the primary and the permanent dentitions;
- Supernumerary teeth may occur singly or in multiples, unilaterally or bilaterally, and in one or both arches;
- The occurrence of one or two supernumerary teeth is most common in the anterior region of the maxilla, followed by the mandibular premolar region;
- The occurrence of supernumerary teeth is less frequent than the congenital absence of teeth, and supernumerary teeth occur twice as often in men as in women;
- Hyperdontia occurs more often in the maxilla than in the mandible, particularly in the maxillary anterior region.

Etiology

- Not fully understood;
- Genetic background is proposed.

Classification of Supernumerary teeth

Classification on the basis of location in the arch

- Mesiodentes
  - A mesiodens is a type of supernumerary tooth that is located between the central incisors.
- Parapremolars;
- Paramolars;
- Distomolars.

Classification on the basis of form:

- Conical types;
- Tuberculate types;
- Supplemental types;
- Odontoms

Effect of Hyperdontia on Occlusion

- Delayed eruption;
- Impaction;
- Ectopic eruption;
- Displacement of adjacent teeth;
- Damage to the tooth structure, including root resorption, malformation, dilaceration, and loss of vitality of adjacent teeth;
- Crowding;
- Spacing;
- Premature contact and occlusal interference;
- Cystic formation.

Clinical features of Hyperdontia

- Abnormal pattern and abnormal sequence of eruption;
- Delayed eruption;
- Absence of eruption;
- Ectopic eruption;
- Asymmetric eruption between the left and right sides of more than 6 months duration;
- Local spacing or crowding;
- Abnormal tooth bulge.

Radiographic examination

If the presence of a supernumerary tooth is suspected, special radiographic techniques such as lateral cephalometric radiographs, orthopantomograms, occlusal radiographs, and computed tomograms are helpful to detect and localize the supernumerary tooth (*Figure 4.25*).

a

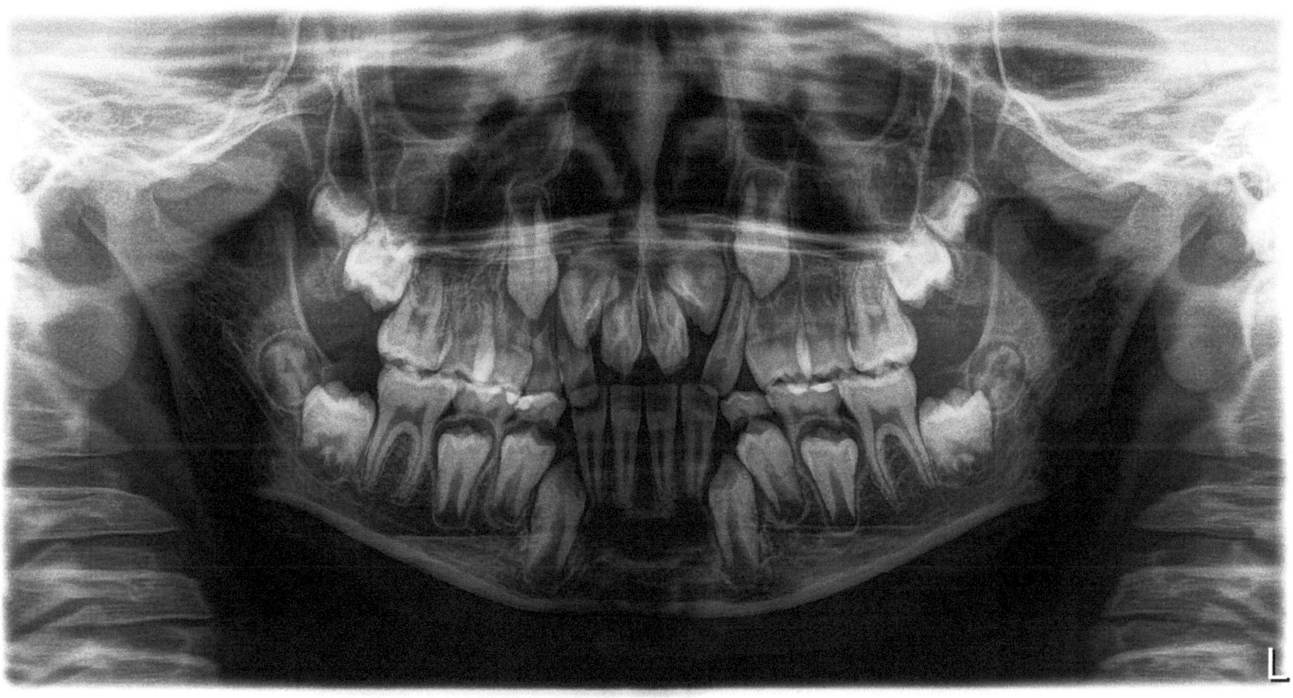

b

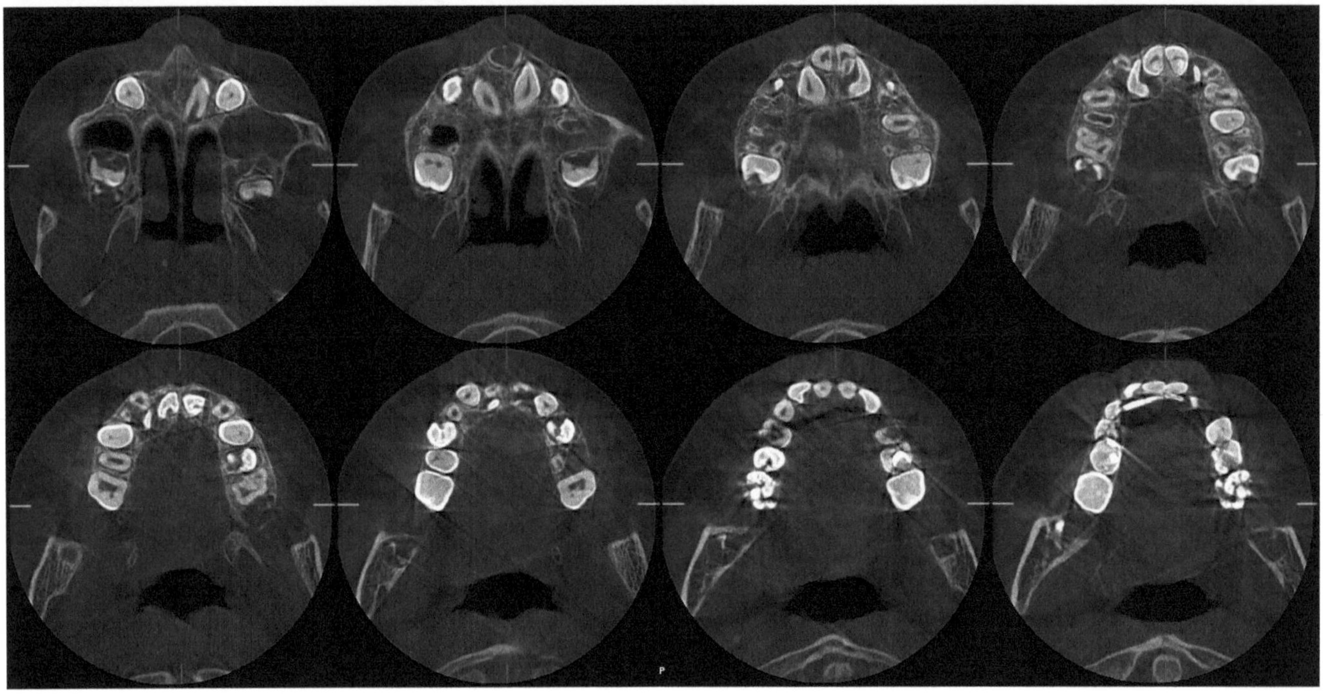

Figure 4.25 Panoramic radiograph of two supernumerary teeth in the upper incisor area (a). Computed tomogram of the same case (b).

Management in the early mixed dentition

Treatment strategies can be:

- Early detection and removal before any damage;
- Early detection and observation for the proper time of removal;
- Late detection and management of damaged situation;
- Supernumeraries that prevent the eruption of adjacent teeth, displace them, and damage tooth structure and occlusion;
- If the supernumerary has not erupted and delayed eruption of permanent teeth is predicted, the space for unerupted teeth must be maintained;
- Long-delayed eruption and the forces of mastication might have caused the formation of fibrous tissue or a bone barrier that will have to be removed to facilitate eruption.

Extract immediately or wait and monitor the condition?

The indications for immediate removal and orthodontic treatment include the following:

- When the supernumerary tooth is erupted and causing space problems for the adjacent teeth;
- When the presence of the supernumerary tooth is preventing or delaying eruption or damaging adjacent teeth;
- When the supernumerary tooth is displacing adjacent teeth;
- When a pathologic lesion such as a cyst is seen;
- When the supernumerary tooth is an obstacle to active orthodontic tooth movement.

The indications for postponed extraction and continued monitoring include the following:

- When the supernumerary tooth is located extremely high in the apex area of permanent teeth and surgical removal can damage root development;
- When the supernumerary tooth is very high and does not interfere with urgent interceptive tooth movement (the extraction can be postponed until after the initial phase of treatment).

Orthodontic management in the early and adult permanent dentition

- In many cases of neglected supernumeraries and delayed eruption of permanent teeth, the adjacent teeth often shift, creating a space deficiency for unerupted teeth. In these situations, besides removal of the supernumerary, space regaining is also recommended;
- If the permanent tooth or teeth are located high in the arch and/or displaced, it is necessary to bond an attachment for orthodontic traction at the time of extraction of the supernumerary tooth;
- We need to consider the existing malocclusion in order to use the space of the extracted supernumerary tooth to our advantage in leveling and alignment;
- If the supernumerary tooth is well aligned and does not interfere with occlusion, we can accept this anomaly.

Retention

- After supernumerary extraction and space closure, we should consider permanent retention because the jaw has grown bigger to accommodate the extra tooth material and spaces tend to reopen.

Late development of new supernumerary teeth

Another important point to consider in the treatment of patients with hyperdontia, especially in cases with multiple supernumerary teeth, is the phenomenon of late development of new supernumerary teeth after removal of the initial supernumerary teeth and even after orthodontic treatment. Careful monitoring is therefore required even after the completion of treatment.

Ankylosis

- Ankylosis is a specific abnormality of tooth eruption and development that is caused by the fusion of cementum with the alveolar bone;
- It is a progressive anomaly of tooth eruption that can occur before, during, or after tooth eruption and usually has a profound effect on occlusion;
- Both permanent and primary teeth may become ankylosed, but primary teeth become ankylosed far more frequently than do permanent teeth; the ratio is about 10 to 1;
- Mandibular teeth are ankylosed more than twice as often as maxillary teeth;
- Almost all infraoccluded primary molars are the result of ankyloses;
- The most frequent ankylosed teeth are mandibular primary second molars, then first molars, and then maxillary primary molars.

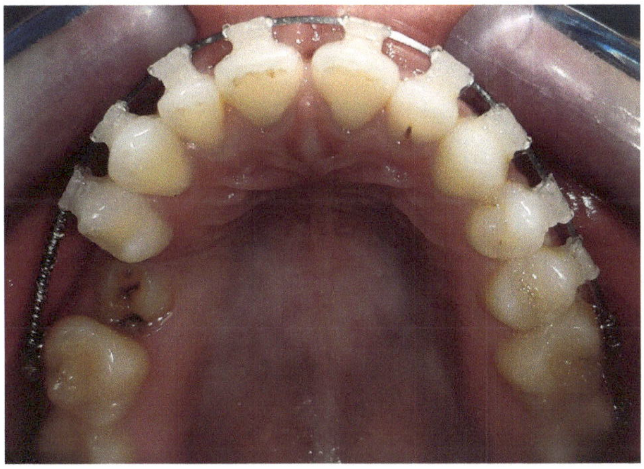

Figure 4.26 Infraocclusion of the upper primary second molar because of ankylosis

Etiology

- Heredity - observation of ankylosis in several members of the same family;
- Trauma;
- Intermittent primary root resorption;
- Disturbed local metabolism;
- Localized infection;
- Chemical or thermal irritation.

Effects on the dentition

- They may interfere with the eruption of succeeding permanent teeth, causing ectopic eruption;
- Arch length loss can result from tipping of adjacent teeth;
- Extrusion of teeth in the opposing arch may occur;
- Submergence of primary teeth damages the occlusion and can be harmful to the jaws and health of the patient;
- Transposition of the second premolar to the place of the missing permanent first molar is a rare consequence of primary second molar ankylosis;
- Submerged primary teeth not only prevent the eruption of the permanent teeth but also can prevent vertical alveolar growth and cause a lateral open bite.

Clinical Features

Ankylosed primary molars show the following clinical signs:

- Ankylosed primary molars often present with infraocclusion relative to adjacent teeth; however, depending on the time of fusion, they may be at the same occlusal level as adjacent teeth;
- On percussion, an ankylosed tooth gives a solid sound, whereas the normal adjacent teeth give a cushioned or dull sound;
- Ankylosed teeth lack mobility even when root resorption is advanced;
- Radiographs can show obliteration of the periodontal ligament space and absence of continuity of periodontal ligament in some areas.

Management of ankylosed primary teeth

Management in the mixed dentition

- If the ankylosed tooth is interfering with the eruption of the successor tooth, immediate extraction is recommended. If the emergence time of the permanent successor is predicted to be more than 6 months later, a proper space maintainer must be provided;
- If the successor is present, the onset of ankylosis in the primary tooth is late, and the permanent successor is usually not affected by the ankylosed tooth, periodic evaluation and removal of the ankylosed tooth at the proper time is recommended;
- If the successor is present, the onset of ankylosis is early, the occlusal level is low, and the possibility of submergence and a disturbed eruption of the permanent tooth is predictable, extraction of the ankylosed tooth and space maintenance is recommended;
- If the successor is missing, depending on the patient's type of occlusion and the situation of the ankylosed tooth, different procedures can be applied;

– If the ankylosed tooth has a good prognosis, it can be left in place. It should be restored with composite resin buildup or a crown if it is below the occlusal level to prevent overeruption of the opposing tooth;
– The ankylosed tooth can be extracted if the patient has crowding and needs extraction in the other segments of the arch. The space can be closed orthodontically;
– If the ankylosed tooth has poor structure and the patient has good occlusion and no need for orthodontic treatment, the ankylosed primary tooth can be extracted at an early age and a provisional bonded restoration can be placed. The permanent tooth should then be replaced by an implant or prosthetic treatment at a proper age.

Management in the early and adult permanent dentition

- If the ankylosed tooth is a permanent tooth and the onset of ankylosis is early, surgical luxation might help;
- If repeated luxation is not useful, extraction is recommended to prevent submergence of the tooth;
- Reimplantation of an ankylosed permanent tooth is another option;
- If the onset of ankylosis in a permanent tooth is late, luxation is not effective, and there is no evidence of submergence, the tooth can be built up later to prevent overeruption of the opposing tooth.

5. Management of Class I Malocclusion

In Class I malocclusions, the major problem is arch length deficiency (except in open bite malocclusions).
There just is not enough room to accommodate all the teeth in their correct positions
Various methods of space gaining include:
1. Extraction;
2. Interproximal reduction;
3. Derotation of posteriors;
4. Uprighting of molars;
5. Proclination of anteriors;
6. Arch expansion;
7. Molar distalization.

Extraction as a method to gain space

Extraction Choice

Upper Central Incisors

- Upper incisors are rarely the extraction of choice to treat a malocclusion;
- In times when incisor prognosis is poor in the long term, the tooth should be considered for extraction as a part of the treatment plan;
- We can position a lateral incisor in the place of central incisor;
- In some cases, the transplantation of a premolar with a developing root into the incisor socket can relieve crowding in the lower arch and provide a useful replacement in the upper labial segment.

Upper Lateral Incisors

- Upper Laterals may be extracted when they are blocked out buccally or lingually, with good contact between central incisor and canines;
- Severe root resorption due to ectopic canines also dictates its extraction.

Lower Incisors *(Figure 5.1)*

a *b*

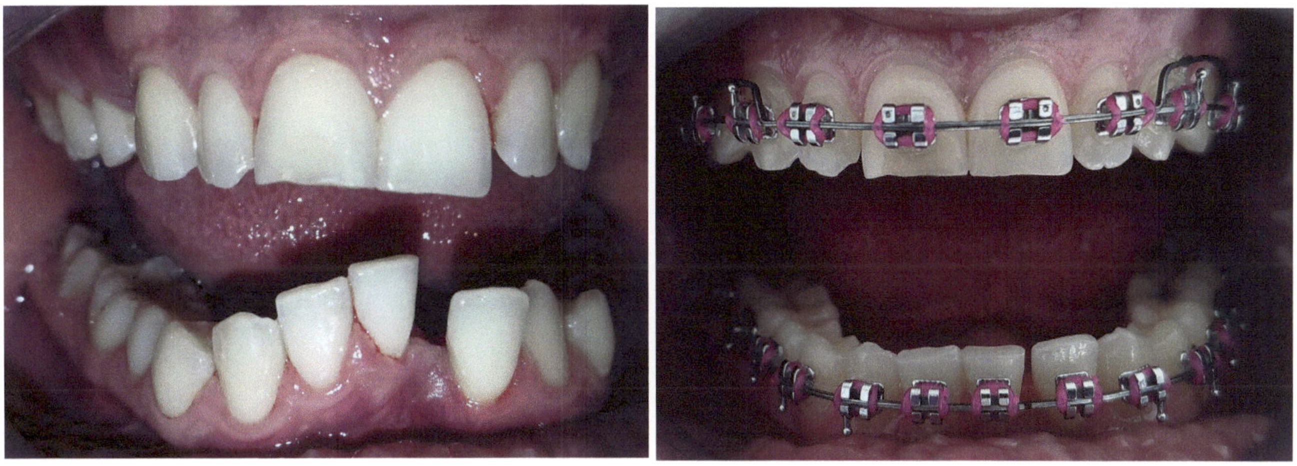

Figure 5.1 Lower incisor extraction in the treatment of Class II malocclusion

Indications

- Class I dental malocclusions with lower anterior crowding with lack of space for almost one lower incisor having normal maxillary dentition and perfect buccal interdigitation (*Figure 5.2*);

a *b*

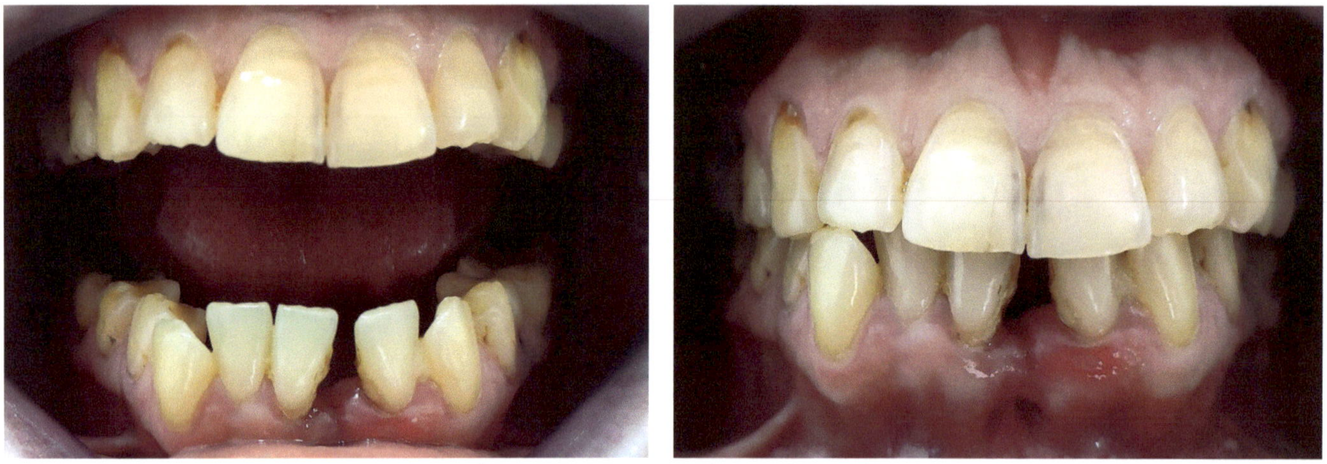

Figure 5.2 Lower incisor extracted to compensate for Bolton discrepancy

- It is also recommended in class I cases with anterior crossbite due to mandibular crowding and incisor protrusion, with adequate posterior intercuspation, acceptable facial esthetics, and absence of skeletal– dental discrepancy in the upper arch;
- In Class I cases with severe anterior tooth-size discrepancy, whether due to agenesis of upper incisors or deficient mesiodistal diameter of an upper incisor or conversely large mesiodistal diameter of lower incisors;
- Moderate Class III malocclusions with an anterior crossbite, or incisors with an edge-to-edge relationship, showing a tendency toward anterior open bite;
- The transposition of anterior teeth, particularly of the canines, or the severe malpositioning of a lower incisor or when one incisor is excluded out of the arch.

Canines

- These teeth are rarely considered for extraction unless very ectopic;
- Ectopic canines in unfavorable positions for alignment, with proper contact between laterals and first premolar, can be extracted.

Premolars

Premolars are often ideal for relieving both anterior and posterior crowding.

First Premolar

The extraction of first premolars has been the most favorable and the most common choice of extraction. The reasons for premolar extraction are:

- For strengthening anchorage;
- Maximum lip retraction;
- Better teeth contact between second premolars and canines;
- The first premolars are closer to anterior crowding.

Second Premolar

- The maxillary first premolar is more esthetic than the second, the contact point of mandibular first molar and first premolar tended to stay closed;
- Second premolar is extracted when the need for anterior space is less;
- In a balanced facial profile when we do not want to flatten the lips.

Comparison between first and second premolar extractions is given in *Table 5.1*

Criterion	Space closure	Space opening
Facial profile	Convex or straight	Straight, Concave
Shape of the canine	Normal shape and color, not too large in comparison with central incisor	Large size, Darker color, high gingival margin
Type of malocclusion	Class I, Class II malocclusions, absence of posterior crossbite. Normodivergent or Hyperdivergent with an anterior open bite or open bite tendency	Class I, Class III malocclusion, anterior or posterior crossbite. Normodivergent or Hypodivergent with a deep bite.
Space available in the upper arch	Less than 8 mm	More than 8 mm
Wisdom teeth	Not erupted in a good position	Absent or extracted
Age	Adolescent patient	Adult patient
Patient`s wish		

Table 5.1 Comparison between first and second premolar extractions

First Molar

Indications for extraction

- During excess molar extrusion;
- Endodontically treated, with caries and/or extensive restorations;
- With pronounced periodontal involvement;
- In the absence of four premolars, in orthodontically re-treated conditions with Angle Class II malocclusion;
- Indicated in severe crowding in patients with a high mandibular plane angle and convex profile as the mesialization of posterior teeth facilitates the counterclockwise rotation of the mandible and helps in cases where molars are missing from the outset;
- Management of open bite cases.

a *b*

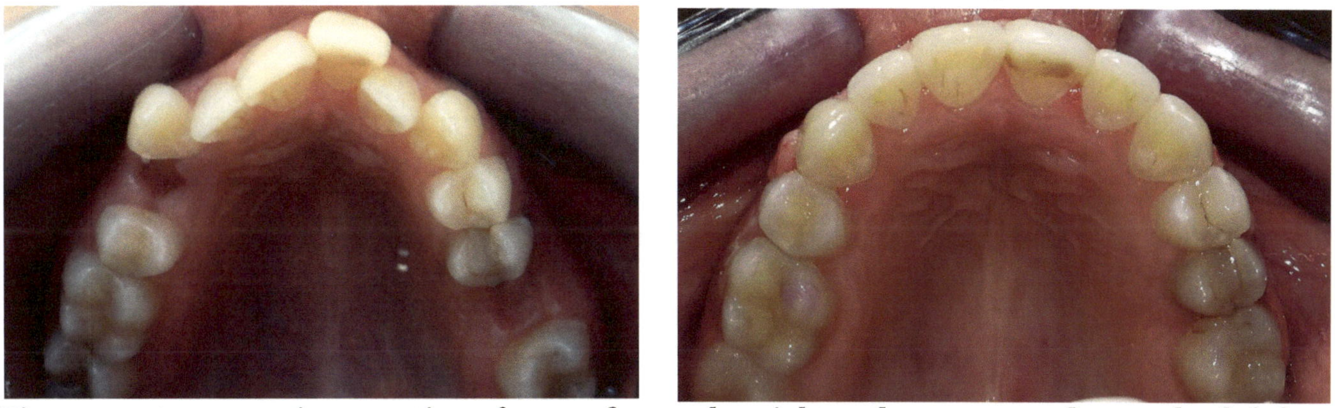

Figure 5.3 Asymmetric extraction of upper first molar right and upper second premolar left for correction of Class II.

Second Molar

The maxillary permanent second molars are an uncommon choice for extraction in orthodontic treatment. They are extracted only in some selective situations.

- Deep overbite;
- Mild anterior or posterior crowding;
- Exceptionally decayed;
- Compromised periodontal status;
- Ectopic eruption of maxillary second molar;
- Class II molar and canine relationship with good facial profile;
- Distally tilted developing maxillary third molars;
- It is sometimes extracted to facilitate the distalization of maxillary first molars;
- Timing of the extractions depends greatly on the position and form of the upper third molars;
- Magness suggests extraction when the third molar has reached the junction of the second molar crown and root;
- Chipman believes the optimum time is when the third molar's occlusal surface is approximately level with the vertical midline of the second molar root. The clinical crown of the third molar should be nearly complete so that a tooth of reasonable size is assured;
- Adequate third molar alignment is not to be expected with second molar extraction after the third molar roots are formed more than one-third.

Third Molar

Indications for extraction

- Effect of the third molar eruption on late mandibular crowding is still controversial;
- Even untreated patients with regular dental arches are affected by late crowding of the anterior teeth in both lower and upper jaws;
- It is believed that third molar is responsible for the relapse after completion of orthodontic treatment;
- According to Schwarze, prophylactic germectomy of the third molar after orthodontic treatment should lessen subsequent crowding of the lower incisors.

Interproximal enamel reduction as a method to gain space

Interproximal enamel reduction (IER) is a clinical procedure involving the reduction, anatomic recontouring, and protection of proximal enamel surfaces of permanent teeth in order to create space for orthodontic treatment.

Indications

1. In 1944, Ballard recommended careful stripping of the proximal surfaces of the anterior teeth when there was a tooth-size discrepancy. Stripping was first used to obtain space for the correction and prevention of crowding of mandibular incisors;
2. Stripping is also carried out for the reshaping of enamel on some teeth, thus contributing to an improved finishing of orthodontic treatment and dental esthetics;
3. Normalization of gingival contour and elimination of triangular spaces above the papilla is also one of the indications, so as to improve esthetics and smile;
4. Stripping can also provide space for flattening the curve of Spee;
5. Interproximal enamel reduction is the common strategy to treat interarch tooth-size discrepancies, like Bolton's discrepancy;

6. Camouflage of Class II and III malocclusions: The use of mandibular stripping can be beneficial in camouflaging slight to moderate Class III conditions and overjet. In orthodontic treatment to camouflage Class II with the extraction of two maxillary premolars, correcting the crowding and inclination of the mandibular incisors with stripping is an ideal solution.

Contraindications

- Stripping would be dangerous to carry out in severe crowding (more than 8 mm per arch as this would lead to excessive loss of enamel;
- IER should not be used when there is active periodontal disease or lack of dental stability. Although little scientific evidence exists linking IER and increased dental mobility, it is prudent to avoid this technique in these situations;
- IER should not be used when there is poor oral hygiene; the orthodontist could be held responsible for all subsequent iatrogenic activity;
- Stripping should not be used in small and hypersensitive teeth, as the risk of the appearance of or an increase in dental sensitivity is great;
- Stripping should not be carried out on 'square' teeth as teeth with straight proximal surfaces and wide bases produce broad contact surfaces, and could potentially cause food impaction and reduced interseptal bone (*Figure 5.4*).

a *b* c *d* *e*

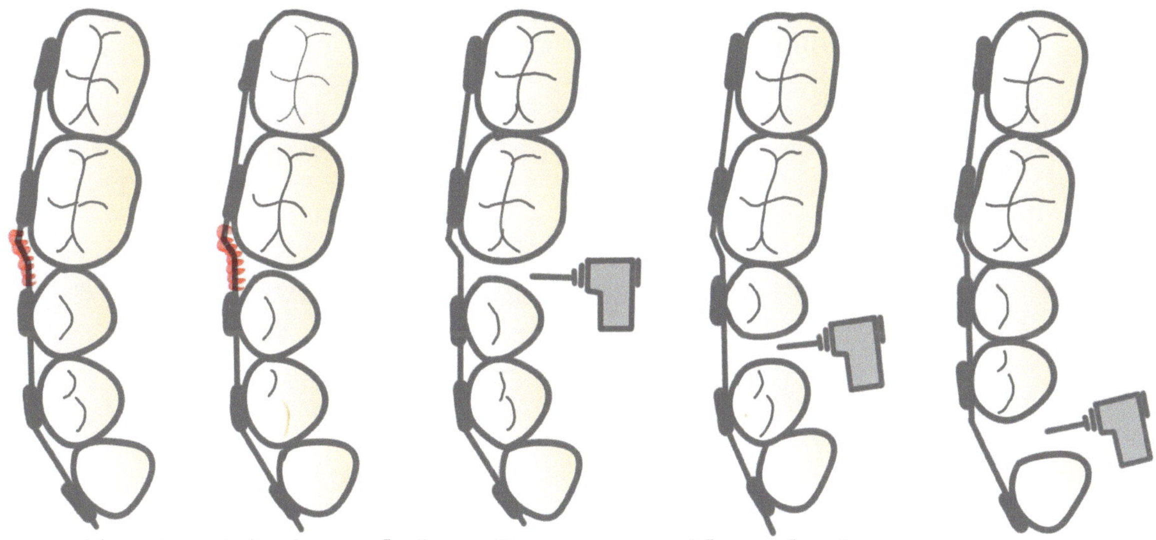

Figure 5.4 Air rotor stripping technique. Open space with an elastic separator or compressed coil spring (a); Space created distal to second premolar (b); Stripping in the opened space (c); Space moved by distalizing of the second premolar and stripping between first and second premolar (d); Stripping between first premolar and canine (d).

Derotation of posterior teeth as a method to gain space

Rotated posterior teeth occupy more space. Derotation of these teeth helps not only in regaining this space but also in preventing caries and periodontal disease. The space regained varies upon the tooth concerned and the extent of rotation.
Derotation can be best achieved using a couple (forces equal in magnitude but opposite in direction) on the lingual and buccal surfaces of the tooth. A rotated tooth occupies less space in the arch and their correction needs space to be created in the arch. *Figure 5.5*
For more information see "Rotation"

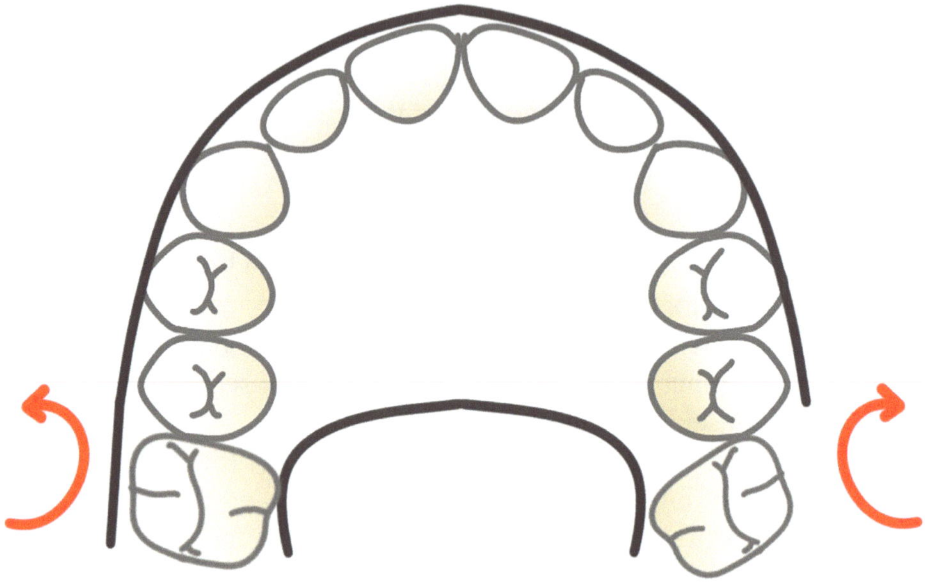

Figure 5.5 Derotation of upper first molars with transpalatal arch.

Uprighting of tilted posterior teeth

- Early loss of second deciduous molar or unrestored caries on its distal surface or extraction of the second premolar causes tipping of first molar.
- Tilted posterior teeth always occupy more space.
- A delayed eruption of the first or the second molar may also cause the posterior teeth to tilt mesially.
- Uprighting of molars can lead to an arch length gain of 1–1.5 mm.

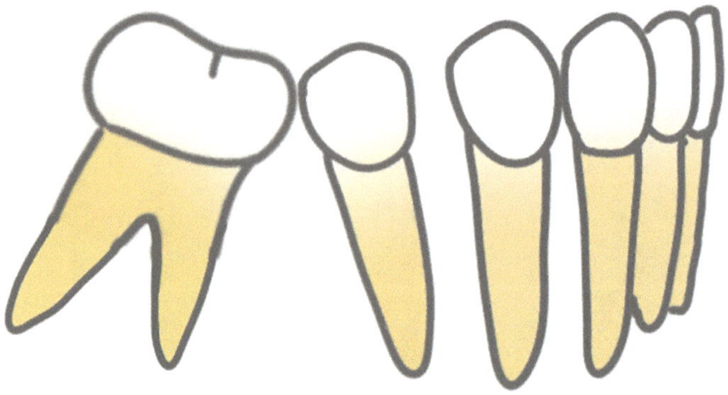

Figure 5.6 Tilted posterior tooth.

Management

- Fixed appliances using uprighting springs;
- Space regainers or the various screw appliances are used frequently;
- The lip bumper and its modifications can also achieve good results in the lower arch.

Details on mechanotherapy are given in the 'Uprighting tilted molars' part of the book.

Proclination of anterior teeth

Proclination of anterior teeth helps in gaining space and relieving crowding. This can be done in cases where these teeth are retroclined or their proclination will not affect the soft-tissue profile of the patient unfavorably or the basal bone relationship.

Management in the mixed dentition

- Retroclination of upper anterior teeth is sometimes responsible for restraining the forward growth of the mandible. In this cases early treatment is recommended;
- Removable appliances with 'Z' spring, screws (medium-, mini-, or microscrews) can be used;
- 2 x 4 fixed appliances in this stage is the preferred choice.

Management in the early and adult permanent dentition

- Treatment can be executed with fixed appliance (*Figure 5.7*);
- Brackets put on the anterior teeth with round wires result in proclination;
- Another way to procline teeth is by using a protrusion arch.

a

b

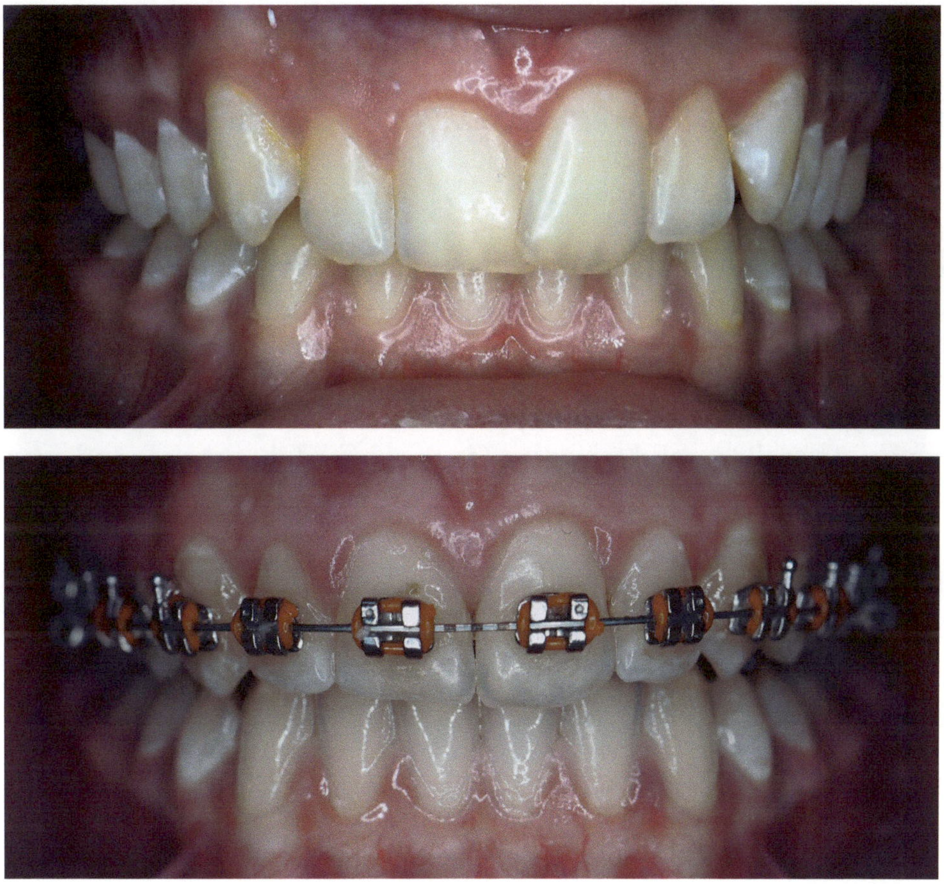

Figure 5.7 Proclination of upper anterior teeth for space gaining and correction of the retruded lower jaw.

Arch expansion

Arch expansion is another method to gain space. Arch expansion is usually more successful in the maxillary arch when compared to the mandibular arch. The different expansion appliances are extensively dealt in the correction of the posterior crossbite section.

Molar distalization

Maxillary molar distalization is commonly indicated for space gaining in the upper arch and/or to correct distal tooth malpositions. Multiple treatment methods and appliances for molar distalization have been described.

- Distalization of the first molars is the fastest (at times exceeding 1 mm/month) and anchorage loss is the least when treated before the eruption of the second molar;
- The distal movement of upper molar roots against adjacent unerupted teeth could cause root resorption of the first molar;
- The effect of distalization on maxillary third molars is variable but in general, no distal movement but 4° of tipping is observed;
- The positional changes of third molars can lead to impaction, especially if there is no space available at the beginning of treatment;
- For this reason, third molars are removed when possible.

Indications and Contraindications for molar distalization are listed in the following lists:

Indications for molar distalization

- Class II malocclusion with mild maxillary dentoalveolar protrusion/crowding (or) mild arch length discrepancy: 4–5 mm discrepancy;
- End-on molar relationship with mild to moderate space requirement;
- No requirement for stability and esthetics;
- Mesially and lingually tipped upper molars;
- In a growing child to relieve mild crowding (as they afford more space and growth with which to work);
- Normal or hypodivergent growth pattern;
- Class II subdivision cases requiring unilateral distal molar movement;
- Regaining the space loss due to mesial drift of first molars following premature loss of deciduous teeth.

Contraindications for molar distalization

Dental Malocclusions

- Class I or III molar relation;
- Dental open bite;
- Maxillary first molar distally inclined;
- Severe overjet and bimaxillary protrusion cases.

Skeletal Malocclusions

- Severe Class II skeletal pattern;
- Skeletal open bites;
- Excess lower anterior face height.

Soft Tissue Considerations

- Convex profile;
- Functional;

- Numerous signs and symptoms of temporomandibular joint;
- Posteriorly and superiorly displaced condyles;

Complications of Molar Distalization

- Anchorage loss;
- Anterior movement of anchor unit;
- Incisor flaring;
- Premolar mesial tipping;
- Overjet increase;
- Distal tipping of molars during distalization,
- Vertical opening of the bite;
- Possible impaction of the second and third molar.

The types of distalizing appliances are observed in 'Methods for the correction of Class II malocclusion'.

Treatment Sequence for Class I Malocclusion Correction

The routine sequence followed in the correction of Class I malocclusion is as follows:
- Alignment;
- Correction of crossbites;
- Alignment of an impacted tooth;
- Closure of diastema or anterior spacing;
- Leveling;
- Space closure;
- Detailing and final settling followed by retention.

Sequence of Class I correction		Space opening
Alignment	Correction of crowding, rotation	• Use of superelastic NiTi wires • Multistranded steel wires • Looped stainless steel archwires
Crossbite correction	Mild to moderate anterior and posterior crossbites	• Correction with archwire • Crossbite elastics • Expansion arches • Heavy labial arches
Aligning of impacted tooth	Orthodontic mechanics to bring the tooth into the arch	• Attachments to main archwire • Soldered attachments • Special auxiliary springs
Anterior space closure	Diastema and generalized anterior space closure	• Part of overall treatment • Timing of frenectomy to be decided
Leveling	Leveling by intrusion	• Segmented arches • Bypass arches • Skeletal anchorage
	Leveling by relative intrusion and extrusion	• Continuous archwires • Class II or III elastics • Bite planes • Reverse curve wires

Sequence of Class I correction		Space opening
Extraction space closure and reduction in overjet	En masse or segmental retraction	• Individual canine retraction followed by four incisor retraction • En masse anterior retraction
	Friction or friction-free mechanics	• Sliding mechanics • Loop mechanics
	Anchorage considerations	• Maximum anchorage situations • Moderate anchorage situations • Minimum anchorage situations
Simultaneous intrusion and retraction	Intrusion and retraction of four Incisors	• Three-piece base arch • Ricketts' utility arch
	Intrusion and retraction of six anterior teeth	• K-Sir arch
Finishing and detailing	Root paralleling	• Uprighting springs • Flexible full dimension archwire
	Minor tooth irregularities	• Rebonding of brackets and flexible wire insertion • Compensatory step bends
	Incisor torque	• Piggyback torquing auxiliary • Use of full-dimension archwire
	Midline discrepancies	• Asymmetric use of elastics
	Maintaining the closure of all spaces	• Passive tie backs
	Coordinating arch widths and arch form	• Cross-elastics
	Bolton's discrepancy	• Proximal slicing • Composite buildup
	Final settling	• Settling elastics • Removal of heavy archwire • Resilient round wire placement

Table 5.2 Treatment steps in Class I malocclusion correction

Alignment

- Correction of severely rotated teeth is done at this stage (Figure 5.8);

a *b*

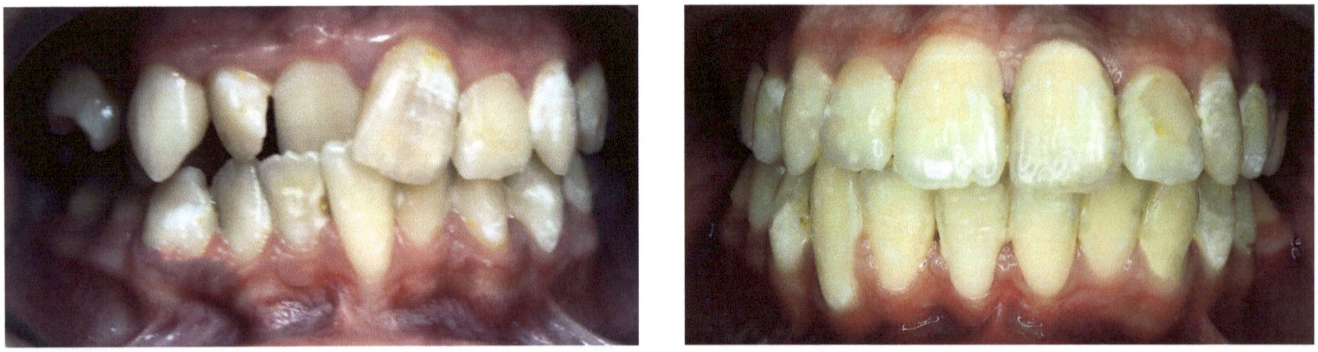

Figure 5.8 Before (a) and after the derotation of canine teeth (b).

- Alignment of a high canine tooth;

Canines are teeth with long radices and the force needed for their extrusion is more than the force to intrude the teeth next to them – lateral incisor;

1) When using the continuous wire technique, ligating of a high canine in the initial stages of treatment will cause open bite because of the intrusion of the lateral incisor;

- To avoid these unwanted side effects we could use the segmented arch technique. The incisors and posterior segments including canines are ligated to different archwires;
- Light delta elastics could be used as an extra anchorage for extrusion of canines; (*Figure 5.9*)

a

b

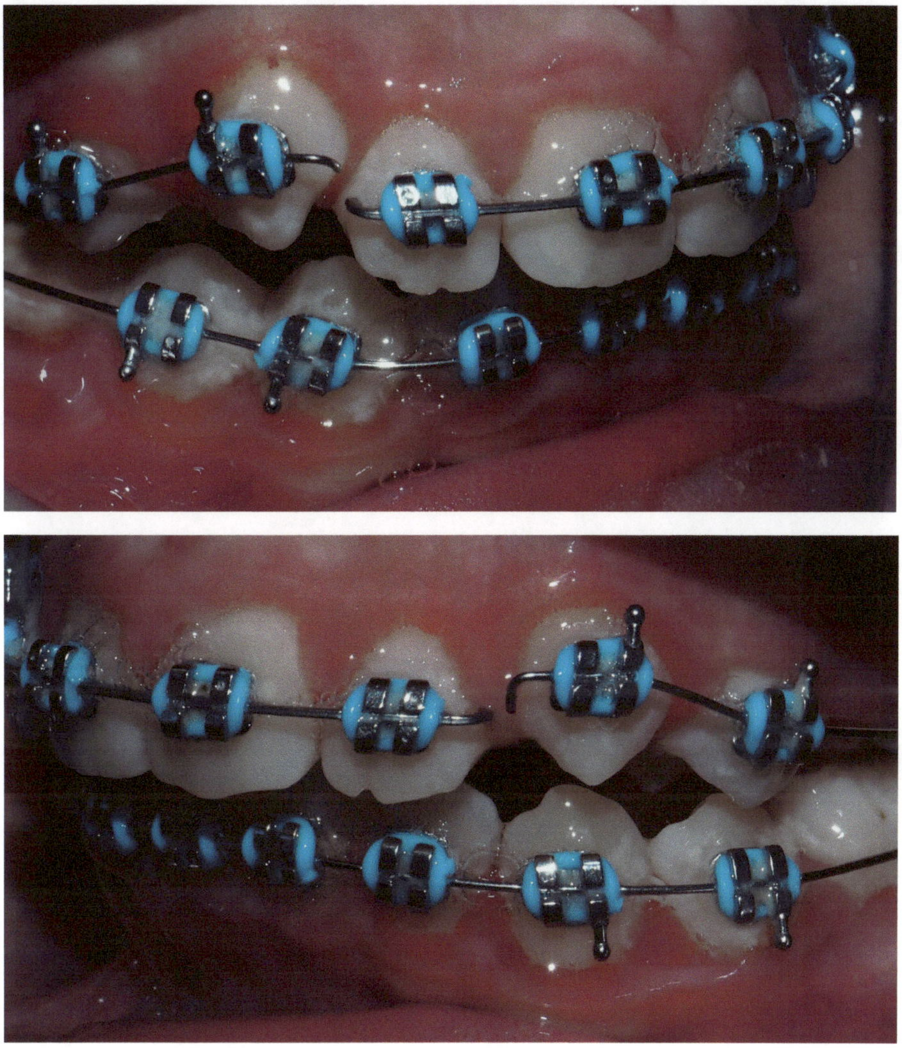

Figure 5.9 Extrusion of the high canine tooth

2) The second method is to align the arch to a stiff wire (last wire depending on the slot used For example 19x25 SS for a 022-inch slot);

- Make step down bend in this main wire in the place of the canine;
- Ligate the canine bracket with a light 016 inch NiTi wire as a second or piggy back wire. (*Figure 5.10*)

Correction of Crossbite

Mild to moderate crossbite problems, either anterior or posterior, should be corrected during the initial stages of treatment. Marked or severe crossbite correction requires either surgical intervention or is corrected later during orthodontic treatment.

a

b

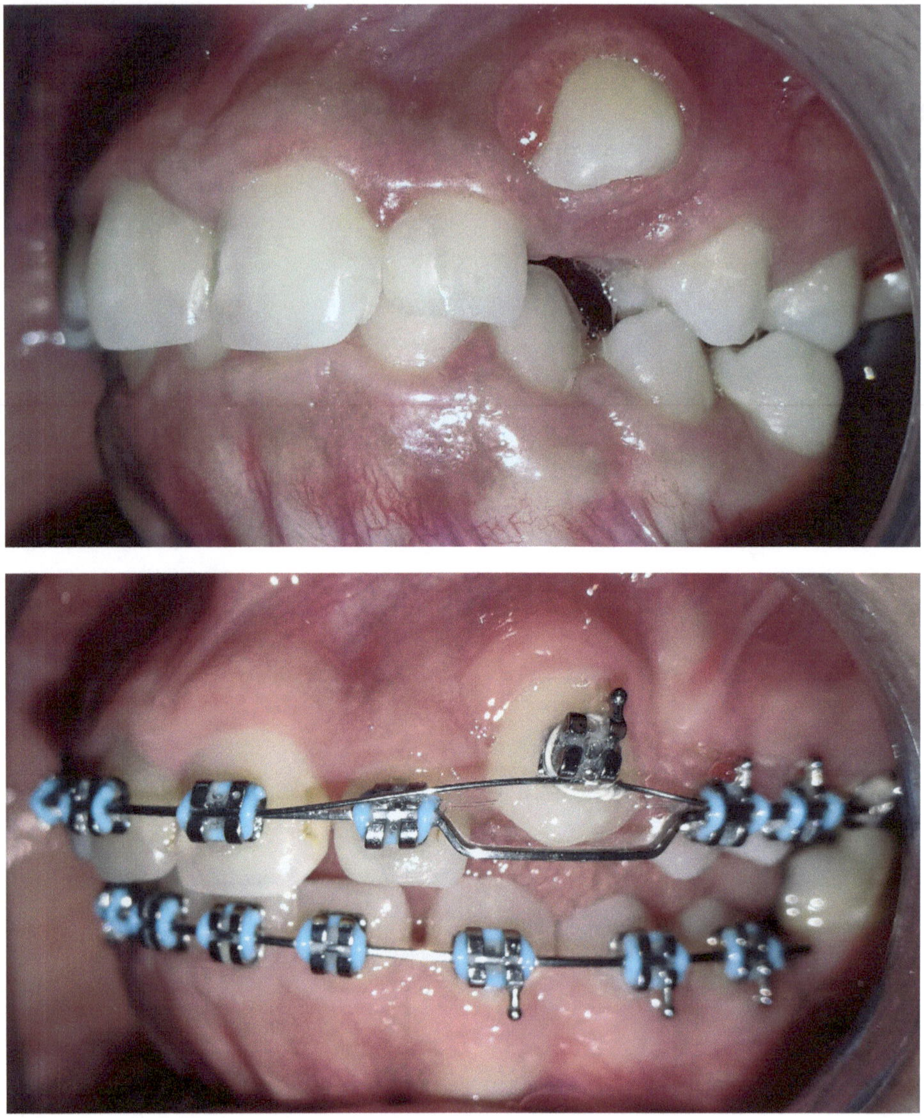

Figure 5.10 Extrusion of the high canine tooth with accessory wire.

Anterior Crossbite

- The methods of correction of anterior crossbites are mentioned in sagittal treatment mechanics;
- Occlusal interferences to crossbite correction necessitate the use of bite plates along with the routine fixed appliance mechanotherapy (*Figure 5.11*).

a b

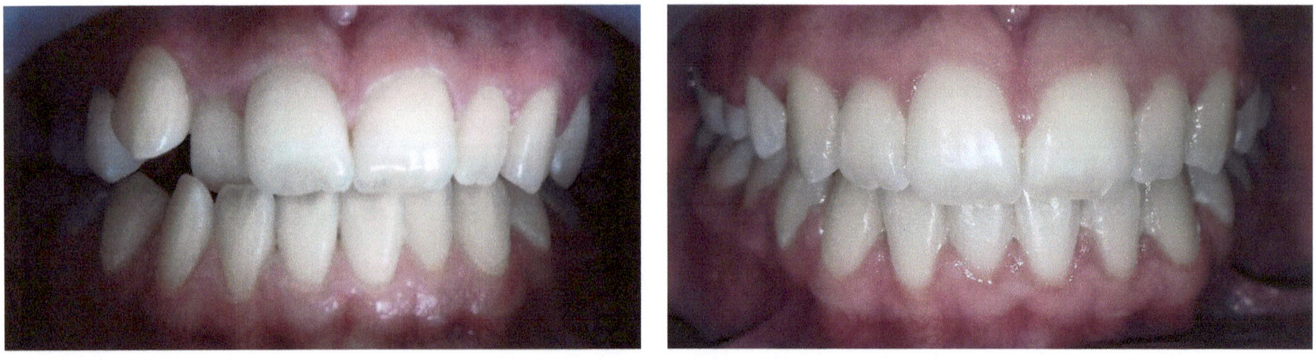

c d

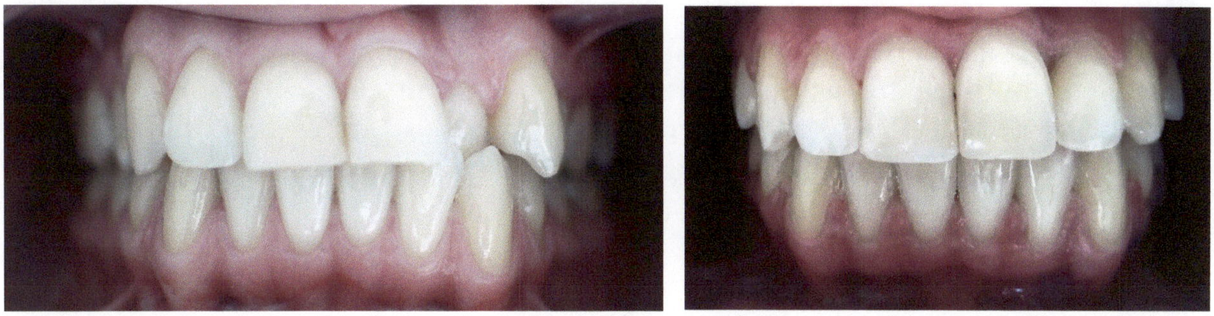

Figure 5.11 Anterior crossbite correction of lateral incisor with posterior bite planes (a,b) and (c,d).

Dental Posterior Crossbites

- Use of crossbite elastics (*Figure 5.12*);
  - Crossbite elastics are dealt with in correction of posterior crossbite section;
- Expansion arches;
  - Involve the use of heavy labial archwire of 36- or 40-mil steel in the headgear tubes to expand or to maintain the expansion achieved by other methods, like expansion arches.

a b c d e f

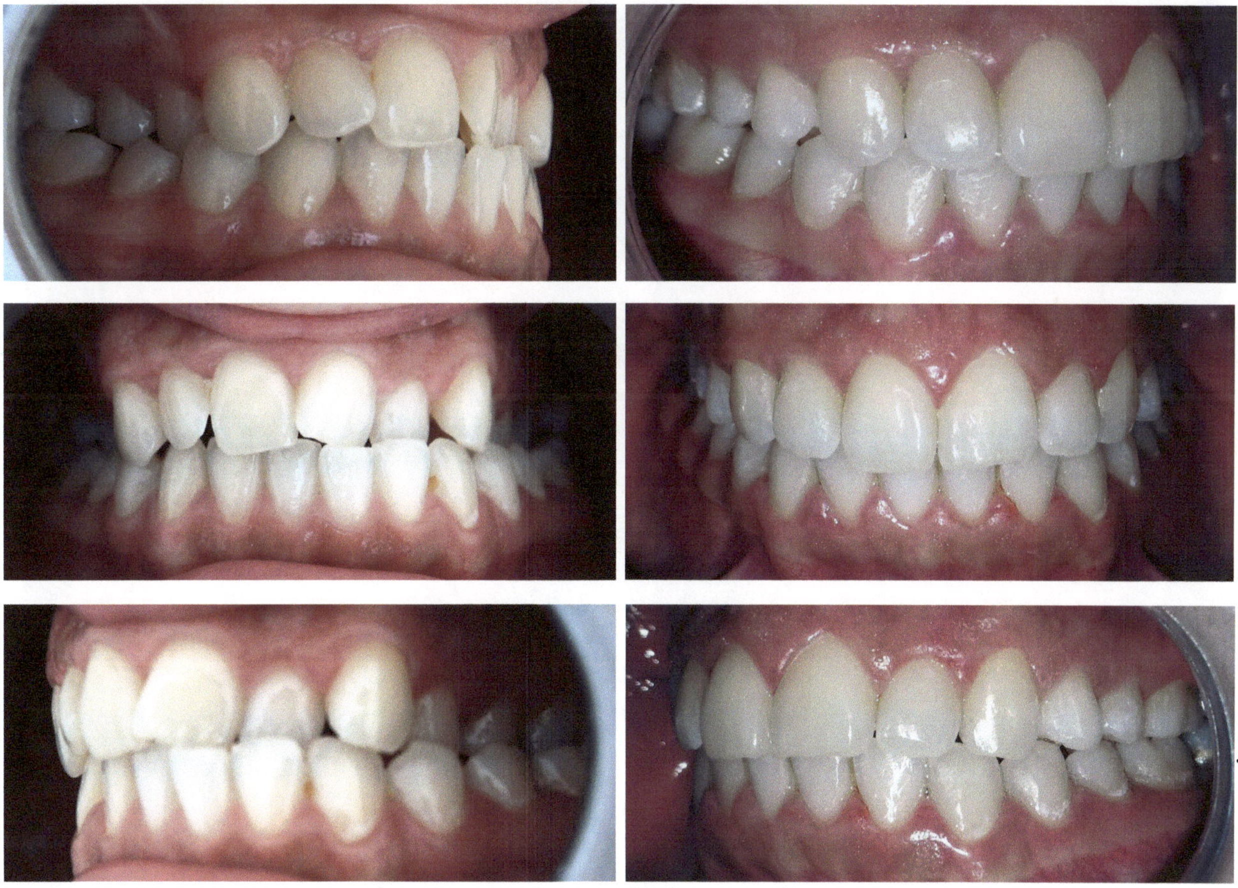

Figure 5.12 Posterior crossbite correction with the use of cross elastics. Before (a,c,e) and after treatment (b,d,f).

Align Impacted Tooth

The management of impacted tooth involves three important steps:

1. Location of the impacted tooth,
2. Attachment to the tooth surface following surgical exposure and
3. Relocation of the impacted tooth into the arch by orthodontic mechanics.

The treatment of impacted teeth is another topic of this book. Hence, this section will be dealing with brief review only the orthodontic mechanics in bringing the tooth into alignment.

Mechanics

- Orthodontic treatment should begin immediately after surgical exposure;
- Sufficient space should be created before surgery and also the alignment of other teeth should be completed;
- The bonded impacted tooth is connected to the main archwire with a ligature wire and brought into alignment;
- The other methods are soldering heavy base wire either palatal or labial (Fig. 42.8) and use of special cantilever springs.

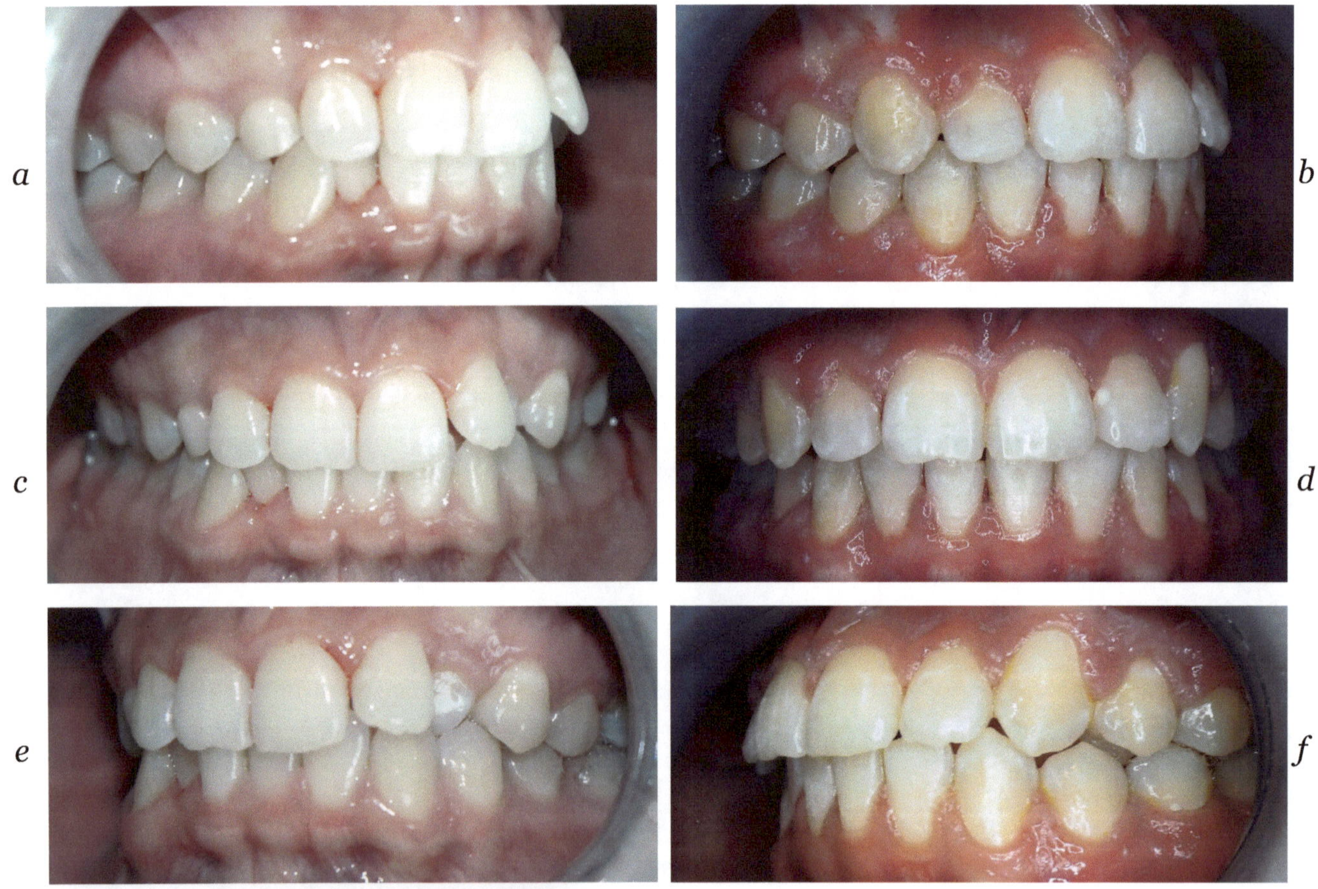

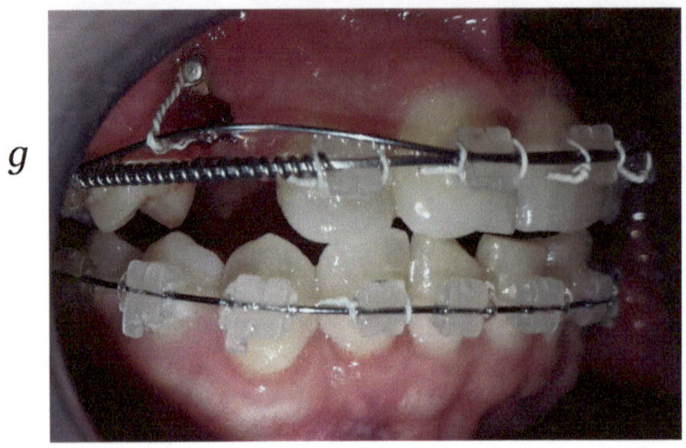

Figure 5. 13 Treatment of vestibularly impacted maxillary canine. Before (a,c,e) and after treatment (b,d,f). Orthodontic extrusion is done with piggy back wire size 0.016 inch NiTi (g).

Anterior Space/Diastema Closure

- This could be done by the use of power chain elastics or open coil springs;
- Important to say is that all space closing should be done after full arch alignment and with heavy stainless steel full dimension archwires *(Figure 5.14).*

a *b*

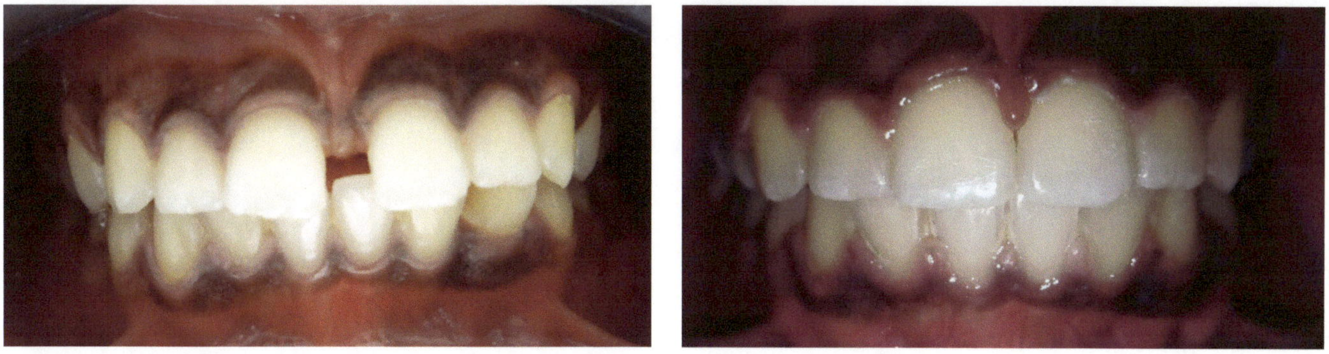

Figure 5.14 Before (a) and after (b) diastema closure with fixed appliance.

Leveling the curve of Spee

Leveling of the curve of Spee can be accomplished by three mechanics:

1. Leveling by intrusion;
2. Leveling by relative intrusion and
3. Leveling by extrusion.

- Leveling by extrusion increases the facial height; it is not ideal in average or high-angle cases;
- Relative intrusion will be successful in growing patients only and intrusion is most widely used in adult patients.

Leveling by Intrusion (*Figure 5.15*)

Intrusion can be achieved in three possible ways:

1. With segmented archwire technique using an auxiliary intrusion arch;
2. Bypass arches (continuous archwires that bypass premolars and/or canines);
3. By using skeletal anchorage unit.

Management in the mixed dentition

Leveling by intrusion

- Begg Stage I Archwire (*Figure 5.16*);
- It is made with 0.018-inch resilient wire on the anterior teeth;
- Anchor bends are incorporated in the archwires in front of the molar buccal tubes.
- 2 x 4 Appliances

The effect produced by stage 1 archwire in Begg's technique can be produced by using the 2 x 4 technique in edgewise appliances also.

Leveling by relative intrusion

- A functional appliance can be used.

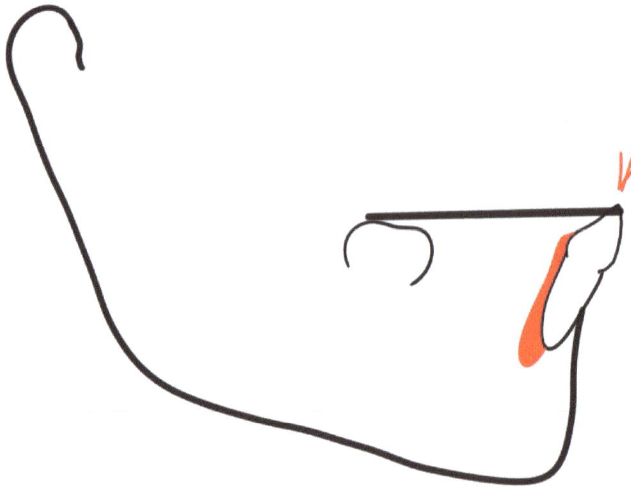

Figure 5.15 Leveling by absolute intrusion

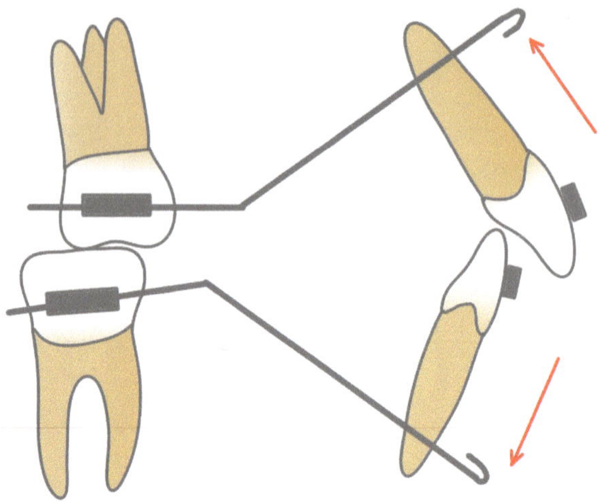

Figure 5.16 Bypass wire with posterior bend used in Begg `s technique.

Leveling by extrusion

- Anterior bite plane fixed or removable.

More details are given in 'Treatment of deep bite'

Management in the early and adult permanent dentition

Leveling by intrusion

Segmented Arch Techniques (*Figure 5.17*).

The basic mechanism for intrusion consists of three parts:

- A posterior anchorage unit;
- An anterior segment;
- An intrusive arch spring;

- The posterior segments in both sides are joined by transpalatal arch and a low lingual arch in maxilla and mandible, respectively;
- The intrusive arch comprises of a 0.018 x 0.022-inch wire with a 3 mm helix looped two and a half times and placed mesial to the auxiliary tube;
- An anterior alignment arch or the anterior segment is placed in the four incisors or the central incisors and the intrusive arch is attached to that wire either labially, incisally, or gingivally. (*Figure 5.18*).

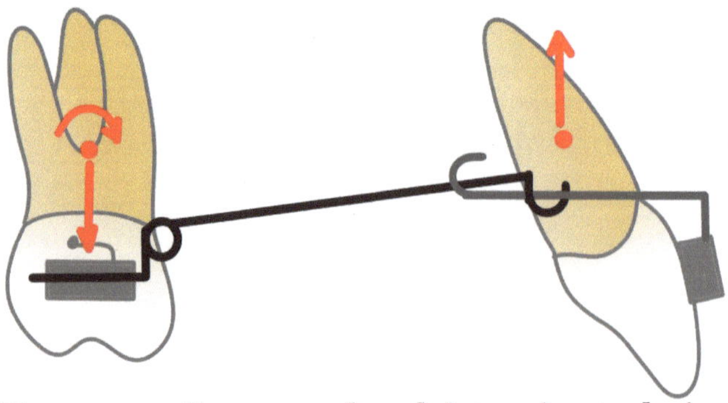

Figure 5.17 Segmented arch intrusion technique

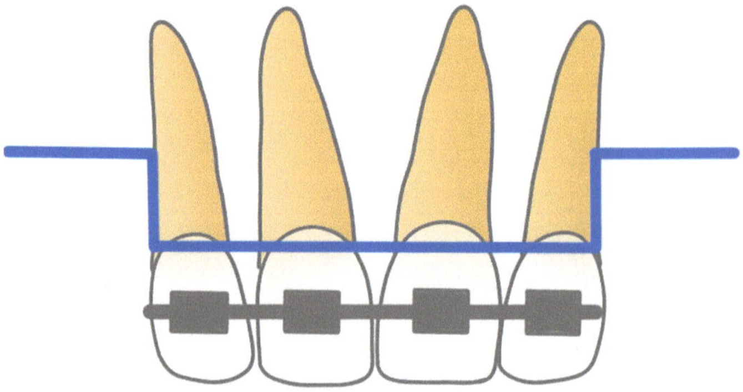

Figure 5.18 Anterior part of the segmented arch appliance

Utility arch

- Bypass arches are effective for patients during mixed dentition or early dentition (i.e. who have some growth);
- Utility Arch engages only the first molars and the four incisors (*Figure 5.19*).

Skeletal Anchorage to Intrude Incisors

Absolute anchorage devices, like bone screws or bone anchors, have provided the opportunity of intrusion of both anterior teeth in deep bite cases as well as posterior teeth in open bite cases *(Figure 5.20).*

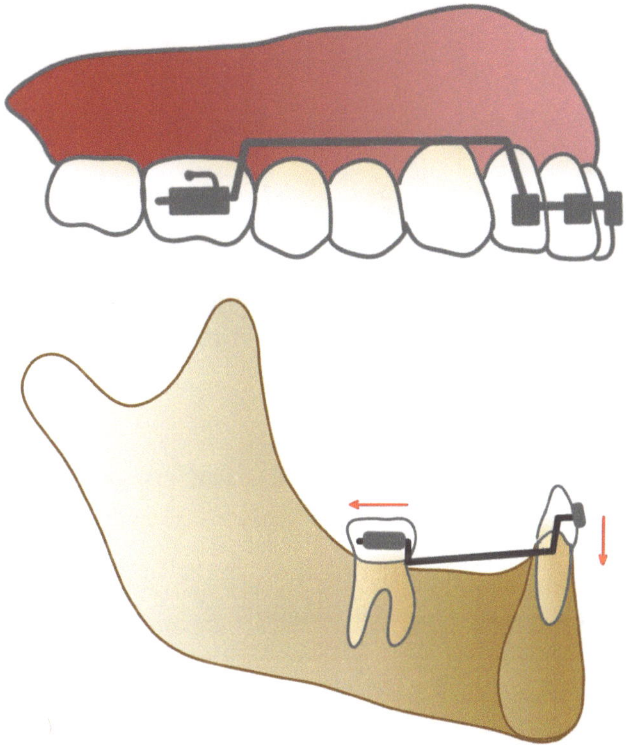

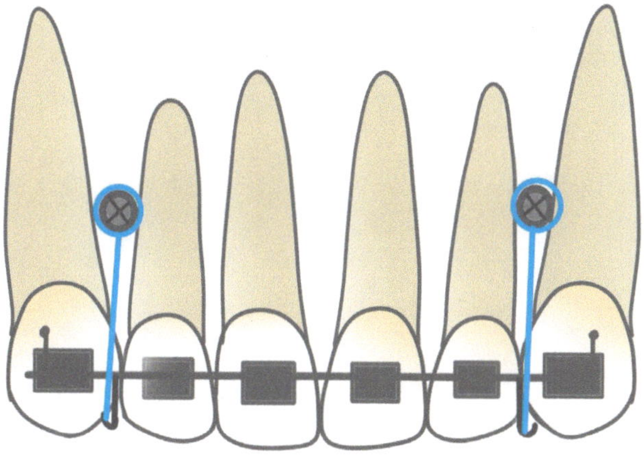

Figure 5.20 Use of two mini-implants in the anterior sector as anchorage for intrusion

Figure 5.19 Utility arch in the upper and lower jaw.

Leveling by Relative Intrusion and Extrusion

- Continuous archwires;
- Use of Class II or Class III elastics;
- Reverse curve archwires (*Figure 5.21*);
- Bite planes.

Details about leveling mechanics are given in 'treatment of deep bite'

Closure of Spaces

Orthodontic space closure is the closure of spaces caused by the extraction of teeth, the congenital absence of teeth, or the excessive space between teeth. It should be individually personalized based on the diagnosis and treatment plan.

Anchorage Planning for Space Closure

Three groups of closure of extraction sites have been described by Nanda (*Figure 5.22*).

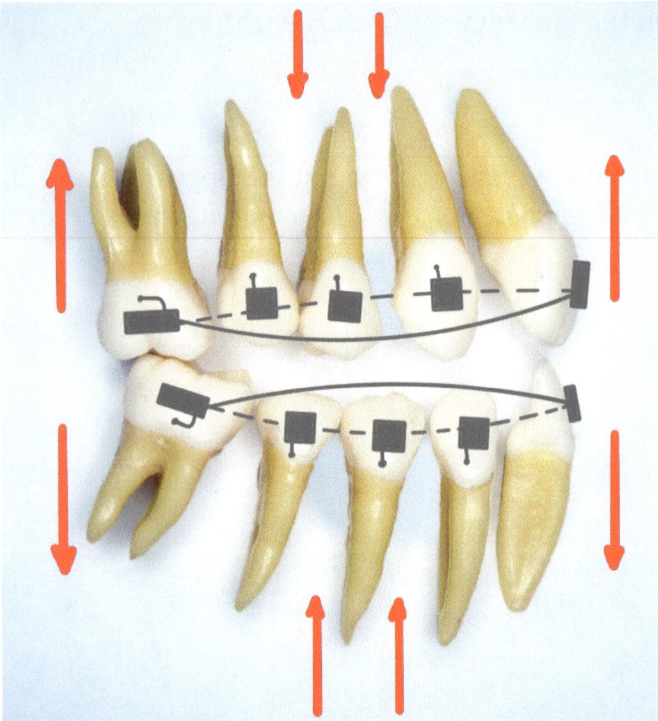

Figure 5.21 Reverse curve archwires before installation in the slots of the brackets.

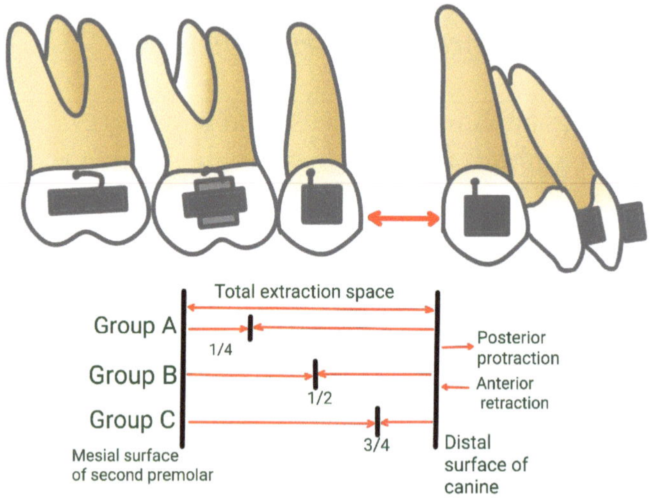

Figure 5.22 Anchorage classification based on the utilization of extraction space.

1. Group A anchorage: This category describes the critical maintenance of the posterior tooth position. About 75% or more of the extraction space is needed for anterior retraction.
2. Group B anchorage: This category describes relatively symmetric space closure with the equal movement of the anterior and posterior teeth to close the space. This is the least difficult of the space closures.
3. Group C anchorage: This category describes noncritical anchorage, where 75% or more of the space closure is achieved through the mesial movement of the posterior segment; this could also be described as critical anterior anchorage.

The types of closure may not necessarily be bilaterally the same in a given arch. In asymmetric malocclusions, one side may have group B while the contralateral side may have group A.
Retraction of anterior teeth can be carried out en masse (six anterior teeth) or retraction of four incisors followed by individual canine retraction.

Orthodontic tooth movement during space closure is achieved by two mechanics
- Sliding mechanics;
- Loop mechanics.

Four suggested ways to accomplish space closure:
1. Elastics;
2. Coils;
3. Loops;
4. Retroligature;

Elastic chains

- The force of the elastomeric chain tends to degrade with time, with 60% force loss after four weeks; 50 % of the force loss took place the first day of use;
- Wong observed a loss of force of 50-70% after the first 24 hours when the chain was kept in water at 37°;
- In a premolar extraction case, the chain will stretch excessively upon the extraction sites; this provokes adjacent teeth rotation;
- If the chain is not stretched, the spaces will not close;
- The power chain is useful for closing one or two small spaces at the end of a treatment and to avoid space reopening in advanced treatment phases.

According to the distance between the center of the eyelets (interlink distance), chains are divided into four types (*Figure 5.23*):

- Closed or continuous chain;
  - Recommended for lower incisor space closure;
  - It should be stretched elastics three times its length in order to obtain the desired force level;
- Short-chain;
  - Recommended for inferior dental arch space closure;
- Long-chain
  - Recommended for upper dental arch space closure;

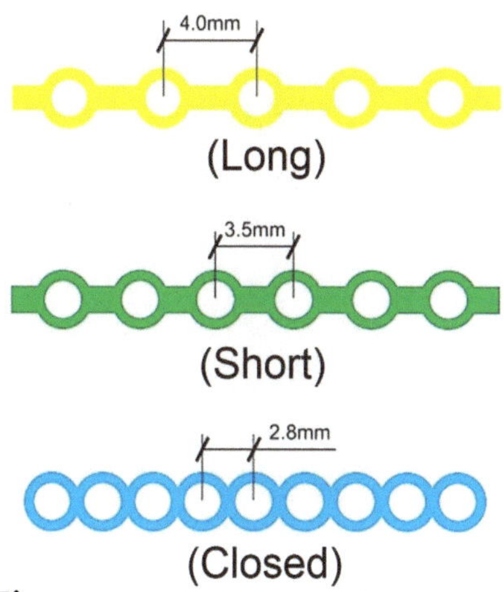

Figure 5.24

Space closure with a molar to molar chain (*Figure 5.24*)

Molar to molar chain treatment effects:

- Space closure;
  - Inclination of teeth next to extraction space toward each other;
- Anterior segment retroclination;
- Deepening of the anterior bite.
  - Chain placed from molar to molar exerts initially 400 g in the upper dental arch and 350 g in the lower dental arch, gradually the force diminishes;
  - Approximately 1mm of space closure per month.

Management

- To avoid unwanted torque or to deepen the Spee curve (roller coaster effect), place a heavy archwire during space closure with an elastomeric chain;
- Be cautious placing molar to molar chain in deep bite patients;
- Do not apply too much pressure during chain placement, because we may debond some braces;
- Replace the chain every 21 days.

Space closure with open coil and power chains *(Figure 5.25)*

We can close extraction sites or diastemas combining two forces: a traction force and a pushing force; for example, a power chain in combination with a NiTi open coil spring.

- Space closure is at about 1.5 to 2 mm per month;
- Use heavy archwires during space closure;
- Place wire ligature on teeth on which the coil is going to lean on.

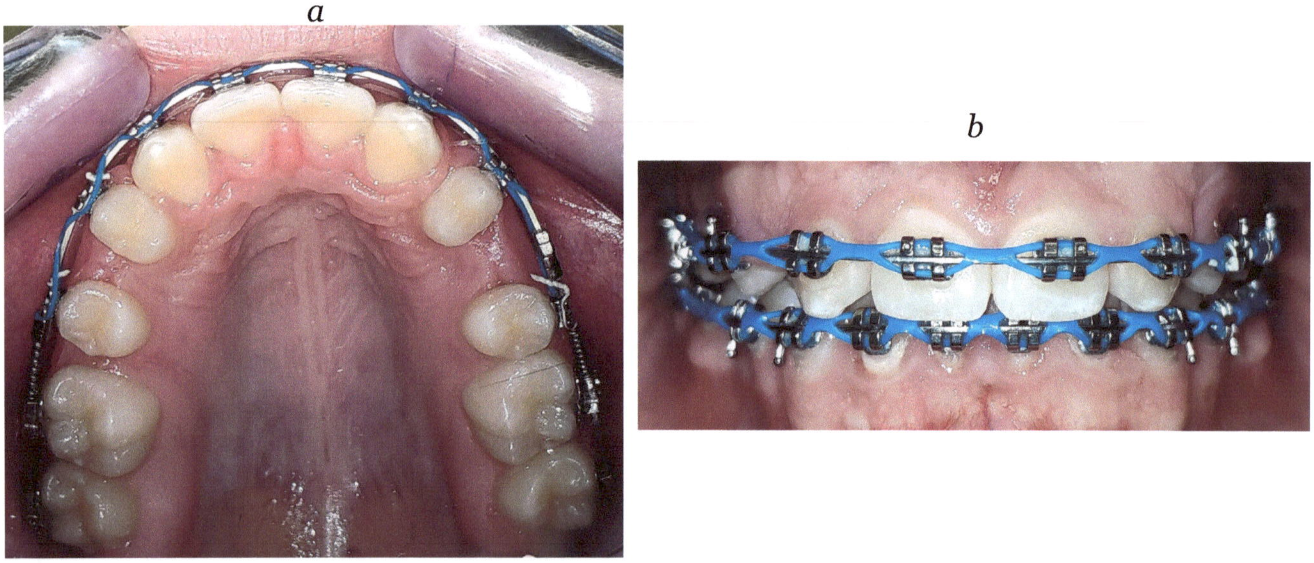

Figure 5.25 Combination of an open coil and elastic chain for space closure

Space closure with two parallel forces

This is done with two simultaneous forces (buccal and lingual). We must place additional buttons or lingual accessories in order to apply a simultaneous force in the lingual aspect of the tooth as well as on the buccal side.

- It is a great force and risk of root resorption is a disadvantage;
- This method should not be used in short rooted teeth.

Closed coil springs *(Figure 5.26)*

- Coil springs are made of nickel-titanium alloy;
- Coils exert physiologic loads, act for longer periods of time, so they do not have to be changed that often;
- The variables that affect the force level produced by the coils are: the caliber of the archwire, the alloy, the size of the spiral, the length and magnitude of the coil activation;
- There are two types of closed coils in the market, with one and two stainless steel eyelets;
- The eyelets are soldered to the coil with a laser and this makes placement on tubes and bracket hooks easier;
- The forces range from 25 g to 300 g depending on the manufacturer.
- NiTi closed coils close spaces faster in comparison with elastic chain (almost double the rate);

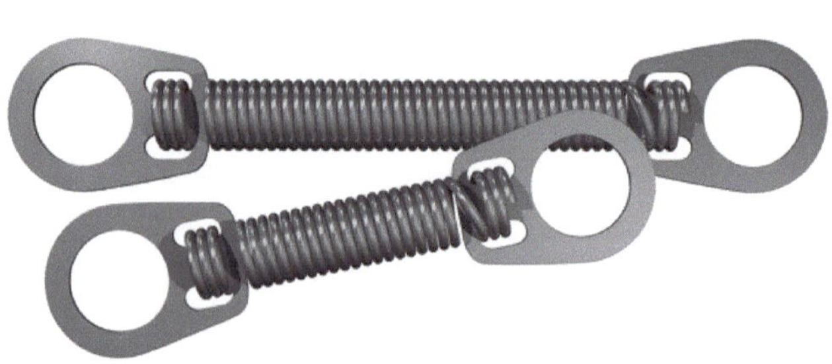

Figure 5.26 Closed coil springs

- They are ideal for large space closure;
- Use 150 g to 200g coils;
- Place the eyelet of the coil at the distal wings of the canine and wire ligature or elastomeric tie on the mesial wings. This will diminish undesired canine rotation.

Space closure with loops

- It is also known as frictionless mechanics
- Loops are divided into horizontal, vertical or mixed loops, and may be open or closed;
- Horizontal loops have a mechanical action expressed in a vertical plane, they are ideal for mesiodistal movement (space closure);
- Vertical loops have a mechanical action expressed in the horizontal plane, they are ideal for intrusive and extrusive movements.
  - The force exerted by a 0.017 x 0.025 stainless steel loop seven millimeters high is approximately 250 g;
  - When we want more flexibility and less force, we can extend the loop and add spirals or helixes.

Loops are designed for space closure and retrusion of the anterior sector

- Open “I” loop (*Figure 5.27*);
  - This vertical loop is 7 mm high and is made on the archwire, Generally located between the canine and the lateral incisor;
  - This loop must be opened to be active.
- Closed “I” loop (*Figure 5. 28)*;
  - Vertical loop, 7 mm high, made on the archwire, the arms inter-cross, and generally is located between the lateral incisor and the canine;
  - This loop activates by being closed.

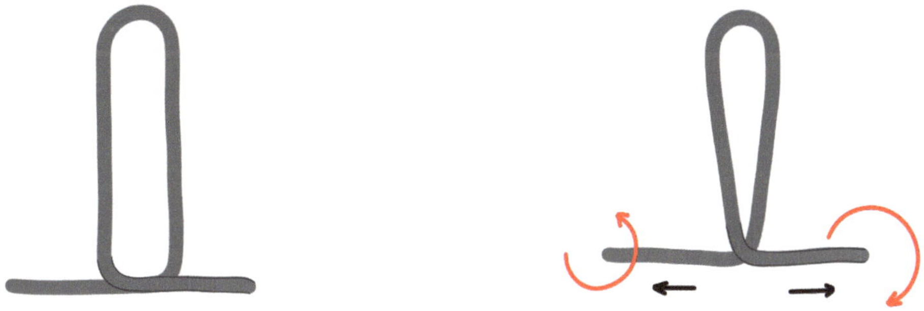

Figure 5.28 Closed “I” loop

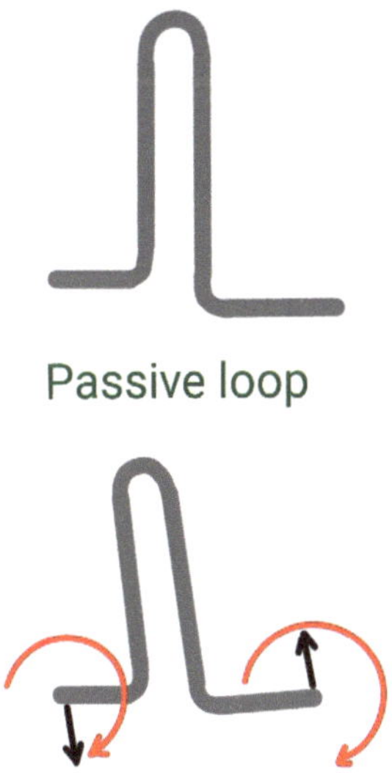

Figure 5.27 Open “I” loop

- Closed helicoid “I” loop (*Figure 5.29*);
  - Vertical loop 7 mm high, the arms intercross, and at the gingival end form a circular loop. Made in the archwire usually between the lateral incisor and the canine;
  - This loop activates by closing.
- Bull or Keyhole loop *(Figure 5. 30)*;

- Vertical loop 7 mm high, the longitudinal arms touch one another and at the gingival end, and forms an open circle that looks like a "keyhole"; done on the archwire, generally between the lateral incisor and the canine;
- This loop activates by being opened.

a *b*

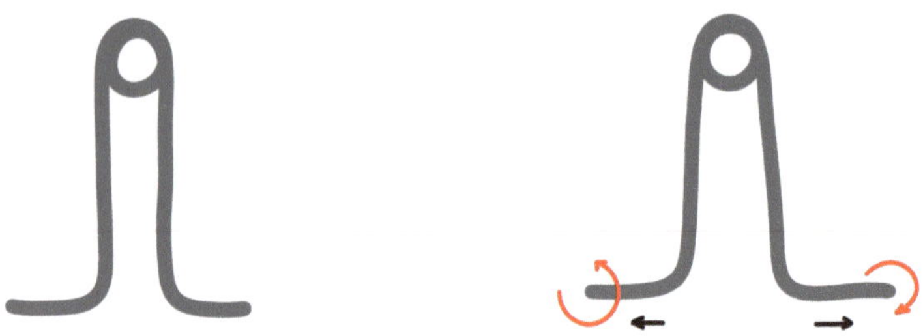

Figure 5.29 Closed helicoid "I" loop. Passive I loop (a) and Active I loop (b).

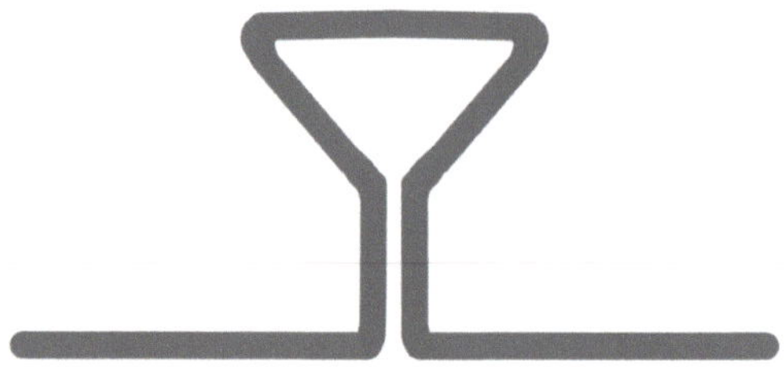

Figure 5.30 Bull or Keyhole loop

- "T" loop (*Figure 5.31*);
  - Mixed vertical and horizontal loop 7 mm high, done on the archwire and usually located between the lateral incisor and the canine or between the canine and the premolar. In TMA arches the "T" loop can be activated 3 mm behind the molar tube, exerting forces ranging between 250 and 300 g.

a *b*

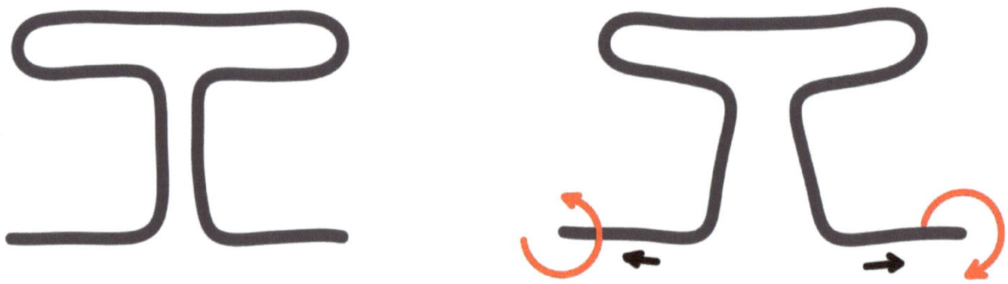

Figure 5.31 "T" loop

- DKL (double key loops) arch (*Figure 5.32*);
  - Mixed vertical and horizontal loop 7 mm high;
  - This loop activates by being opened;
  - This is a steel wire with two loops on each side of the wire and is used for sagittal movements of the anterior or posterior sectors in order to close extraction sites.

Figure 5.32 DKL (double key loops) arch

Retroligatures (lace backs)

Drs. McLaughlin, Bennett, and Trevisi (MBT) suggest the use of stainless steel 0.019" x 0.025" archwires in a 0.022" slot, in combination with retrologatures for space closure

According to the MBT technique, there are three ways to close spaces:

- Active distal ligature type 1 (distal elastomeric ligature);
- Active distal ligature type 2 (mesial elastomeric ligature);
- Active distal ligature with NiTi coils.
- Active distal ligature type 1 (distal elastic ligature):
  - The 0.019" x 0.025" steel wire is placed on the brackets with a metallic or elastomeric ligature;
  - We put the elastic ligature on the hook of the first or second molar;
  - We use a 0.010" steel ligature to ligate the elastic to the hook of the canine bracket or to a soldered hook on the arch.
- Active distal ligature type 2 (mesial elastomeric ligature):
  - The elastomeric ligature is hitched to the hook soldered to the arch;
  - The arch is a 0.019" x 0.025" stainless steel wire;
  - We hitch a 0.010" steel ligature to the hook of the first or second molar and the other end to an elastomeric ligature that is stretched to the hook of the arch.

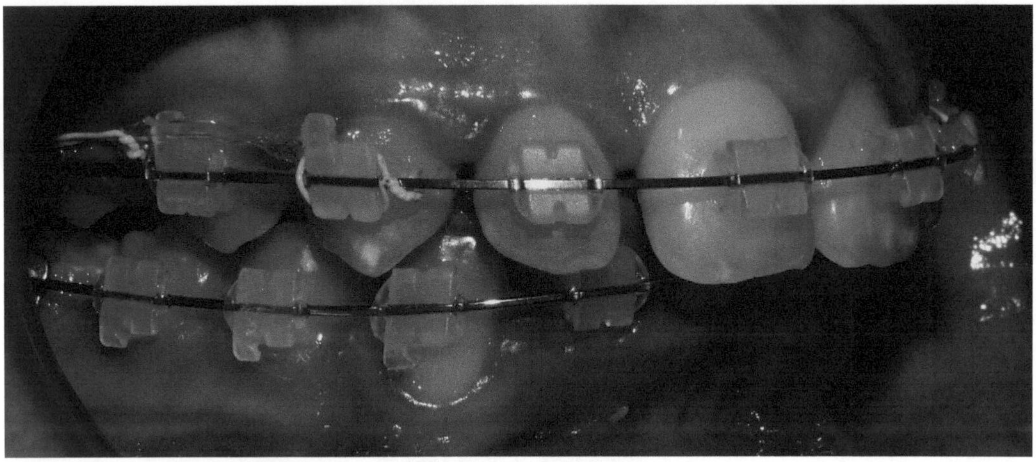

Figure 5.33 Distal ligature with mesial elastic

Finishing and detailing stage of treatment

The final wire in a 0.018 slot will be 0.017 x 0.025 inch steel or beta-titanium and, in 0.022 slots it will be 0.019 x 0.025 inch SS or 0.021 x 0.025 inch beta-titanium.

- Root Paralleling

The required root paralleling is produced by 0.017 x 0.025 inch SS or 0.021 x 0.025 inch beta-titanium in 0.018 and 0.022 slots, respectively.

- Adjustments of minor tooth irregularities
  - Poor bracket positioning can result in minor tooth irregularities;
  - After the brackets are rebounded, a flexible wire must be placed to bring the tooth to the correct position (0.017 x 0.025 beta-titanium in 0.018-inch slots and 0.021 x 0.025 M-NiTi in 0.022-inch slots);
  - Minor irregularities in first order (in-out) and vertical (up-down) are corrected either by incorporating horizontal/vertical offsets (step bends) or by rebounding brackets and inserting flexible wires.

- Incisor Torque
  - It can be accomplished with an auxiliary appliance;
  - Torqueing auxiliary is a piggyback arch that makes contact with the labial surface of

incisors near the gingival margin;

- Additional torqueing springs can be used (*Figure 5.34*);

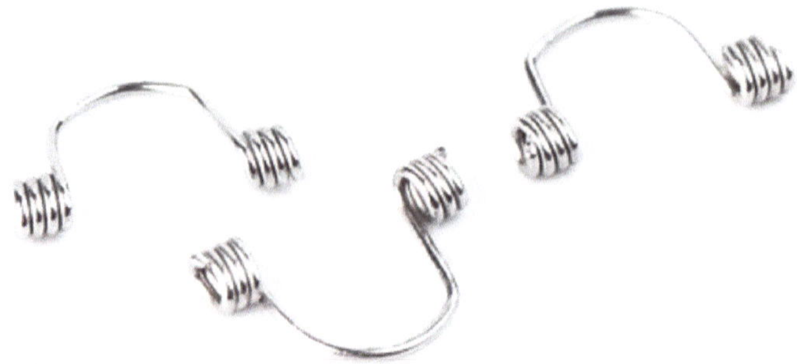

Figure 5.34 Torqueing springs

- Correction of Midline Discrepancies

McLaughlin and Bennet have suggested five methods of elastic wear for specific situations:

1. A single Class II elastic on one side and a double Class II elastic on the other, for cases with a bilateral Class II component; Figure 5.35 (a).
2. A single Class II elastic on one side only, when the overjet results in a slight Class II relationship on that side and the opposite side is in a Class I position; Figure 5.35 (b).
3. Class III elastics on one side and Class II elastics on the other, for cases with the corresponding dental relationships; Figure 5.35 (c).
4. A single Class III elastic on one side only, when that side is in a Class III position and the opposite side has a Class I dental relationship; Figure 5.35 (d).
5. An anterior cross-elastic, when the discrepancy occurs primarily in the anterior segments. Figure 5.35 (e).

a

b

c

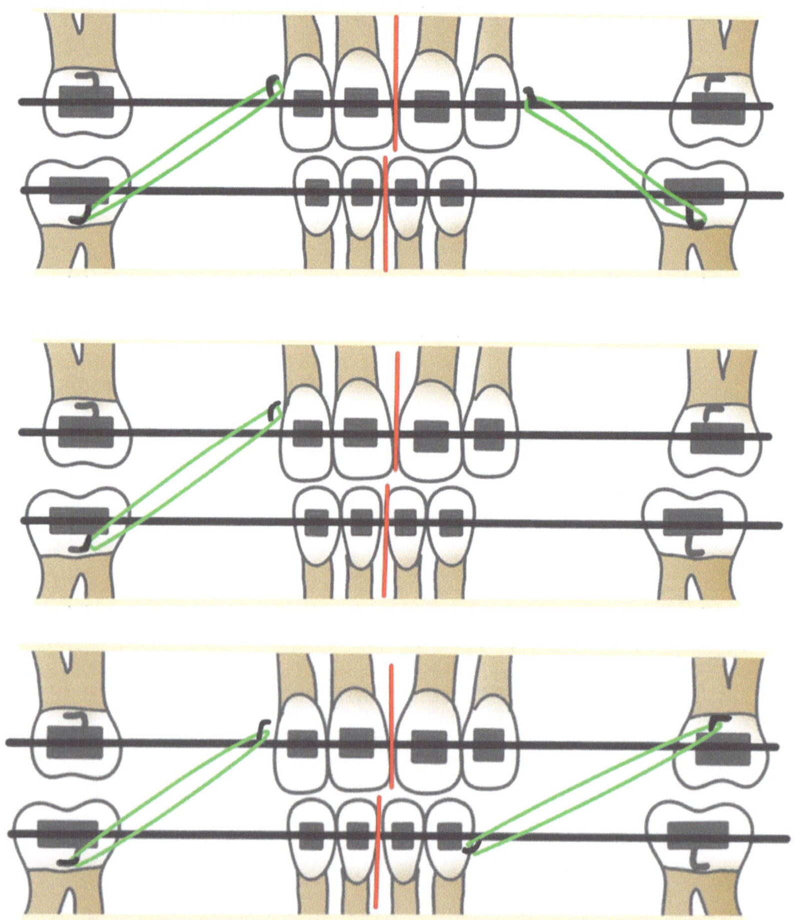

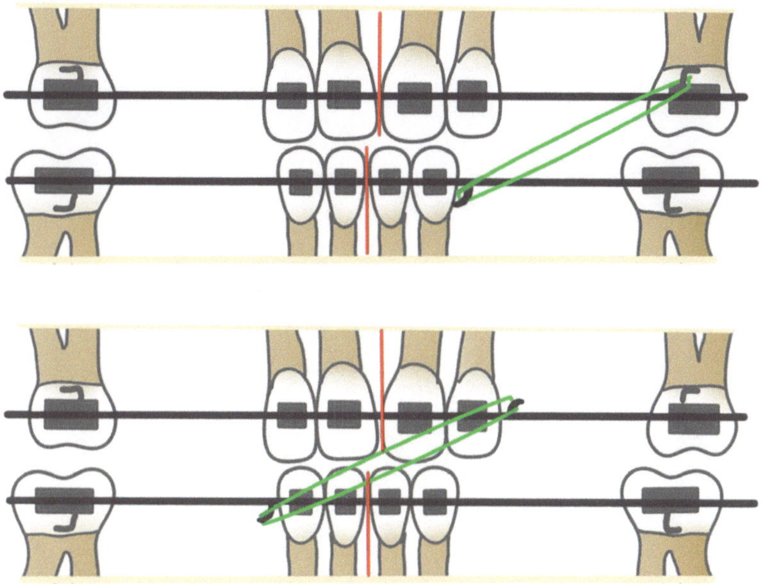

d

e

Figure 5.35

- Asymmetrical elastics should be used for a minimum period of time, and only with rectangular archwires, because of their tendency to cant the occlusal plane;
- The archwires should be tied back while these elastics are worn so that the wires do not slide around the arch, causing unwanted space opening and distortion of the arch form;
- Maintaining the Closure of all Spaces
  - It is done with power chain elastics;
  - Long ligature wires can be ligated around all brackets;
- Coordination of Arch Widths and Arch Forms.
  - Coordination of archwires from the beginning of treatment through the rectangular wire phase will prevent unwanted and troublesome crossbites from developing.
- Bolton's or Tooth Size Discrepancy

- Any tooth size discrepancy should be corrected either by proximal slicing or by composite buildup.

Final Settling of Teeth

In final settling teeth should be brought into full occlusal interdigitation without heavy archwires present.

- Before debonding put 0.014 or 0.016-inch round archwire is in place including the first and second-order compensatory bends;
- The second option is to put 0.016-inch round sectional wire from lateral incisor to lateral incisor (*Figure 5.36*);
- Vertical triangular elastics should be used;
- Discontinuation of interarch elastics and headgear 4–8 weeks prior to debonding is in order.

Retention

- When we have expanded the arch as a method to gain space, we need to retain using removable acrylic Hawley appliance;
- Rotated teeth can be retained with fixed or removable retainers;
- Corrected crossbite retains itself.

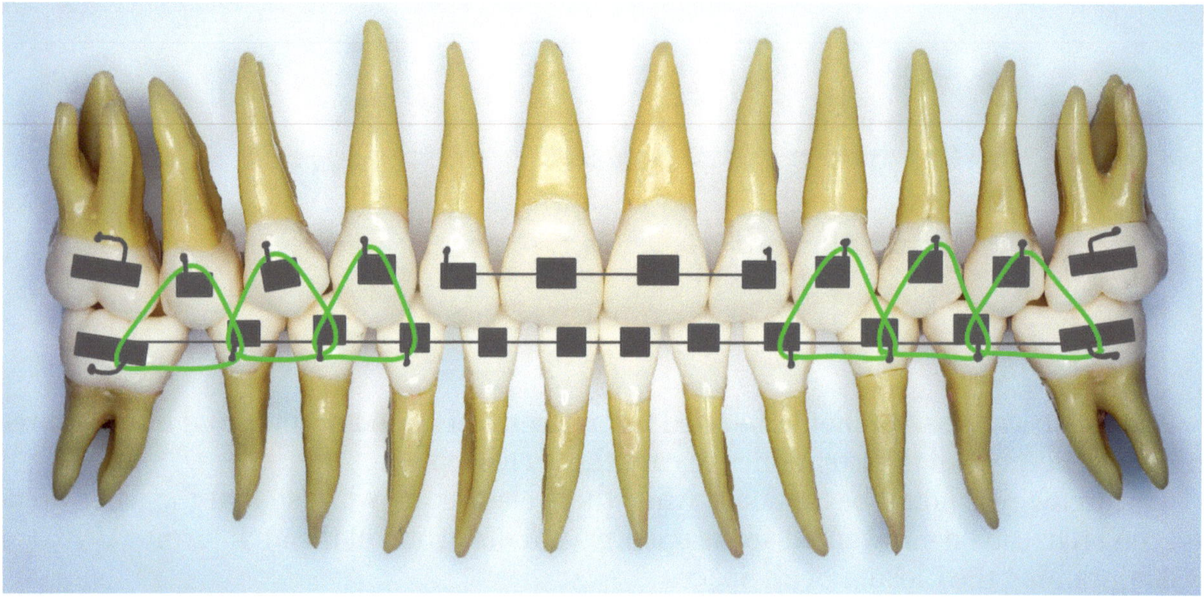

Figure 5.36 Vertical triangular elastics used for settling

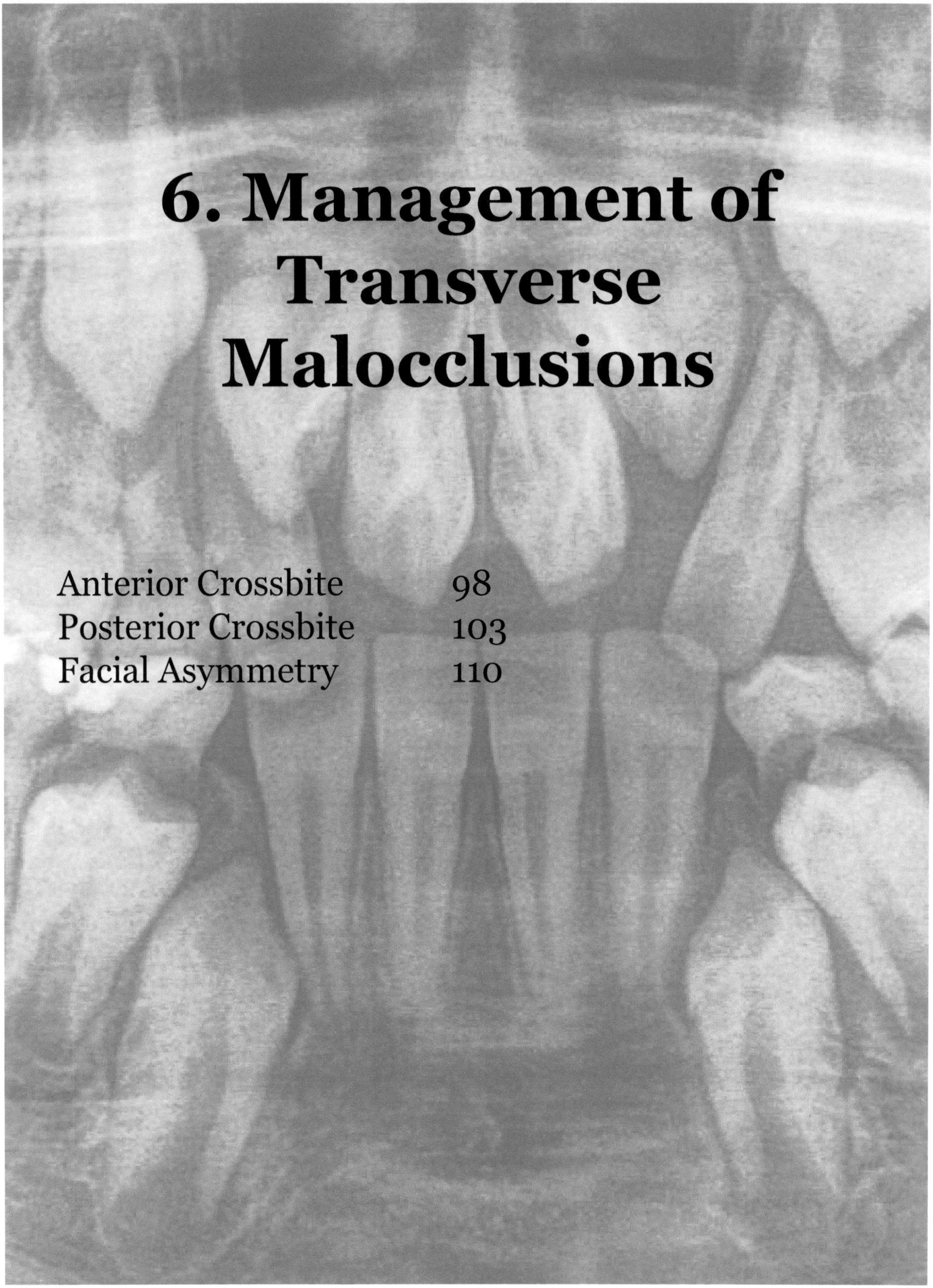

6. Management of Transverse Malocclusions

Management of transverse malocclusions

Transverse malocclusions are induced of constriction or expansion of one arch compared to the other. Transverse malocclusions are evaluated in the sagittal plane.
'Crossbite' refers to a condition where one or more teeth may be abnormally malposed buccally or lingually or labially with reference to the opposing tooth or teeth.

Classification of crossbites

- Anterior crossbite:
  - Single tooth;
  - Multiple teeth;
  - A segment.
- Posterior crossbite:
  - Unilateral;
  - Bilateral;
  - Single tooth crossbite.

Another classification:

- Dental: anterior and posterior;
- Skeletal: anterior and posterior;
- Functional crossbite
  - Anterior crossbite. This is a condition in which one or more primary or permanent maxillary incisors are lingual to the mandibular incisors;
  - Buccal crossbite. Condition in which the maxillary posterior teeth is buccal to the mandibular antagonist;
  - Lingual crossbite. Condition in which the maxillary posterior teeth is lingual to mandibular antagonist;
  - Scissors bite or telescopic bite. Mandibular teeth are entirely lingual to the maxillary arch.

Anterior Crossbite

Anterior crossbite is a condition in which one or more primary or permanent maxillary incisor teeth are lingual to the mandibular incisors (*Figure 6.1*).

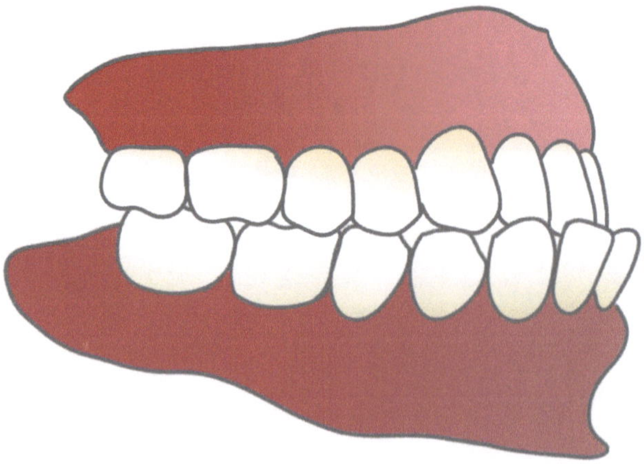

Figure 6.1 Anterior crossbite

Etiology

The etiology of anterior crossbite can be studied under dental, skeletal, and functional factors.

Dental Factors

A dental anterior crossbite is because of abnormal axial inclination of the maxillary incisors.
The reasons for abnormal axial inclination are:

- Trauma to primary teeth or to the permanent tooth bud ;
- Over retained primary tooth;
- Labially positioned supernumerary tooth;
- Inadequate arch length which causes a lingual eruption of a permanent tooth;
- Repaired cleft lip.

Skeletal Factors

- Skeletal crossbite results due to excessive mandibular growth;
- It is genetic or inherited malocclusion;
- In children with cleft palates where there is retrognathic maxilla.

Functional Factors

- A dental crossbite also occurs due to functional interference of the mandible during the closure (*Figure 6.2*);
- This is because of premature tooth contact;
- This results or leads to pseudo-Class III malocclusion.

a *b*

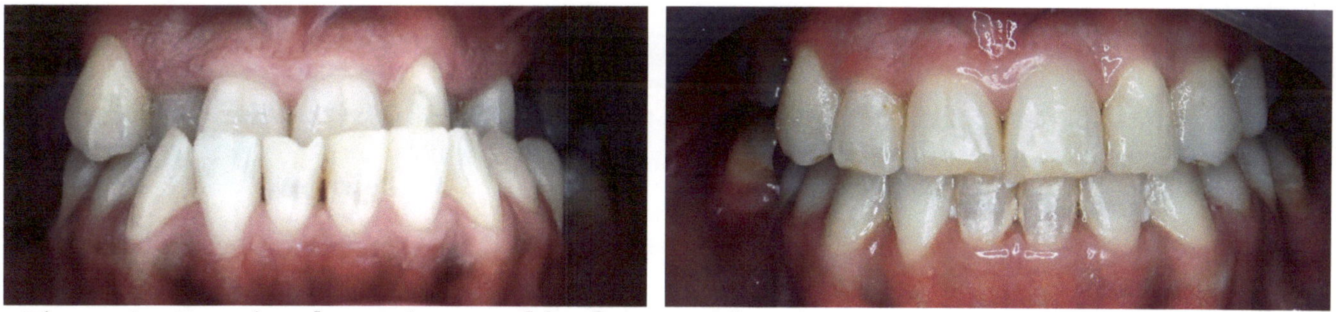

Figure 6.2 Functional anterior crossbite due to tooth contact.

Consequences of Anterior Crossbite

- Excessive wear of anterior teeth;
- Traumatic occlusion of the unlocked tooth;
- If not treated in time, it could lead to overgrowth of the mandible and restriction of the maxilla.

Clinical features

The factors to be considered in diagnosis are:

- The number of teeth involved.

1. Single tooth crossbite—usually local origin and dental crossbite or functional (*Figure 6.3*);

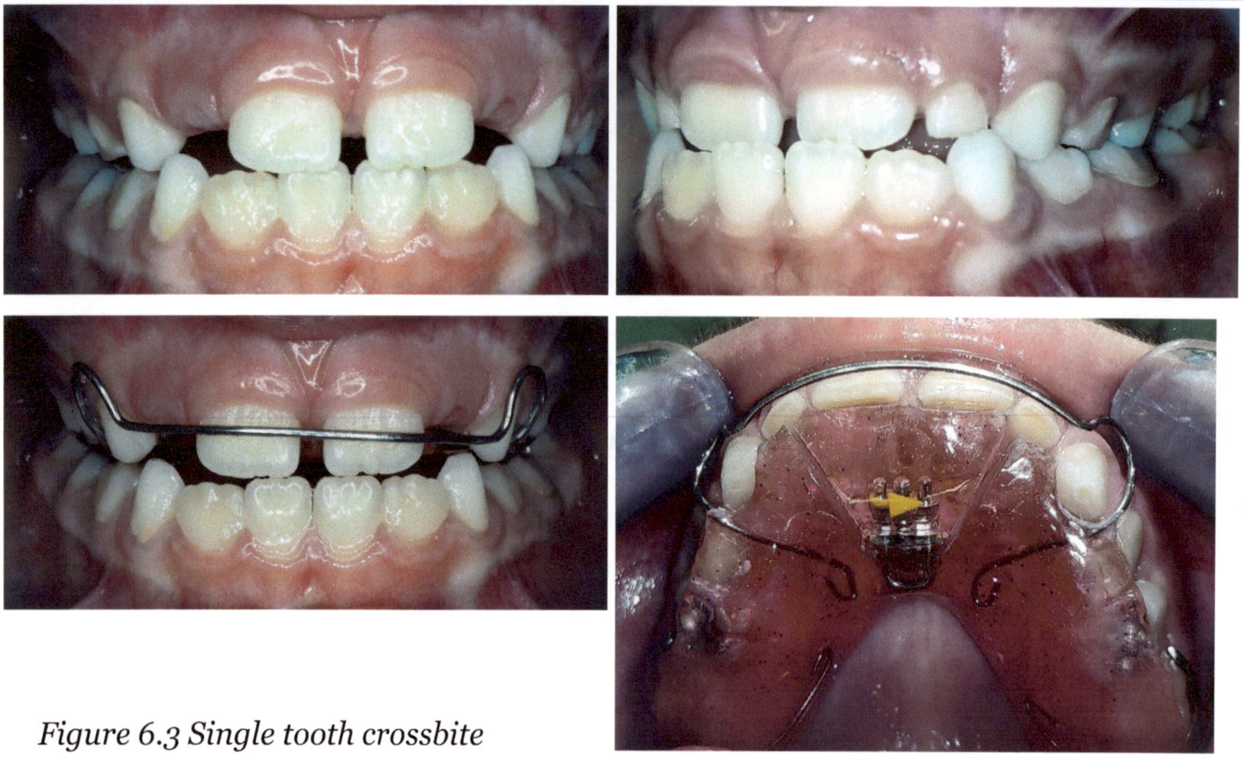

a b c d

Figure 6.3 Single tooth crossbite

2. Segment crossbite—usually skeletal.

- Functional path of closure:

We should evaluate teeth contacts for prematurities. In initial or developing stages of crossbite, simple occlusal grinding will eliminate the development of crossbite;

- Molar and canine relationship:

In dental crossbite, in centric occlusion, molar and canine relationship will be Class I.
In true skeletal crossbites, the molar and canine relationship will be Class III.

- Radiographic findings:

Lateral cephalogram is useful to find out skeletal discrepancy and axial inclination of the incisors relation to the skeletal.

Management of Anterior Crossbite

Factors to be considered for the treatment of anterior crossbite

- Availability of mesiodistal space to correct them in locked tooth;
- Sufficient overbite;
- Position of the tooth;
- Occlusion—whether it is in Class I or Class III.

Management of anterior crossbite in the mixed dentition

- Occlusal equilibration for anterior crossbite:
  - It is done to unlock the blocked upper jaw;
  - Most common we need to abrade primary canine teeth because of premature contacts.

- Inclined plane (*Figure 6.4*):
  - It is a functional appliance;
  - It can be removable or bonded to the upper or lower anterior teeth;
  - It should be used for less than three weeks;
  - It is used full day;
  - Best suited for a single tooth anterior crossbite case.

a *b*

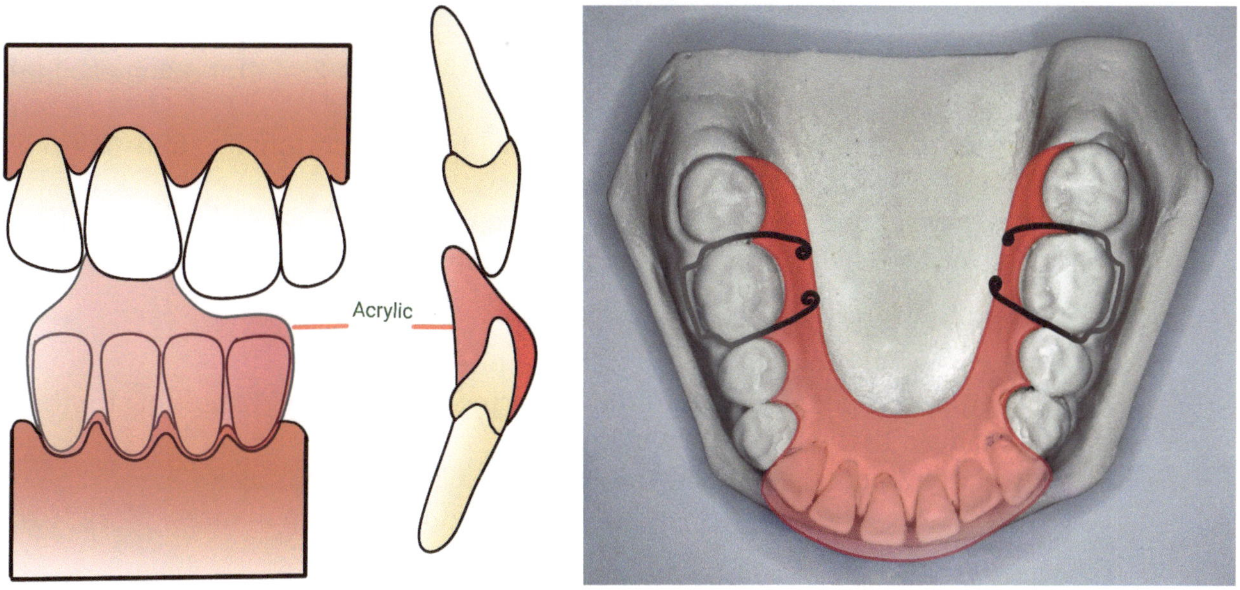

Figure 6.4 Fixed lower inclined plane (a); Removable lower inclined plane (b).

- Face mask
  - The face mask is an option for the correction of skeletal anterior crossbites due to maxillary hypoplasia in young patients that are growing and present primary or early mixed dentition;
  - The maxillae bone responds to orthopedic and functional stimulus because it is of intramembranous ossification origin;
  - The face mask could be used in the permanent dentition stage, but during that phase, it can cause only dentoalveolar changes;
  - A face mask is primarily used to correct Class III skeletal malocclusion due to maxillary retrognathism in young children (Nanda);
  - After surgical correction of the skeletal Class III malocclusion, a face mask is indicated as a retaining device.

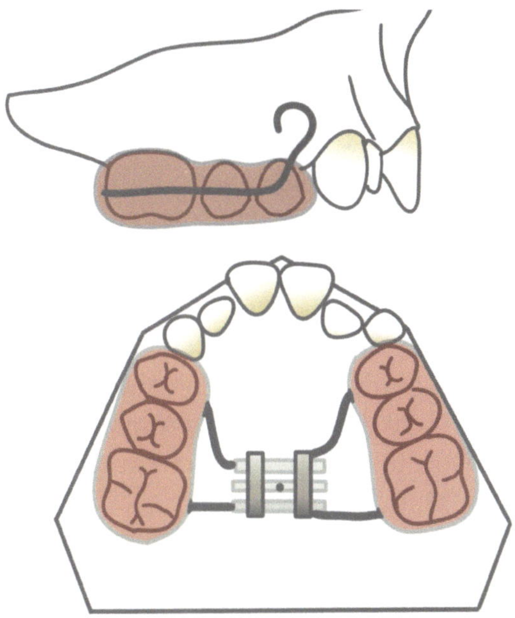

Figure 6.5 Intraoral appliance used with face mask

Parts of the face mask:

o Intraoral appliance
  - The maxillary splint can be either banded or bonded maxillary rapid expansion device (*Figure 6.5*);
  - Turn the midline jackscrew of the appliance once daily, generally before bedtime;
  - The maxillary splint is expanded until the desired transverse change is achieved;

- The two hooks, lying adjacent to canines or first primary molars, used for attaching elastics are soldered to the wire framework.

o Elastic Traction

- The facial mask is secured by stretched elastics from maxillary splint hooks to the facial mask crossbow;
- Heavy forces are generated with 5/16 inches, 14 oz elastics used bilaterally;
- The patient is instructed to wear the facial mask on a full-time basis except during meals full-time wear will last only 3–5 months;
- The facial mask is usually worn until a positive overjet of 2–4 mm is achieved interincisally;
- Part-time or night-time wear is recommended for an additional 3- to 6-month retention period;
- The maxillary splint is then removed, and a removable palatal stabilization plate, with arrow clasps between the first and second deciduous molars, is worn full-time.

• Expansion appliances: used in these situations are:
  - Schwarz type expansion plate with posterior bite plane;
  - Upper Hawley's appliance with cantilever spring to move the in-standing tooth. Posterior bite plane is added to the Hawley's appliance;
  - Removable appliances with Z springs or double cantilever springs;
  - In class III cases due to retrognathic maxilla, functional appliances, like FR III, are used;
  - Fixed appliance: The in-locked tooth or teeth is pulled into the correct labial position by fixed appliances.

Management in the early permanent dentition

Appliances used to correct a dentoalveolar anterior crossbite

Forward arch

- It consists of a 0.018" or 0.020" stainless steel wire main arch that must be separated 2 mm from the slots of the upper incisor brackets;
- Two stops or omegas are made mesial to the tubes of the molar bands that will impede the main arch from slipping;
- We should use posterior bite planes to disarticulate the bite;
- There is no torque control of the upper incisors with this method.

Bite block

- It is an appliance that can be useful to open the bite in order to uncross an anterior tooth or a group of teeth that are in a palatal position;
- It can be a fixed or a removable appliance and can be placed on the upper or lower dental arch on the occlusal aspects of molars and premolars;
- Made of acrylic;
- It is used in combination with fixed appliance therapy.

Management in adults

- Dental crossbite is managed with a fixed appliance in the same manner as in early permanent dentition;

- Skeletal correction in the permanent dentition is done with orthognathic surgery;

Retention

Corrected anterior open bite retains itself with occlusal contacts.

Posterior Crossbite

A posterior crossbite is an abnormal buccolingual relationship of a tooth or teeth between maxilla and mandible when they are brought into centric occlusion (*Figure 6.6*).

Posterior crossbite presents as any one or combination of the following ways:
1. Lingual crossbite (unilateral or bilateral);
2. Buccal crossbite (unilateral or bilateral);
3. Complete lingual crossbite (unilateral or bilateral);

The classification of crossbites is shown in *Figure 6.7*.

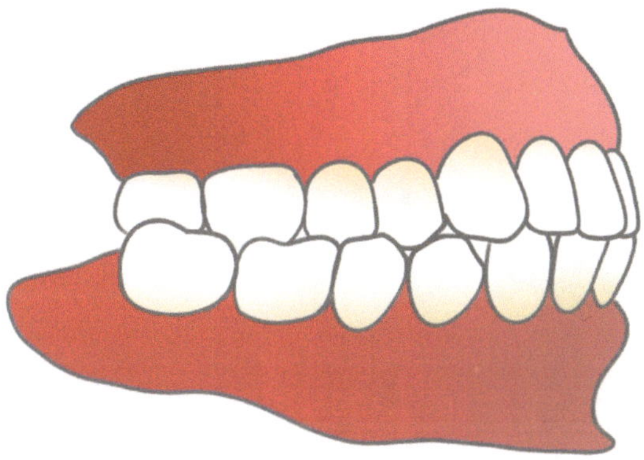

Figure 6.6 Posterior crossbite

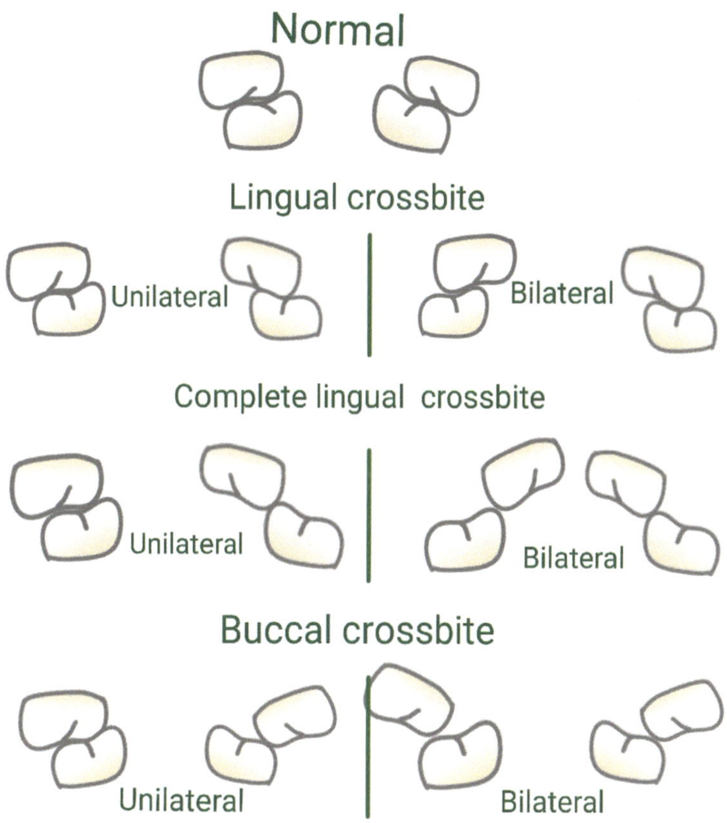

Figure 6.7 Classification of crossbites

Etiology

Dental Factors (Dental Crossbite)

The dental factors responsible for posterior crossbite are:
- Faulty eruption pattern, where the tooth erupts out of position;
- Insufficient arch length: This leads to lingual or buccal deflection of teeth during the eruption;
- Over retained primary tooth: This leads to a lateral shift of the mandible;
- Ectopic eruption;

- Prolonged thumb or finger sucking: This causes narrowing of the arches and lingual tipping of the posterior teeth;

Skeletal Factors (Skeletal Crossbite)

Skeletal crossbite occurs due to two reasons:

- Asymmetric growth of maxilla or mandible due to: (a) inherited growth pattern, (b) trauma, (c) longstanding functional problem;
- The difference in basal width of the maxilla and mandible due to:
  - (a) constricted maxilla;
  - (b) cleft palate.

Functional or Muscular Crossbite

- This is due to functional adjustments to tooth interferences;
- In this condition, muscular adjustment is more when compared to dental crossbites.;
- Functional analysis has to be done.

Consequences of Posterior Crossbite on the dentition are:

- Abnormal wear of the dentition;
- Interference with normal growth and development of dental arches;
- Pain due to muscle spasm;
- Possible damage to periodontium.

Clinical features

- Study models using wax bite in centric relation is a useful diagnostic aid;
- A dental crossbite will exhibit an abnormal buccal or lingual axial inclination;
- A skeletal crossbite may not exhibit abnormal axial inclination of teeth;
- Study models will show which tooth is at fault in the dental crossbite whether maxillary tooth or mandibular tooth;
- The symmetry of the dental arches can be assessed using grids, symmetroscope, Boley gauge or divider;
- This helps in diagnosing the arch at fault in skeletal crossbite;
- Assessment of midlines by (posteroanterior) PA view radiographs or frontal cephalograms should be done;

Midline should be assessed both in rest and centric positions.

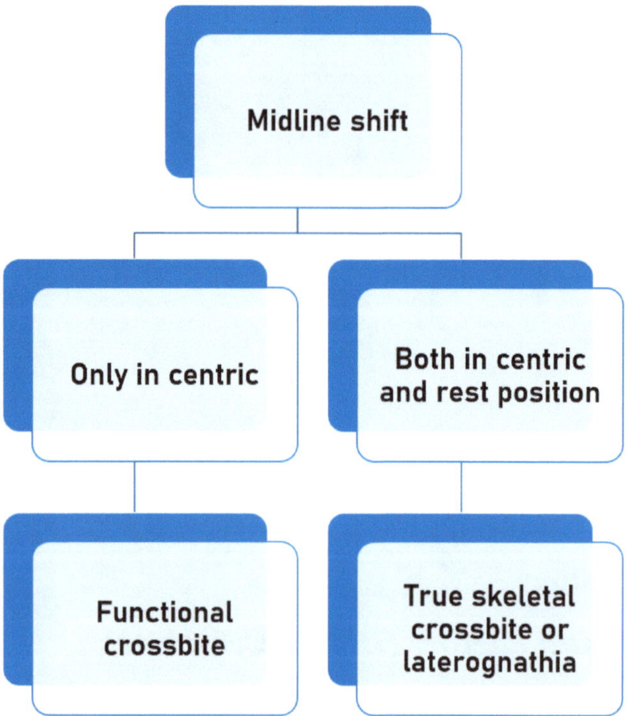

Figure 6.8 Differential diagnosis of midline shift

Differential diagnosis of midline shift is as described in *Figure 6.8*.

Management of Posterior Crossbite

Factors to be considered are

- Availability of space to correct the crossbites;
- Position of the apical portion of the tooth after treatment. This should be in the same position as that of the tooth in normal occlusion;
- Types of tooth movement required, either tipping or bodily movement.

Management in the mixed dentition

- It could be done with removable Hawley appliance with expansion screw;
- Expansion van be symmetric or asymmetric;
- We could use fixed expansion devices like Quad helix, Rapid maxillary expander, W – arch (*Figure 6.8*).

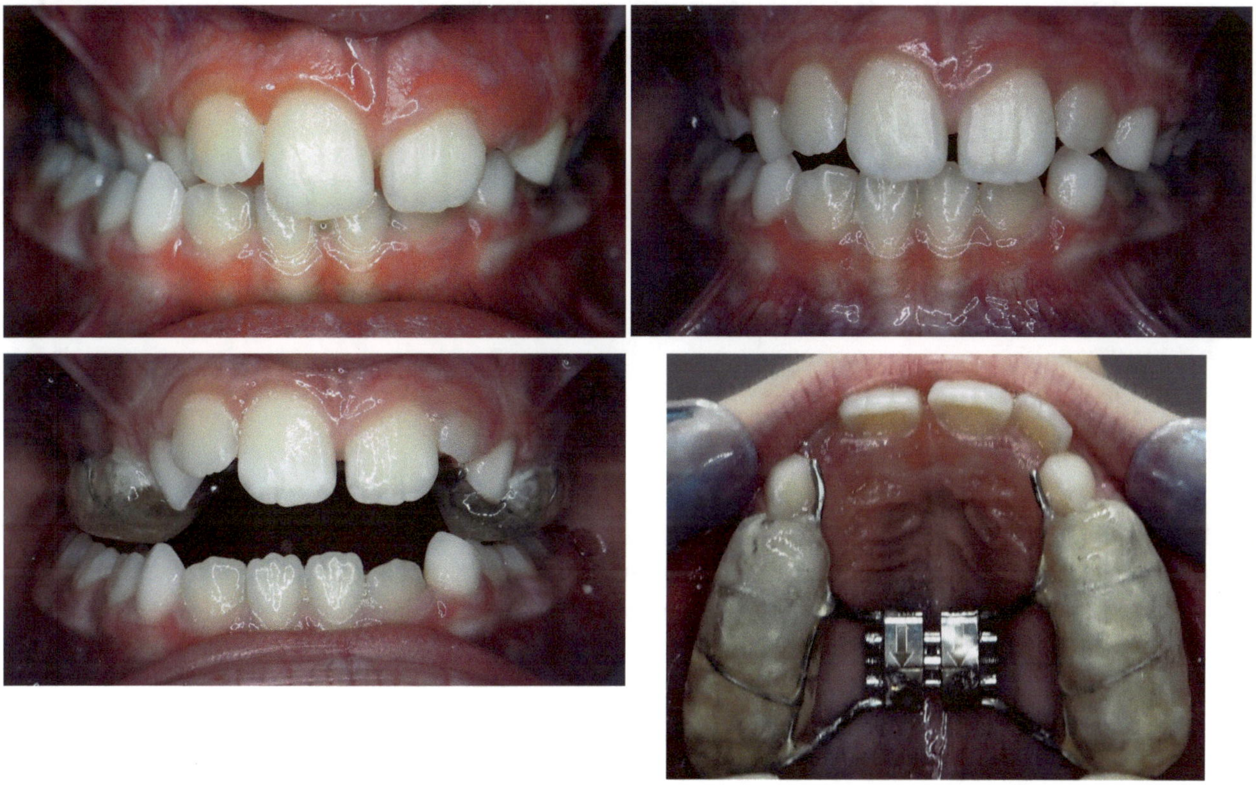
a b c d

Figure 6.9 Functional posterior crossbite (a); Rapid palatal expansion appliance in place (c,d). After debonding (b);

Management in the early permanent dentition

- Single Tooth Dental Crossbite

Usually, in single tooth crossbite, both the antagonist teeth are tipped out of position. Simple through the bite elastics or cross-bite elastics are effective in such cases (*Figure 6.10*).

- It requires patient co-operation;
- Requires bonding of the teeth.

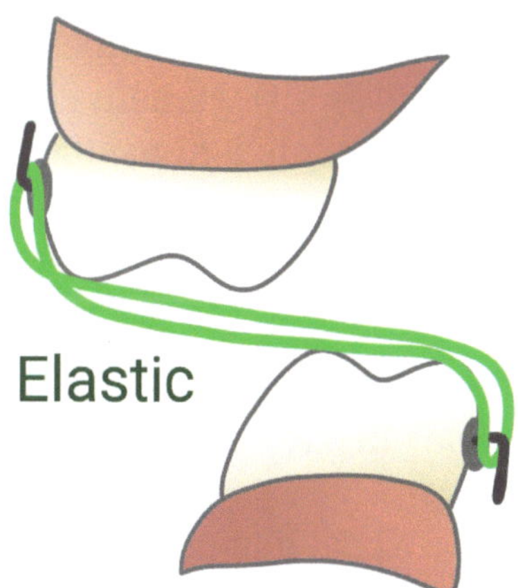

Figure 6.10

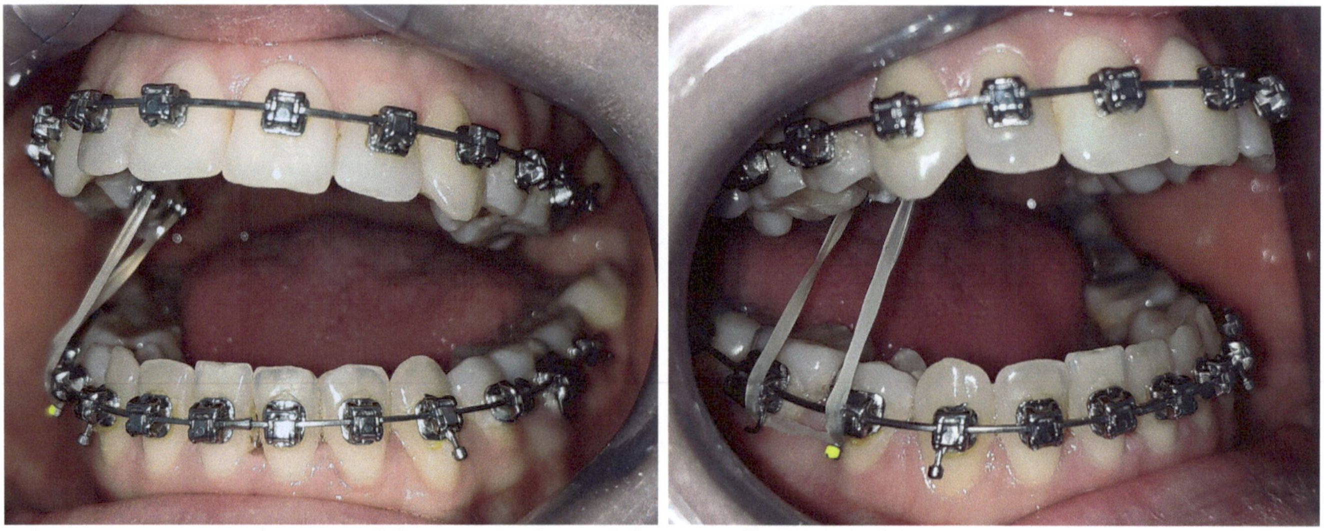

Figure 6.11 Posterior crossbite correction with cross elastics (a,b).

Management of dentoalveolar crossbite in the maxilla

Appliance used

Fixed expanders

Fixed expanders available for rapid or slow expansion include the W-arch, quad helix, Haas, and hyrax expanders, among others.

W-arch (*Figure 6.12*)

- The W-arch is efficient for the correction of posterior crossbites;
- Ideal for bilateral expansion;
- Includes two bands for the permanent first molars or any distal teeth in the arch (primary or permanent).
- 0.036- or 0.040-inch stainless steel archwire soldered to the bands;
- It can be activated in the center of the palatal bow for expansion of the molars;
- Activation of the U-loop close to the bands to activate the arms for expansion of buccal segments;
- The appliance can be activated unilaterally or bilaterally;
- It should be activated about 3 to 4 mm before fixation;
- The appliance is activated approximately every 4 or 5 weeks until the cross-bite has been corrected;
- Remains in the mouth, inactive, for 4 to 6 months to provide retention;
- Requires little patient cooperation and therefore has better patient compliance;
- Provides efficient palatal expansion or accelerates the rate of normal expansion of the midpalatal suture.

Quad helix expander (Figure 6.13)

- It is fabricated from 0.036-inch stainless steel wires soldered to molar bands;
- Four helixes are incorporated in the arch, the range and springiness of the appliance are increased;
- The distal helixes are about 2 to 3 mm distal to the molar bands;
- Activation of the anterior helixes produces posterior expansion, while activation of the

distal helixes produces buccal segment expansion;

- Reactivation can be performed to some extent intraorally by bird beak pliers;
- It is recommended that the appliance be removed for correct activation every 6 to 8 weeks;
- The quad helix can also work unilaterally;
- The combination of a posterior crossbite and a finger-sucking habit is the best indication for this appliance;
- A tongue crib can be added to the anterior bow.

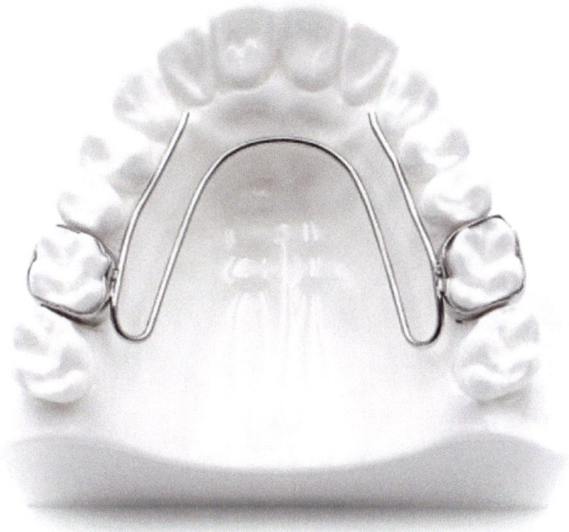

Figure 6.12 W-arch

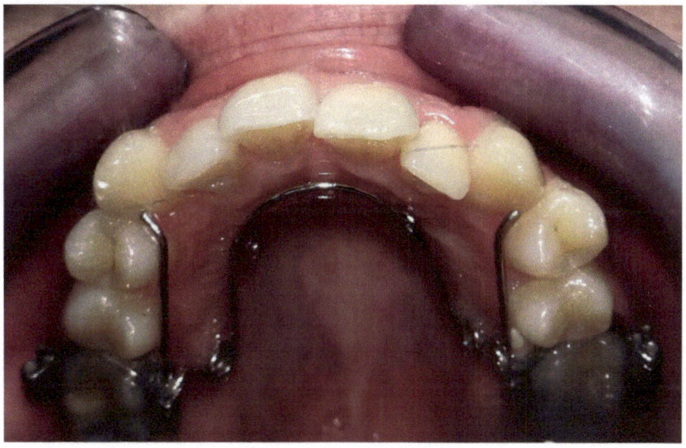

Figure 6.13 Quad helix expander

Haas expander (Figure 6.14)

- The Haas expander is also a fixed expander but is attached to both the left and right buccal segments of the arch as anchorage;
- A is screw embedded in the palatal acrylic resin.
- The screw can be activated once or twice a day for rapid force;
- Rapid palatal expansion is a specific type of expansion that can increase the palatal width skeletally;
- Rapid palatal expansion has several indications in orthodontic and orthopedic treatments, such as skeletal crossbite and constricted maxilla, maxillary protraction, and maxillary deficiency;
- This type of expander has been used during the primary or early mixed dentition with good results.

Hyrax expander (Figure 6.15)

The Hyrax expander is also a type of fixed rapid expander, but the screw is not embedded in acrylic resin and is separated from the palate. Thus, the Hyrax is more hygienic than the Haas expander.

Bonded expander (Figure 6.9 c,d)

- The bonded expander was introduced by McNamara;
- This appliance is a combination of a Hyrax expander and two acrylic resin parts covering the buccal segments.

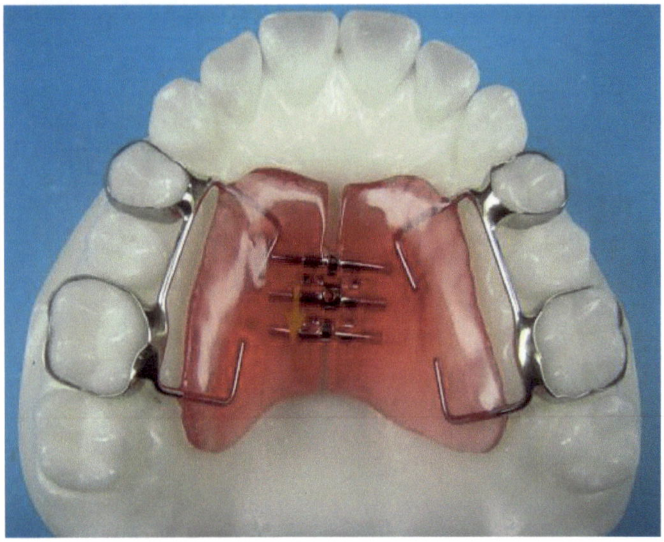

Figure 6.14 Haas expander

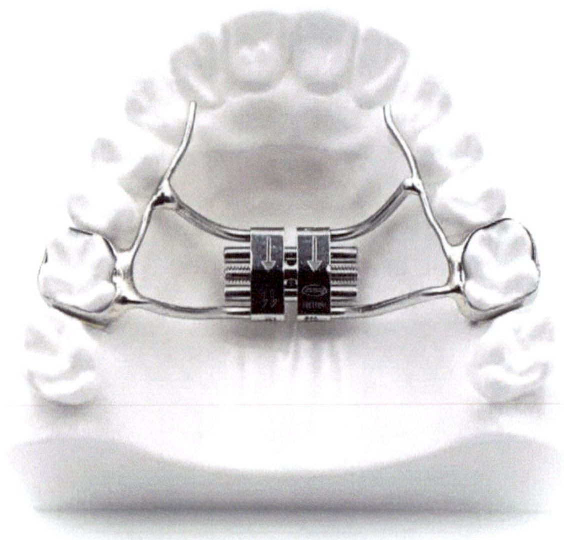

Figure 6.15 Hyrax expander

Removable expanders *(Figure 6.16)*

- Removable expanders are also available for palatal and mandibular expansion;
- They are a slow type of expander and usually are applied for dental or dentoalveolar expansion, not palatal expansion;
- In slow expansion, the screw is opened every 3 to 5 days, in contrast to rapid expanders, which are opened once or twice a day;
- The removable expander is constructed with the screw on the center of the appliance.

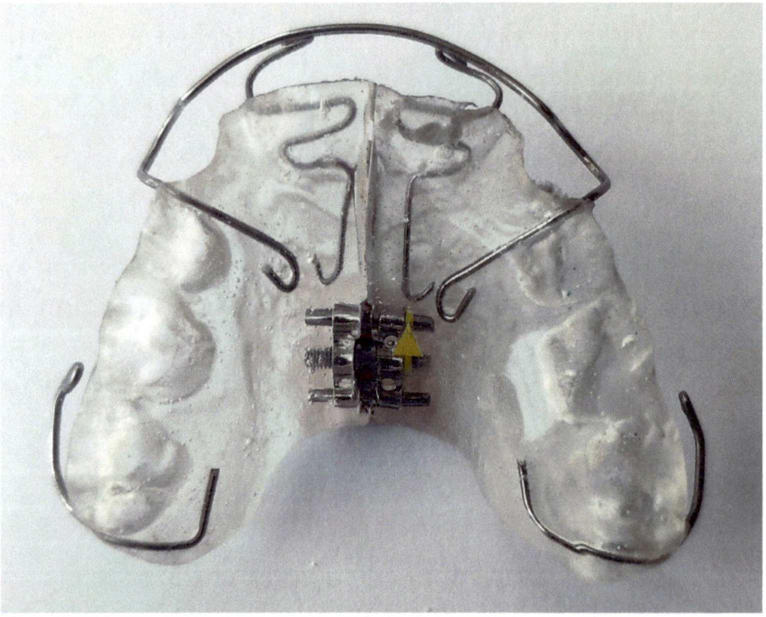

Figure 6.16 Removable expander

Management in the adult dentition

- A dental posterior crossbite can be treated using expansion appliances like hyrax, quad helix;
- Cross elastics;
- Fixed appliance therapy (*Figure 6.17*).

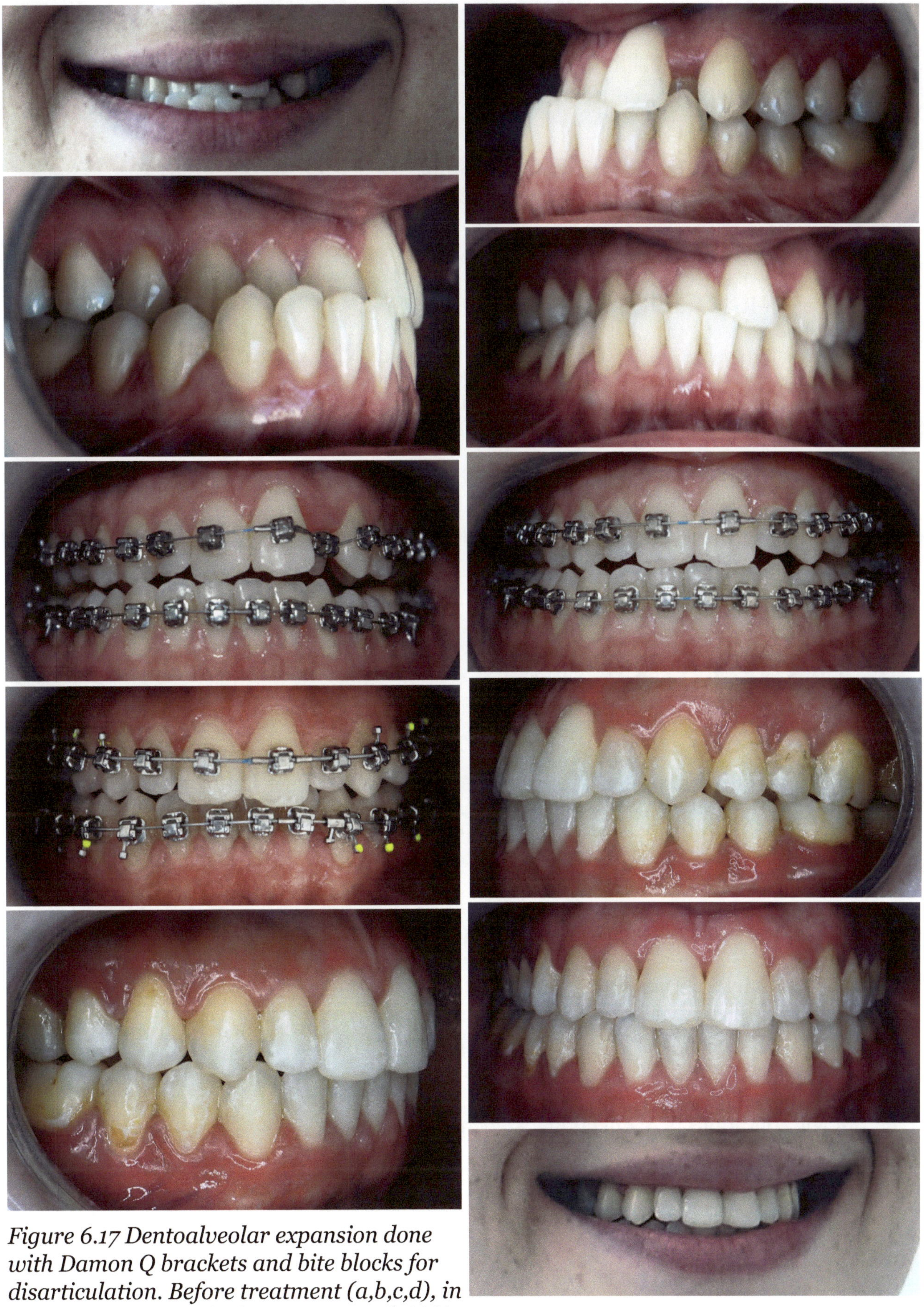

Figure 6.17 Dentoalveolar expansion done with Damon Q brackets and bite blocks for disarticulation. Before treatment (a,b,c,d), in progress (e,f,g), and after treatment (h,i,j,k).

Management of Mandibular dentoalveolar contraction

- It can be done with quad helix spring;
- Removable appliance.

Skeletal Crossbite
This could be due to narrow maxilla or narrow mandible.
Narrow maxilla

Management in the Mixed and early permanent dentition
- Quad helix or W arch;
- Severe cases—RME expander.

Management in adults
- Surgical disjunction.

Narrow mandible

Usually associated with retrognathic mandible;

Management in the mixed and early permanent dentition

- Functional appliances.

Management in adults
- Very severe cases are treated by surgery.

Facial Asymmetry

Facial Asymmetry is defined as "Dissimilarity of parts on either side of a straight line or plane or about a center or axis". Although almost everyone has some facial asymmetry, this is usually mild.

Etiology

Bishara (1994) has classified into genetic/congenital and environmental causes for facial asymmetry.

1. Genetic Causes:
- Craniofacial macrosomia;
- Unilateral cleft lip and palate.
2. Environmental Causes:
- Condylar hypertrophy;
- Condylar fracture;
- Pathologic conditions, like infection, osteochondroma;
- Oral habits;
- Functional mandibular deviation, e.g. premature contacts;
- Retained or missing teeth.

Classification

The facial asymmetry could be any one or combinations of the following types:
- Skeletal;

- Muscular;
- Functional;
- Dental.

Clinical Features

The patient should be assessed in three planes:

Skeletal assessment:

- Assess the facial proportion in all three planes;
- Soft tissue: Assess for bilateral symmetry and for deviation of dorsum and tip of the nose and the philtrum.

Dental assessment:

- Assess for functional displacement;
- Check occlusion in centric occlusion and rest position;
- Look for open/deep bites, crossbite, rotations, midline, and sagittal relation.

Management in the mixed and early permanent dentition

- Occlusal equilibration to correct functional disturbance;
- Early correction of crossbite;
- Space maintenance;
- Skeletal asymmetry can be managed by surgical intervention prior to adolescence. It is done with the main goal to create an environment in which growth is possible;
- Surgery is indicated only when an abnormal growth is making the problem worse;
- Hybrid functional appliances can be given for example asymmetrically activated jasper jumper.

Management in adults

Correction of unilateral molar rotation (*Figure 6.18*);

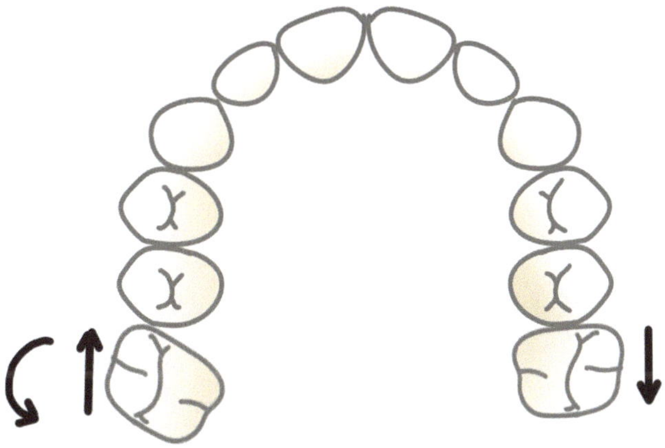

Figure 6.18 Force system used in the correction of rotated molar

- The correction of a unilateral molar rotation can be efficiently achieved by using a transpalatal arch producing a statically determinate force system;
- Clinically, after the alignment of the teeth using light flexible archwires, a rigid segment of

wire (0.017"× 0.025" stainless steel) is placed from the premolar area on the right side of the dental arch extending to the left molar;

- A transpalatal arch (0.032" × 0.032" titanium molybdenum alloy [TMA] or 0.030" stainless steel) is then placed with the unilateral first-order activation.

Canted anterior occlusal plane (in the transverse direction)

- One method of treatment is the use of vertical interarch elastics to extrude the side of the occlusal plane that is farthest from the treatment occlusal plane;
- In patients with a canted maxillary anterior occlusal plane and a deep bite, the cant can be corrected in combination with overbite correction;
  - This can be performed with a one-piece intrusion arch of 0.017 × 0.025-inch titanium molybdenum alloy (TMA) (Ormco Corp., Glendora, Calif.), which is tied to that side of the anterior segment requiring intrusion;
  - The intrusive force level should be approximately 60 gm for four maxillary incisors and approximately 50 gm or less for four mandibular incisors. A diagram of the appliance is presented in *Figure 6.19*.

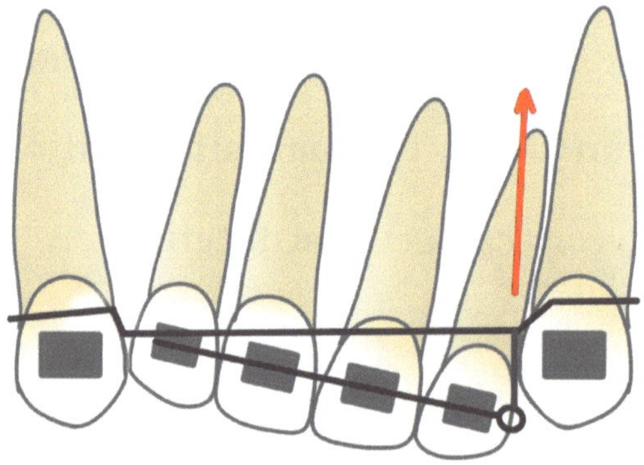

Figure 6.19 Intrusion arch tied to one side

- If the canine also requires intrusion, this is better performed in a separate stage after the incisor intrusion;
- A simple cantilever (0.017 x 0.025-inch TMA) exerting a force of 20 to 25 gm (*Figure 6.20*) can be used;
  - When there is no deep overbite problem and only one side requires extrusion, a unilateral cantilever can be used to correct the occlusal cant;
  - The cantilever, 0.017 × 0.025-inch TMA, comes out of the auxiliary tube of the first molar on the side where the extrusion is to take place and is hooked around the anterior segment.
  - A force of approximately 30 gm is sufficient

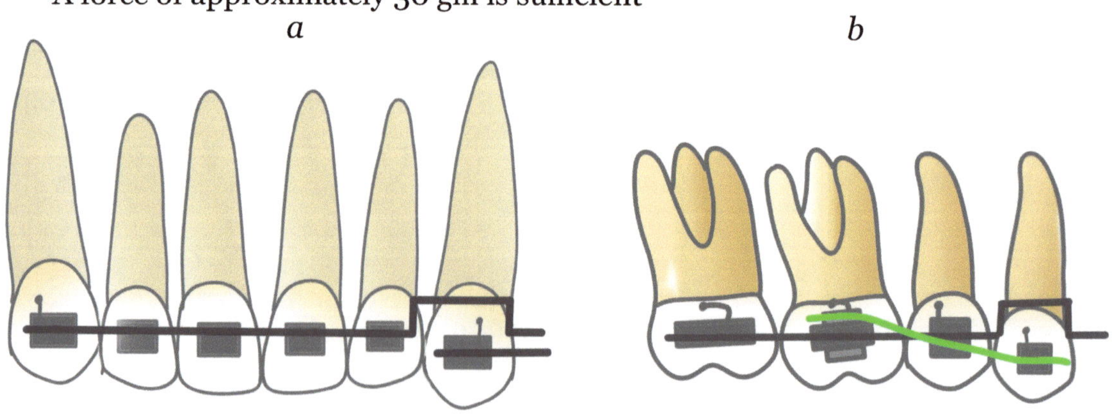

Figure 6.20 Intrison of canine with cantilever spring. Frontal view (a); Buccal view (b).

Canted posterior occlusal plane (in anteroposterior direction)

- A variation of the intrusion arch can also be used to correct a cant of the posterior occlusal plane in patients who have a deep overbite;
  - The magnitude of the force is increased to 150 gm that causes a large tip-back moment on the buccal segment, thereby, flattening the occlusal plane;
  - This appliance (*Figure 6.21*) delivers appropriate force to the area of the arch in need of correction. The side effects are minimal in contrast to the undesirable side effects when using interarch elastics for this problem;
- Occlusal canting can be treated by the use of a mini implant.

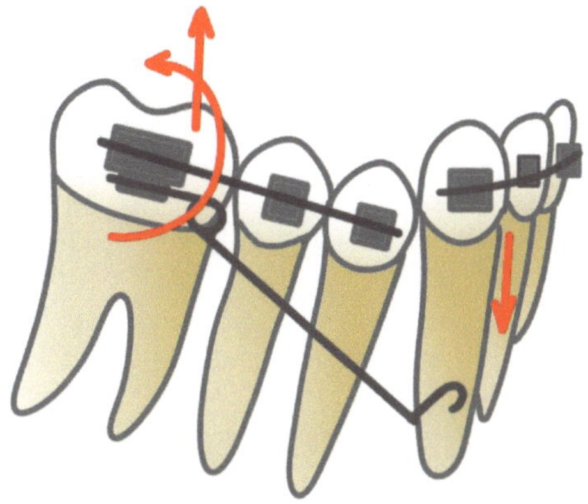

Figure 6.21

Unilateral dental crossbite

- The treatment of a unilateral dental crossbite can be performed with lingual arch (0.032 x 0.032-inch TMA) in the mandible and transpalatal arch (TPA) in the maxilla, expansion activation should be built into the transpalatal arch;
- After the crossbite has been corrected, the wire should be removed, made passive, and reinserted. A diagram of the appliance is shown in *Figure 6.22*.
- In adult patients, surgical correction of severe asymmetry is advised.

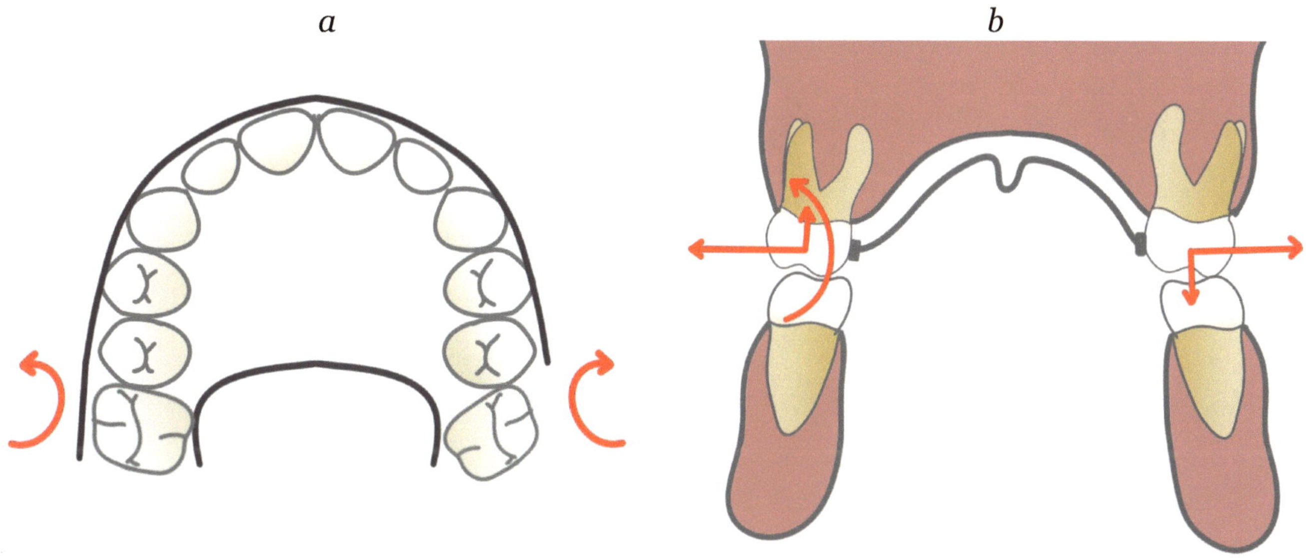

Figure 6.22 Transpalatal arch for derotation of a posterior tooth (a); Activation of transpalatal arch for expansion (b);

Retention

- Retention protocol after asymmetry correction includes removable appliances – Hawley type when treatment included expansion of the arches;
- Essix retainers are best for retaining de-rotated anterior and posterior teeth.

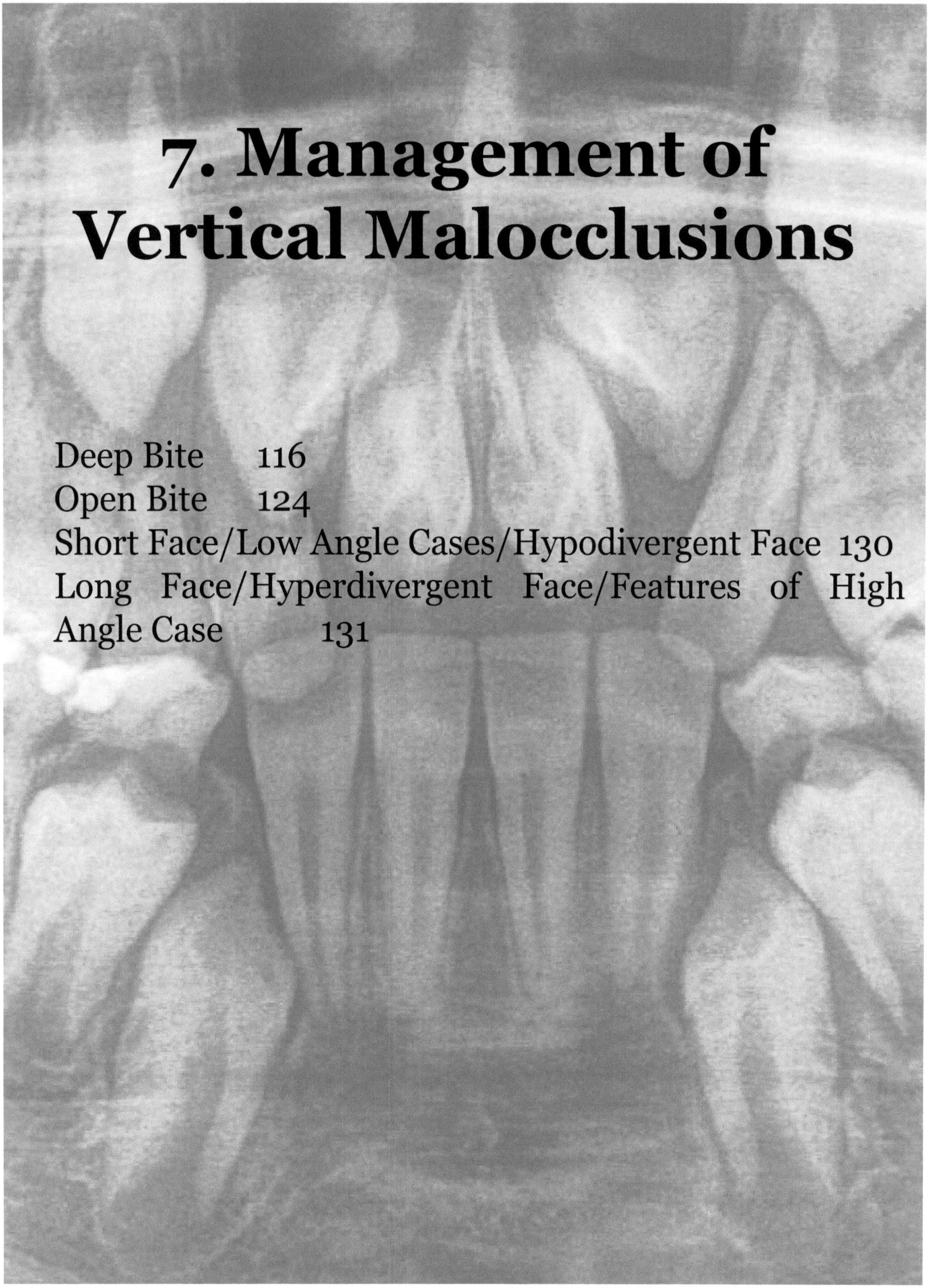

7. Management of Vertical Malocclusions

Deep Bite

Deep bite describes a condition of an excessive overbite, where the vertical measurement between the maxillary and mandibular incisal margins is excessive when the mandible is brought into habitual or centric occlusion.

- In a normal overbite, the upper incisors slightly overlap the lower incisors. It is usually expressed in millimeters;
- The overbite is measured quickly by marking a short line on the labial surface of the lower incisor with a sharpened lead pencil;
- The distance from the incisal edges to the mark is then measured with the use of the Boley gauge or divider (*Figure 7.1*);
- The normal value of overbite: 1–3 mm;
- The overbite is also described as the percentage of the mandibular incisor crown length overlapped by maxillary central incisors;
- 5–20% of overlap of the mandibular incisors is considered normal.

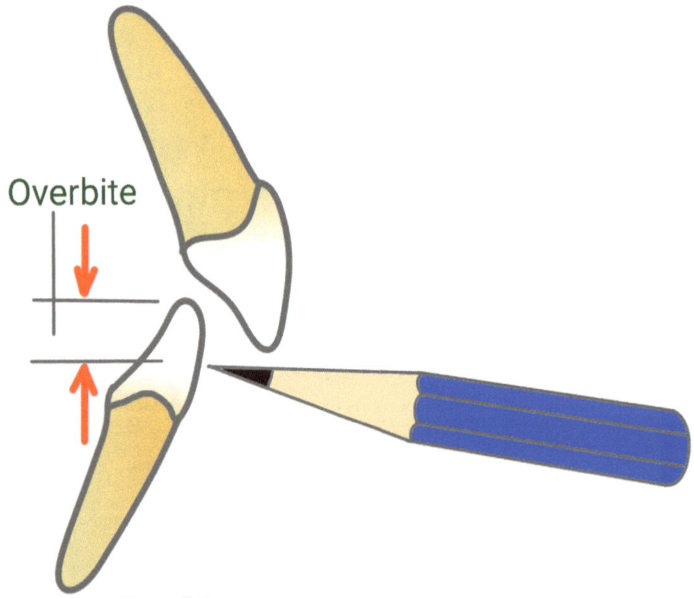

Figure 7.1 Overbite measurement

Unfavorable consequence of a deep bite

- Deep bite affects the facial esthetics;
- Excessive overbite where the lower incisors hit the lingual of maxillary incisors or gingival tissues results in periodontal destruction;
- There will be anterior migration of maxillary anterior teeth;
- Wear of mandibular incisors;
- Spacing in the maxillary anterior region;
- Can lead to problems in the temporomandibular joint.

Classification

A deep bite can be divided into dental and skeletal deep bite following proper diagnosis.

- Skeletal deep bite: May be due to malrelationship of alveolar bones and/or underlying mandibular or maxillary bone;
- Dental deep bite: In this type of deep bite, the problem lies in the dentition.

Etiology

Causes for Dental Deep Bite

- Premature loss of permanent teeth causing lingual collapse of anterior teeth;
- Anterior tipping of posterior teeth;
- Infraocclusion of posterior teeth due to tongue thrusting;
- Supraocclusion of anterior teeth;
- Occasionally deep bite is caused due to large sized teeth.

Causes for Skeletal Deep Bite

- Horizontal growth pattern;
- Short anterior facial height (AFH);
- Posterior facial height (PFH) is long;
- Upper facial height (UFH): Lower facial height (LFH) is reduced;
- Less interocclusal clearance;
- Convergent rotation of skeletal jaw bases;

Clinical features of skeletal deep bite

- Deep curve of Spee in mandibular dentition (*Figure 7.2*);

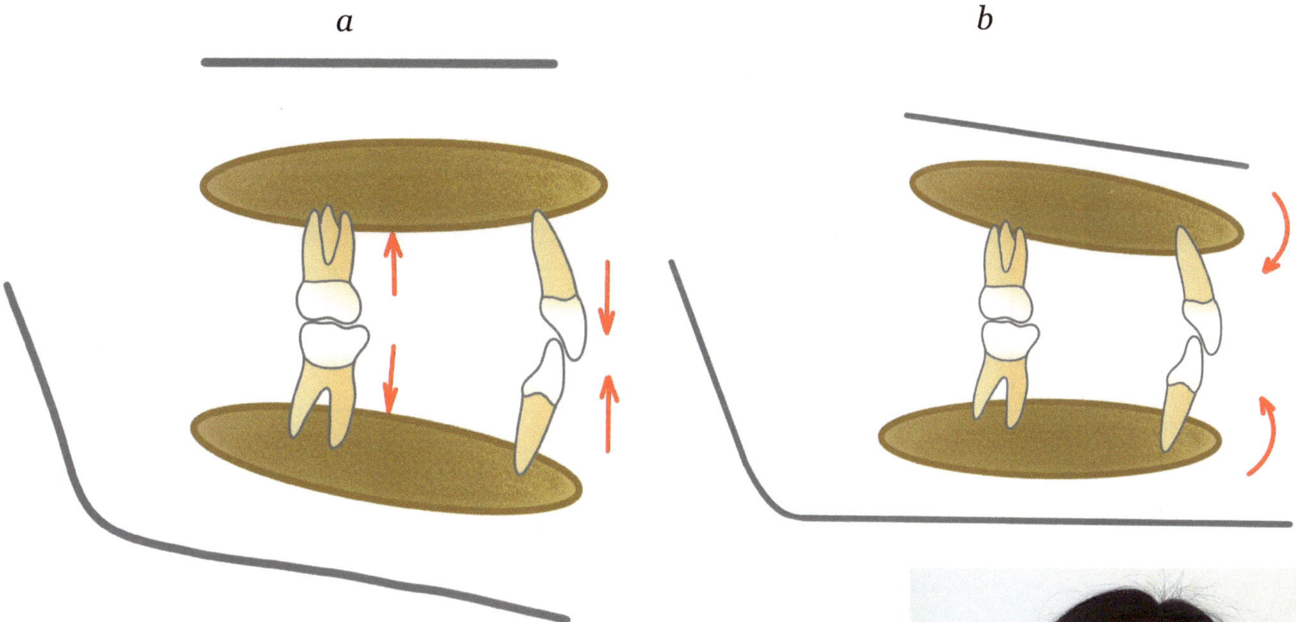

Figure 7.2; Dentoalveolar deep bite due to infraocclusion of molars and supraocclusion of incisors (a). Skeletal deep bite due to rotation of the jaws (b).

- A reverse curve of Spee in maxillary dentition;
- When there is maxillary excess—gummy smile (*Figure 7.3*);
- Lower facial height is less.

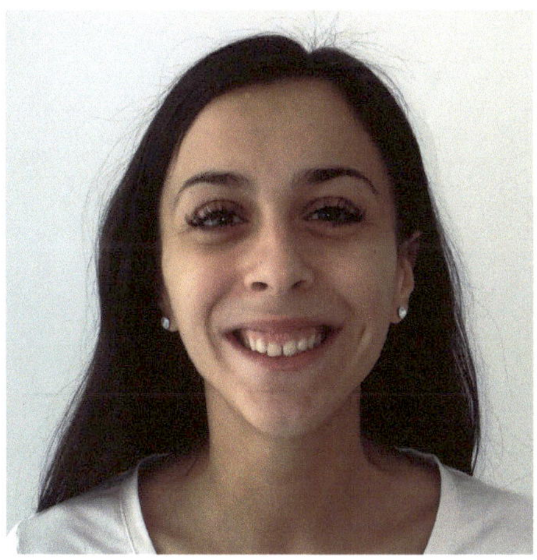

Figure 7.3 Maxillary excess results in gummy smile.

Management

The primary determining factor in treatment planning is to decide whether deep bite correction is achieved by intrusion or extrusion.
There are five important factors to obtain a stable relationship.

Lip relationship

- When lips are incompetent we can observe:
  - Deep bite with large interlabial gap;
  - Increased distance between incisal edge of incisors and upper lip (gummy lip);
  - Bite opening by the intrusion of anterior teeth is done.
- With Competent lips
  - Deep bite with less interlabial gap;
  - Normal or reduced distance between incisal edges of incisors and upper lip;
  - The extrusion of posterior teeth is done.

Vertical facial relationship

- Extrusion of 1 mm of posterior teeth results in an increase in anterior facial height by 2.5 mm;
- Extrusion mechanics has to be avoided in patients with increased facial height or high mandibular plane angle;
- In patients with Class II division 2 malocclusion, extrusion of posterior teeth may be the treatment of choice;
- When we have Increased AFH or increased FMA—treatment would be an intrusion of anterior teeth;
- When we have reduced AFH or reduced FMA—treatment would be extrusion.

Occlusal plane

One of the objectives in the correction of a deep bite is to obtain a flat occlusal plane. Flat occlusal plane or leveling of the curve of Spee can be obtained by the intrusion, extrusion or relative intrusion (*Figure 7.4*).

a *b*

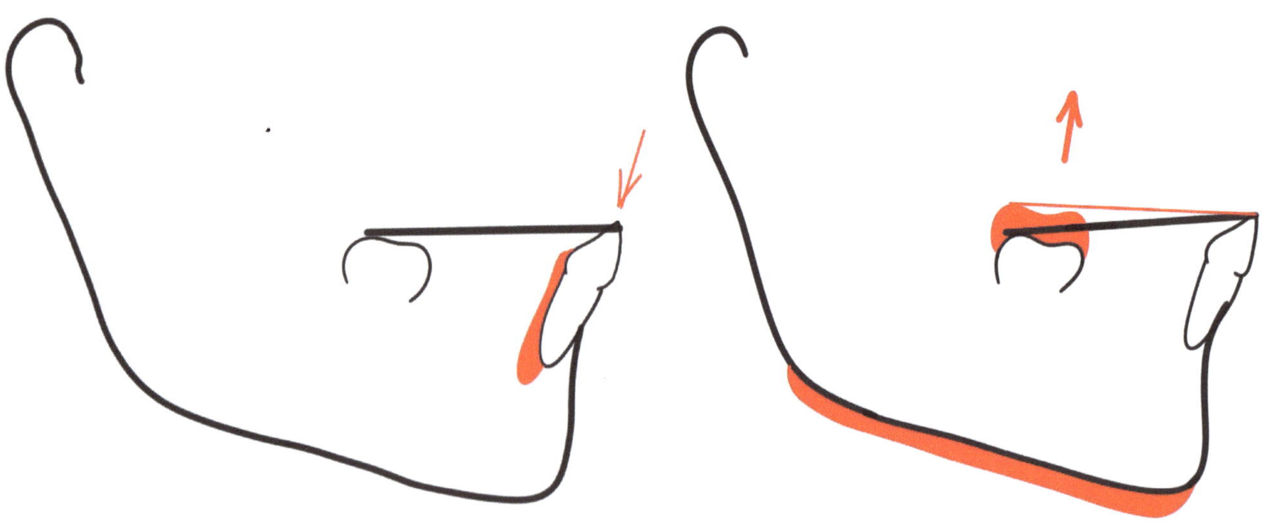

c

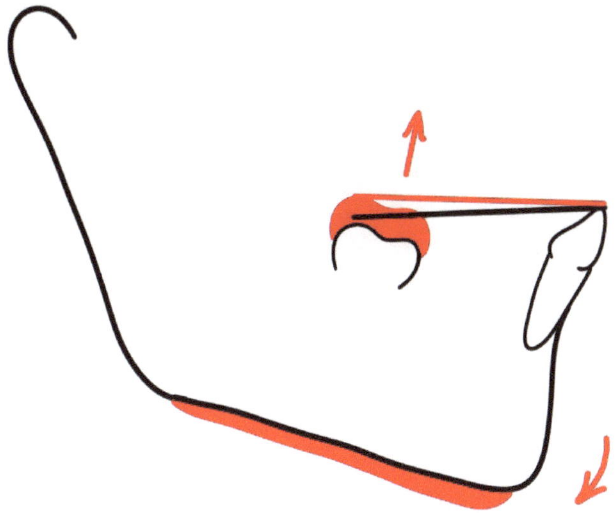

Figure 7.4 Deep bite correction with absolute intrusion (a), Relative intrusion (b), Extrusion (c)

Interocclusal space

- Normal freeway space is 2–4 mm. This should be maintained even after bite opening by extrusion;
- If the interocclusal or freeway space is intruded, the results will not be stable.

Age of patient and duration of treatment

- In young patients, bite opening can be achieved through orthodontic mechanism;
- In adults with a skeletal problem, the surgical approach is the preferred method of treatment.

Treatment Mechanics/Appliances Used

This can be broadly classified into three types:
1. Intrusion mechanics;
2. Relative intrusion technique;
3. Extrusion mechanics.

Intrusion can be achieved by three possible ways:
1. With segmented archwire technique using an auxiliary intrusion arch;
2. Bypass arches (continuous archwires that bypass premolars and/or canines);
3. By using skeletal anchorage unit.

Leveling by extrusion.
- Leveling by extrusion increases the facial height; hence, it is not ideal in average or high-angle cases.

Relative intrusion will be successful in growing patients only and intrusion is most widely used in adult patients.

Management in the mixed dentition

Treatment by intrusion

• ***Begg Stage I Archwire***

The typical bypass version of the archwire is used in the Begg technique in the first stage to achieve leveling (*Figure 7.5*). The light force delivered by the 0.016-inch resilient wire on the anterior teeth is the optimal force necessary to depress upper and lower anteriors without distal tipping of anchor molars.

- Anchor bends are incorporated in the archwires in front of the molar buccal tubes;
- The amplitude of the anchor bend should be sufficient to deflect the anterior portion of the archwire to the mucobuccal fold when the archwire is engaged in the buccal tubes.

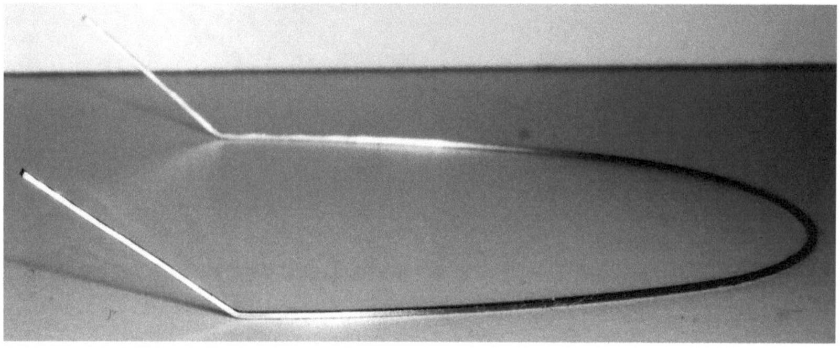

Figure 7.5 Archwire with anchor bends.

• ***2 x 4 Appliances***

The effect produced by stage 1 archwire in Begg's technique can be produced by using the 2 x 4 technique in edgewise appliances also.

Treatment by relative intrusion

• Functional appliance: Functional appliances used during the growth period cause relative intrusion. In this, the lower incisors are prevented from erupting. The posteriors are allowed to erupt. This causes opening of the bite.

Treatment by extrusion

• Anterior bite plane: Both fixed and removable anterior bite plane causes supraeruption of posterior. When the appliance is given, there should be posterior clearance by 1.5 mm. The bite opening by supraeruption of posterior teeth should not encroach upon the normal freeway space.

Treatment in the permanent dentition

Leveling by intrusion

• *Segmented Arch Techniques*

The basic mechanism for intrusion consists of three parts:

1. Posterior anchorage unit;
2. Anterior segment;
3. Intrusive arch spring (*Figure 7.6*).

- The posterior teeth are aligned together and joined by a buccal stabilizing segment of at least 0.018 x 0.018-inch;

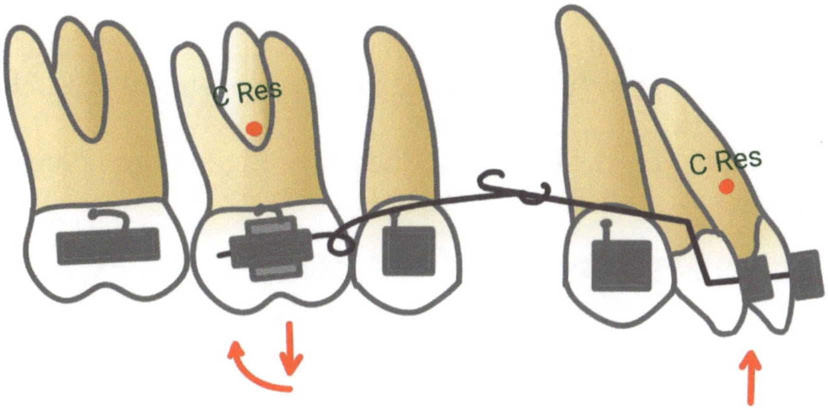

Figure 7.6 Three piece appliance for intrusion

- The posterior segments in both sides are joined by transpalatal arch and a low lingual arch in maxilla and mandible, respectively;
- A special bracket-tube or triple-tube combination is fixed on the upper or lower first permanent molars;
- The intrusive arch normally comprises of a 0.018 x 0.022 inch or 0.018 x 0.025 inch edgewise wire with a 3 mm helix looped two and a half times placed mesial to the auxiliary tube;
- The curvature is placed in the intrusive arch for the incisal portion to lie gingival to the central incisors;
- An intrusive force develops when the arch is tied to the incisor level;
- The intrusive spring is not directly attached to the incisor brackets;
- An anterior alignment arch or the anterior segment is placed in the four incisors or the central incisors and the intrusive arch is attached to that wire either labially, incisally or gingivally;
- Burstone recommends a force value of 100 g for the intrusion of four maxillary incisors (25 g per tooth) and lesser value for lower incisors (10–15 g per tooth);
- The common side effect of the intrusion arch is it causes flaring of the incisors. This can be prevented by not placing the intrusive arch directly into the brackets of the anterior teeth;
- The intrusive arch is tied distal to the midline between the central and lateral incisors or distal to lateral incisors;
- When the canine lies bilaterally occlusal to the premolar, the canine must be intruded separately following anterior intrusion;
- When the canines have not erupted symmetrically, a canine intrusion is required only on one side;
- A canine-intrusion spring, fabricated from 0.018 x 0.025 inch SS wire is activated to produce 50–75 g of force and is inserted into the auxiliary tube of the first molar and into the vertical tube of a canine bracket, will produce separate canine intrusion.

• *Utility arch*

- Bypass arches are effective for patients during mixed dentition or early permanent dentition (who have some growth left);
- The success of bypass arches requires that the force should be kept minimum and light;
- The drawback of bypass arches is poor posterior anchorage as only molars are available;
- Significant extrusion of molars is a possible and hence adequate measure to prevent molar extrusion has to be taken:
    - o High-pull headgear;
    - o Use of transpalatal arches;
    - o Nance holding arch;
    - o Incorporation of a second molar tooth.

- Utility arch engages only the first molars and the four incisors;
- With a 0.018 inch appliance, the recommended wire for the mandibular arch is 0.016 x 0.016 inch or 0.016 x 0.022-inch blue Elgiloy (not heat-treated). For most maxillary arches, 0.016 x 0.022-inch blue Elgiloy is recommended;
- With a 0.022 inch appliance, 0.019 x 0.019-inch blue Elgiloy can be used in either arch. A 0.016 x 0.022 inch TMA wire is a modern alternative (*Figure 7.7*);

a *b*

c

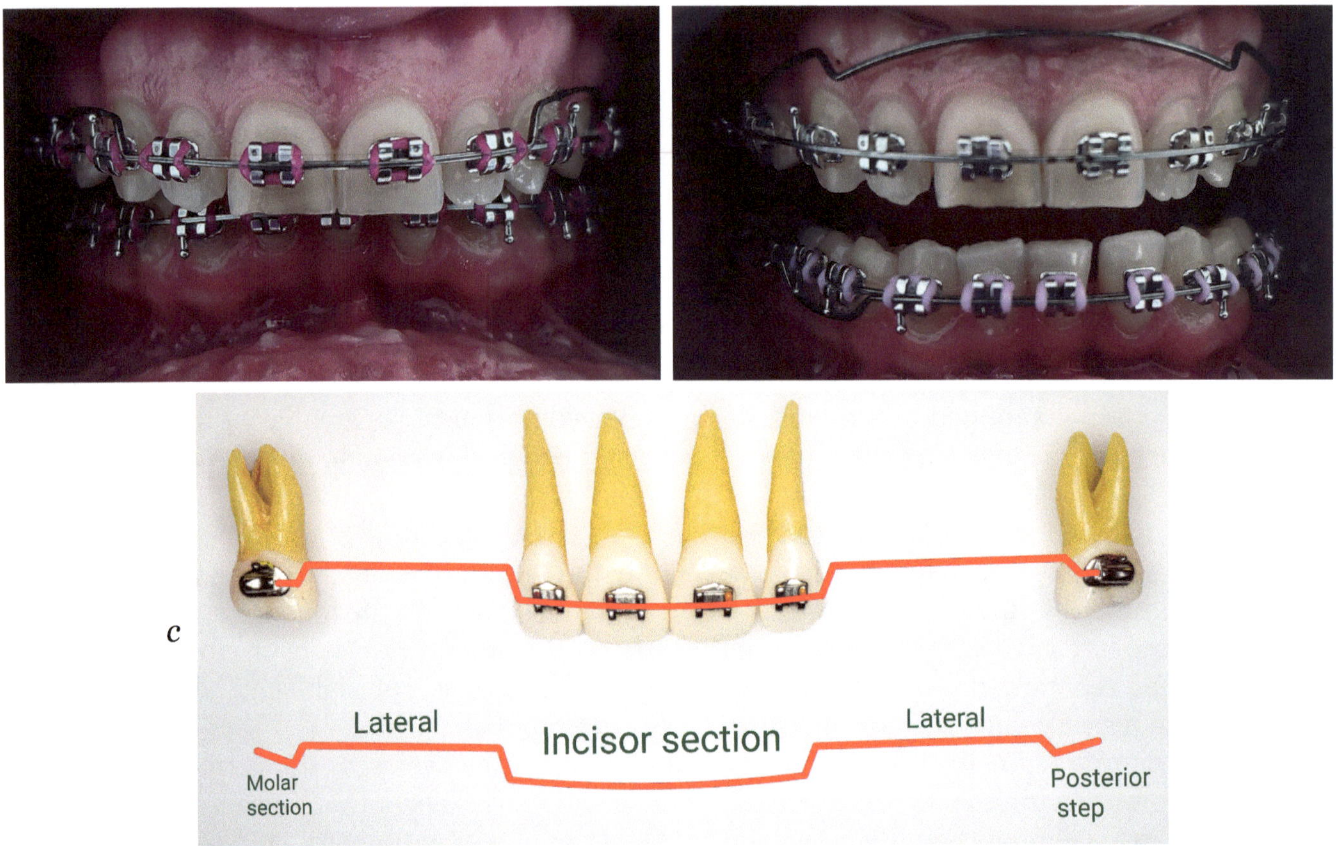

Figure 7.7 Intrusion done with Utility arch (a,b), parts of the utility arch (c)

- Utility arch initiates in the auxiliary tube on the first molar;
- The molar segment of the archwire is cut flush with the distal aspect of the auxiliary tube. Immediately 5–6 mm anterior to the tube, a 90° bend is placed with arch-forming pliers, and a posterior vertical step, usually 3–4 mm long, is formed;
- Another right-angle bend is then placed in the wire so that the horizontal or vestibular segment travels anteriorly parallel to the occlusal plane;
- At the embrasure between the canine and the lateral incisor, another right-angle bend redirects the wire toward the occlusal surface;
- After an anterior vertical step of 5–8 mm, a final 90° bend creates the incisal segment, which should lie in the brackets of the lower anterior teeth;
- A sectional leveling arch is used for correcting any irregularities in the position of the lower anterior teeth before the placement of the utility arch;
- The archwire continues in a similar fashion to the opposite molar;
- Utility arch can be activated for intrusion by placing the gable bend directed occlusally in the vestibular segment;
- Engaging the utility arch produces approximately 25 grams of force on each of the incisors, the force considered ideal for the intrusion of lower incisors;
- The total effect is tipping back the molars along with possible intrusion and torqueing of the incisors.

- *Skeletal Anchorage to Intrude Incisors*

Absolute anchorage devices, like bone screws or bone anchors, have provided the opportunity of intrusion of both anterior teeth in deep bite cases as well as posterior teeth in open bite cases.

Leveling by relative extrusion

- *A reverse curve of Spee arches.*

Preformed archwires that are bent in the direction opposite to curve of Spee are called reverse curve wires. They are made from resilient wires. They are used to flatten the curve of Spee (*Figure 7.8*).

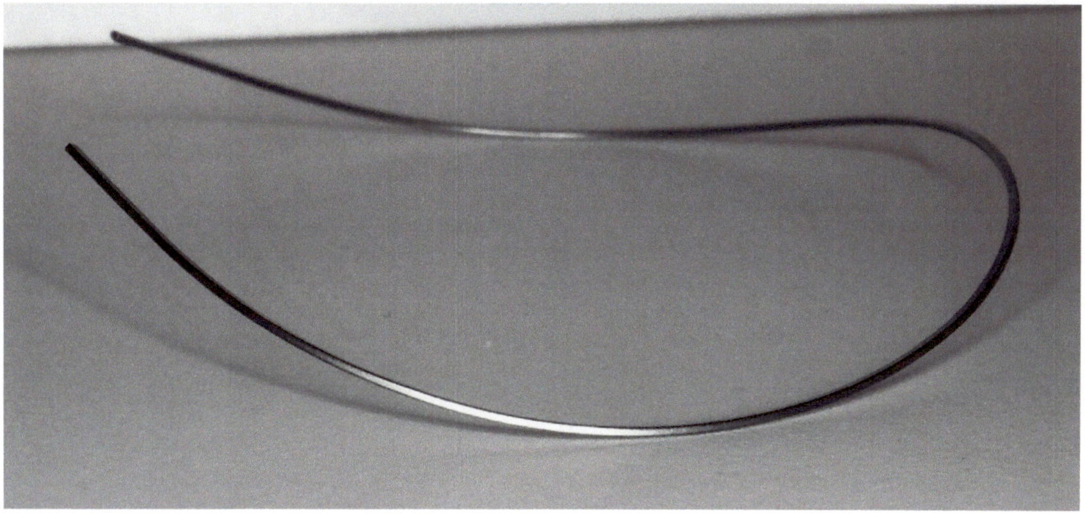

Figure 7.8 Reverse curve arch

- Archwires with anchor bends or tip back bends.

Tip back bends or anchor bends are placed in continuous archwire mesial to the molar tube. This causes intrusion of the anterior and slight extrusion of posterior teeth.

Leveling by Extrusion

- Anterior bite plane: fixed or removable (*Figure 7.9*).

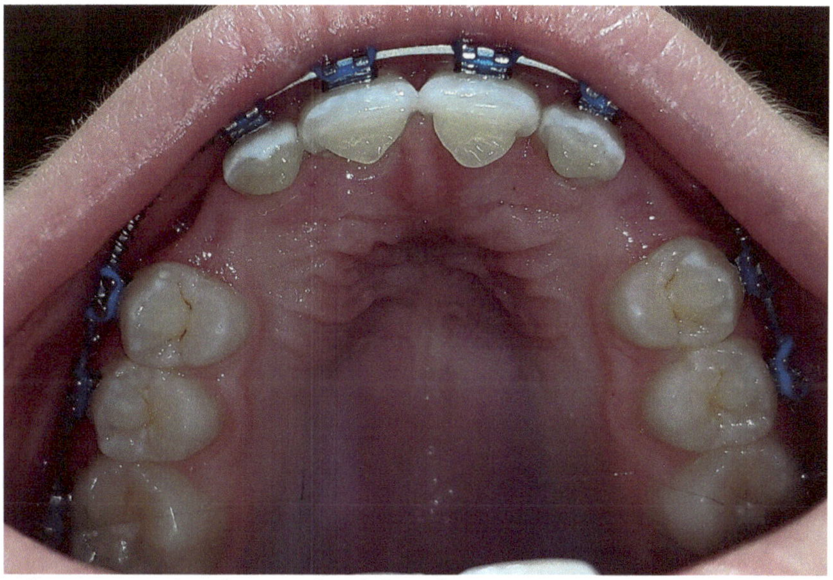

Figure 7.9 Fixed anterior bite plane

Retention

- Retention after deep bite correction is done by providing good anterior contacts;
- Removable retainer Hawley type with anterior bite plane is advisable;
- Retention should be discontinued after the vertical growth is final;
- In adult patients, a skeletal deep bite can be camouflaged by dental movements, but the result is not stable and there is a tendency for deepening of the bite after treatment;
- The muscles of mastication tend to intrude the posterior teeth if we used extrusion or relative extrusion method of treatment;
- For dental deep bite in an adult patient, we can use removable retainer with an anterior bite plane;
- For skeletal correction in adults, the method of treatment should be surgical.

Open Bite

'Open bite' is a condition where a vertical space exists between the occlusal or incisal surfaces of maxillary and mandibular teeth in the buccal or anterior segments, when the mandible is brought into habitual or centric occlusion.

Open bite tendency is a condition, where there is overjet present but not vertical overlap. This is called incomplete overbite and is also called open bite tendency (*Figure 7.10*).

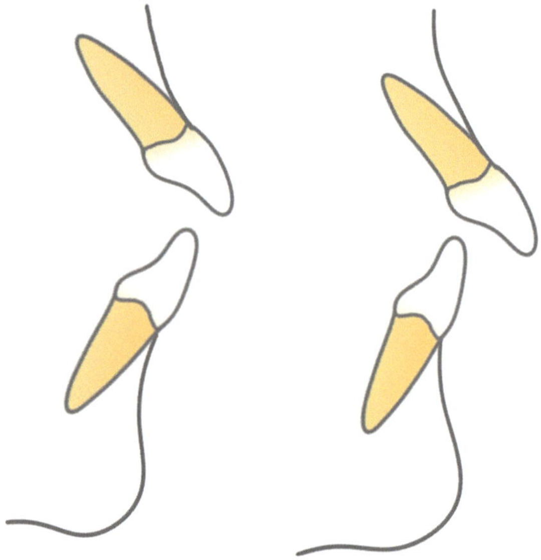

Figure 7.10. Open bite and incomplete overbite

Etiology of Open Bite

Etiology can be classified under two headings (Fletcher, 1975):

- Epigenetic factors:
  - Altered morphology and size of the tongue;
  - Disharmony in the skeletal growth pattern of maxilla and mandible;
  - The vertical relationship of the jaw;
  - Tongue posture.

- Environmental factors:
  - Abnormal function, like thumb sucking habits;

- Improper respiration (Linder- Aronson, 1972);
- Tongue dysfunction;
- Protracted tongue posture which is either: - Endogenous—retained infantile swallow or - Acquired adaptation—adaptation to inflamed tonsils.

Classification

Different forms of an open bite may be observed:

1. Incomplete overbite: In this condition, there is overjet present but not vertical overlap;
2. Simple open bite: the problem is confined to the teeth and alveolar process.
- More than 1 mm of space is seen between the incisors;
- The posterior teeth are in occlusion.
3. Complex open bite: there is disharmony in the skeletal components of the anterior face height. Open bite extends from premolars or deciduous molars on one side to the corresponding teeth on the opposite side (*Figure 7.11*);

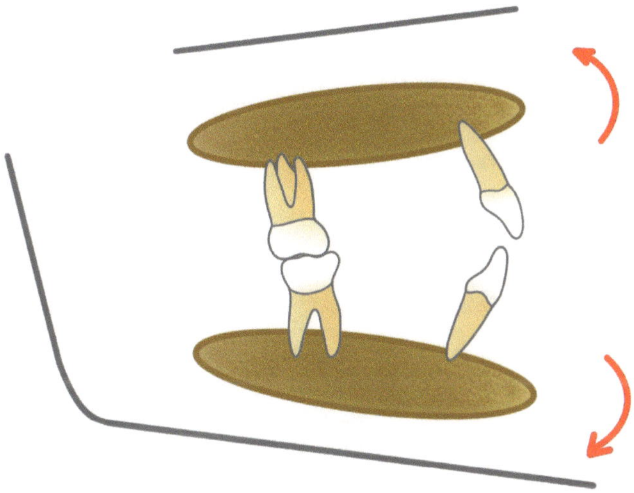

Figure 7.11 Complex open bite. Disharmony of skeletal basis

4. Compound or infantile open bite: Compound or infantile open bite is completely open up to the molars;
5. Iatrogenic open bite: Iatrogenic open bite is due to orthodontic treatment.

According to the position in the dentition we have
- Anterior open bite;
- Posterior open bite.

Clinical features

- The palatal plane is tipped upward;
- Steep mandibular plane;
- Increased anterior facial height;
- Obtuse gonial angle;
- Narrow maxillary arch;
- Excessive gingival display;
- Decreased freeway space.

Management

Factors to be considered:

- The balance between the nose, lip, and chin;
- Nasolabial angle:
    - Acute—retraction of incisors will improve esthetic;
    - Obtuse—proclination of incisors will improve esthetic;
    - Lip configuration;
- Length of the lower third of the face;
- Chin prominence.

Management in the mixed dentition

- Simple anterior open bite;
    - Habit breaking should be the primary objective of treatment during mixed dentition;
    - Along with habit breaking, an open bite can be corrected;
    - In mixed dentition, functional appliances, like Activator, Bionator or Frankel are indicated;
    - Fixed appliances are used to close the open bite along with habit breaking appliance in late mixed dentition;
    - Tongue spikes, either removable or fixed type are used to prevent tongue thrusting or digit sucking (Figure 7.12);

a *b*

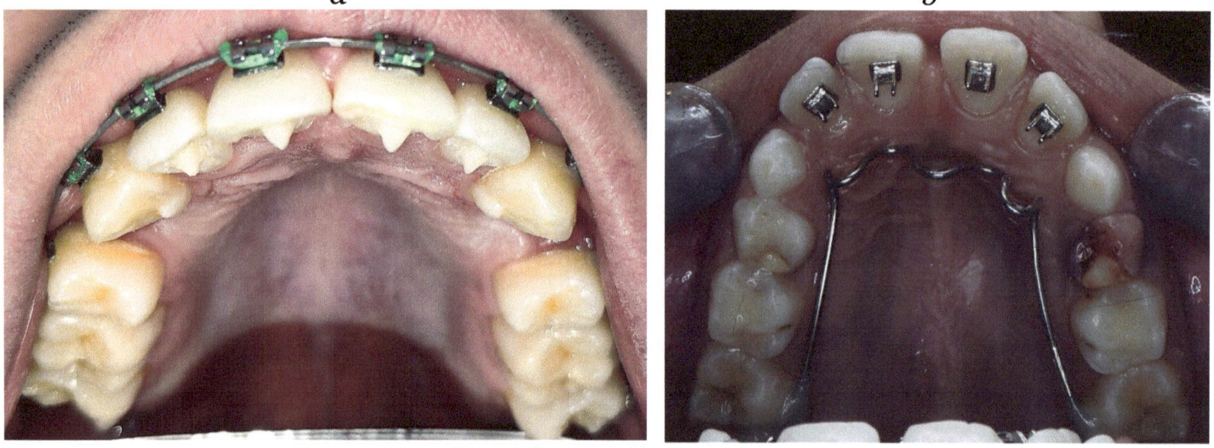

Figure 7.12 Composite tongue spikes (a) Metal bonded tongue spikes (b).

- Simple Posterior Open Bites
    - Causes for posterior open bite include ankylosed primary molars, lateral tongue thrust;
    - Early treatment: is done with:
        - o Bionator or activator with flanges is used to prevent lateral tongue thrust;
        - o Removal of an ankylosed primary tooth;
        - o Posterior open bite is difficult to treat if the tongue reflex gets fixed. A permanent type of retention is required after correction;
        - o Tongue spikes can also be used.

- Complex or skeletal open bite is a symptom of serious skeletal dysplasia. Early diagnosis of the skeletal open bite is crucial—since it helps to minimize the problem.
    - Bionator or Frankel for open bite correction is indicated for early management;

- Complex open bite is difficult to treat orthodontically.

Treatment in the early permanent dentition

Simple anterior open bite

1. Habit braking should have been achieved;
2. Treatment is mostly done with a fixed appliance.

Single tooth open bite treatment (*Figure 7.13*)

- Extrusion bend can be used;
- 016 x 016-inch stainless steel wire is used;
- A step down with an amplitude of less than 0.5 mm is made;
- A wire is inserted into the brackets.

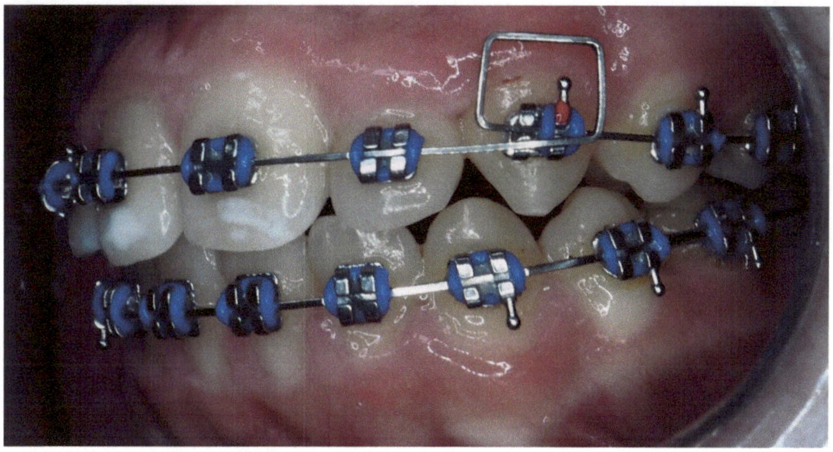

Figure 7.13 Treatment of single tooth anterior open bite

Extrusion of the incisor segment

- Extrusion arch
  - It is made of rectangular stainless steel wire;
  - It is inserted after alignment of the teeth;
  - A vertical I loop is made in a gingival direction between the lateral incisors and canines;
  - The anterior segment of the wire is bent more incisally than the posterior segments with a step of 0.5 to 1 mm;
  - After extrusion is done, the wire should be left in place for 2 to 4 months.

- Combination of an upper and lower reverse curve

This type of wire is very useful for space closure in the anterior segment. We just have to place a reverse curve on the upper maxilla and in the lower maxilla, we place a curved wire. This will provoke an extrusion and a palatal movement of the upper and lower incisors
  - The wire used is 0.017x 0.025" rectangular NiTi or TMA.

- Inverted tip back

- This is done by placing two 45° bends at the ends of the archwire;
- These bends are introduced in the tubes of the molars, provoking rotation in the posterior segment and extrusion in the anterior segment;
- When inserted in posterior teeth only, the wire is deflected incisally and pushed into the

anterior brackets;

- Use of intermaxillary elastics
  - These elastics are used for bite closure, occlusion detailing, etc;
  - This type of elastic must be worn 24 hours a day and must be replaced every 12 hours due to memory and elasticity;
  - The force can vary from 2 to 6.5 ounces (1 ounce=28.35 g) and they can be placed in many configurations (box, trapezoid, delta, etc.);
  - The size of the elastic can vary from 1/8" to 5/16';
  - To close an anterior open bite with intermaxillary elastics use rectangular wires (0.017" x 0.025");
  - To close a posterior open bite with intermaxillary elastics use round elastic wires (0.016").

- Brackets bonding closer to the gingival margin (*Figure 7.14*)

Bonding the anterior brackets 0.5 mm or 1 mm closer to the gingival margin (central 4.5 mm or 5 mm and the lateral 4 mm or 4.5 mm) and the posterior brackets near the occlusal aspect of the tooth, will aid in the closure of the anterior bite, because there will be an anterior extrusion and a posterior intrusion when ligating continuous wire.

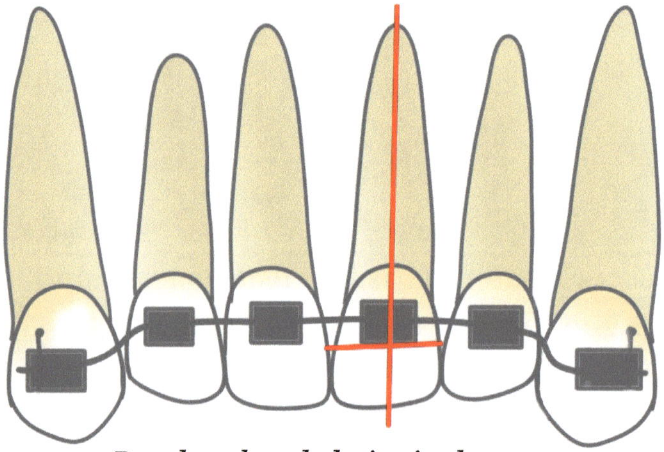

Figure 7.14 Brackets bonded gingival

Intrusion of posterior teeth

- Posterior bite blocks
  - One of the functions of bite blocks is the intrusion of the posterior segment which provokes a mandibular autorotation that successfully closes open bites;
  - These blocks can be placed in the upper and lower dental arches, and they can be fixed or removable.

- High Pull headgear
  - It is used to intrude molars or to redirect maxillary growth *(Figure 7.15)*;
  - A high or parietal traction force, as vertical as possible, will have molar intrusive action, that added to the anterior teeth extrusion will provoke the closure of the anterior bite;
  - Orthopedic force directed over the center of resistance of the maxilla will cause the palatal plane to incline, the mandible will rotate in a counterclockwise manner favoring the correction of the anterior open bite.

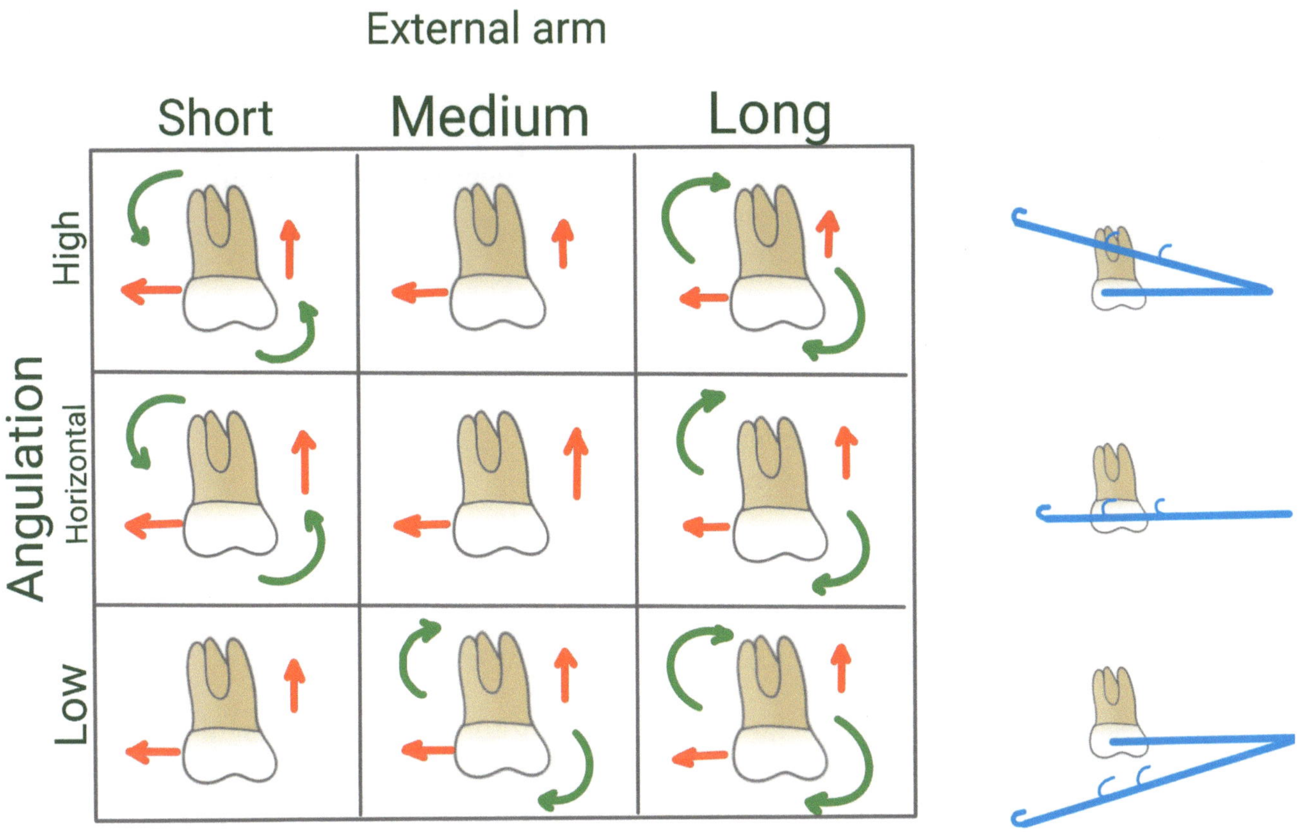

Figure 7.15 High pull (High), Medium pull (Horizontal), Low pull (Low), Short external arm (Short), Medium external arm (Medium), Long external arm (Long)

- TPA or Chromosome arch with bands on molars

Another way to intrude molar and to close an anterior open bite is by placing a TPA or a chromosome arch with an acrylic intrusion Button (*Figure 7.16*).

- The tongue will lean on the disc while swallowing, intruding the molars;
- The intrusive force is approximately 80 g;
- This disc must be 2 mm to 3 mm separated from the palatal vault so the intrusive forces do not impinge the disc.

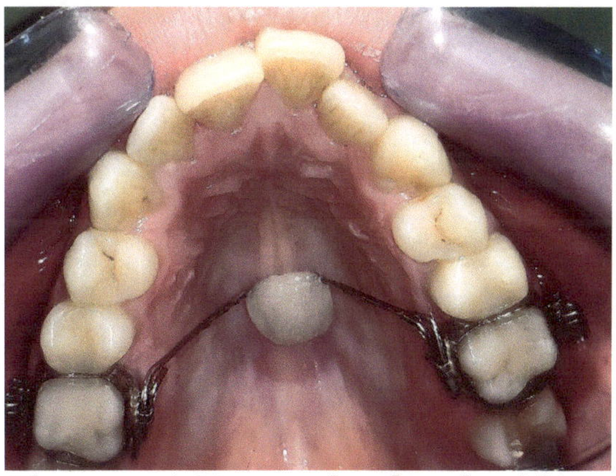

Figure 7.16 Transpalatal arch with an acrylic button for slow intrusion.

Management of Adult Skeletal Open Bite

- Orthognathic surgery

Adult skeletal open bite is best treated by orthognathic surgery. The greater the skeletal elements contribute to the etiology, the poorer the prognosis for treatment (Mizrahi, 1978).

- A Lefort I type surgery is performed in the upper maxilla in which the maxilla is impacted and as a result the mandible autorotates;
- Segmentary surgeries (anterior or posterior) can be combined with this surgery.

- Glossectomy

Macroglossia is an increase of the size of the tongue that provokes a functional and cosmetic problem. Practically swallowing is not altered but chewing is difficult.

According to Moyers, macroglossia has local and general etiology.

Local factors include
1. Congenital: Hemangioma, lymphangioma;
2. Inflammatory: Tuberculosis, actinomycosis, subgingival calculus, syphilis, ranula;
3. Traumatic: Irritation, post-operatory edema;
4. Neoplastic: Gland cell tumors, lipoma, leiomyoma.

General:
1. Congenital: Idiopathic, hemangioma, cretinism;
2. Inflammatory: Chronic glossitis;
3. Traumatic: Due to post-operatory edema;
4. Metabolic: Acromegaly, proteinosis, Steroid therapy.

Classification

1. True macroglossia: when there is a true enlargement of the tongue;
2. Relative macroglossia: When there is insufficient space in the oral cavity.

Both pathologies can be congenital or acquired and the symptoms are proportional to the degree of macroglossia and the age of the patient.
The clinical diagnosis of macroglossia can be done on this basis of

- Tongue protrusion;
- Speech;
- Swallowing;
- Breathing.

- When the patient presents true macroglossia, one of the alternatives is surgery to reduce the dimension of the tongue (glossectomy).

Retention

- Retention after correction of an open bite can be done with a fixed and removable appliance;
- The removable appliance can be made with posterior bite blocks if we used posterior intrusion as a method of treatment;
- The removable appliance can be made with tongue guard if we have corrected tongue trust habit;
- Retention should continue until vertical growth has stopped.

Short Face/Low Angle Cases/ Hypodivergent Face

Hypodivergent vertical dysplasia is clinically termed as a short face. Generally, facial pattern with a mandibular plane angle less than 20° are considered as hypodivergent. The following are the clinical features of low angle cases.

Extraoral Features

- Brachycephalic head form;
- Euryprosopic facial form;
- Wide set eyes;

- Prominent cheek bones;
- Low mandibular plane angle;
- Horizontal or orthognathic growth pattern;
- Prominent chin;
- Straight or dished in soft tissue profile;
- Small gonial angle;
- Large and broad ramus;
- Reduced lower facial height;
- Thin lips;
- Strong masseter muscles.

Intraoral Features

- Flat palatal plane;
- Broad arch;
- Crowded mandibular incisors;
- Deep overbite.

Cephalometric findings

- FMA is less than 25°;
- SN to MP is less than 32°.

Long Face/Hyperdivergent Face/Features of High Angle Case

Hyperdivergent vertical dysplasia is clinically termed as long face syndrome. Generally, facial patterns with a mandibular plane angle of more than 30° are considered as hyperdivergent.
The clinical features of high angle case are as follows:

Extraoral Features

- Dolichocephalic head form;
- Leptoprosopic face;
- Long sloping forehead with heavy glabella;
- Long and thin nose;
- Large gonial angle;
- Short ramus;
- Long anterior face height;
- Short posterior face height;
- Downward and backward;
- Convex soft tissue profile position of mandible;
- Vertical mandibular growth;
- Ectomorphic;
- Weak temporal muscles;
- Incompetent lip.

Intraoral Features

- Open bite relationship;
- High and narrow arched;
- Arch length discrepancy;

- Over erupted incisors s Impacted third molars.

Cephalometric Findings

- Prognathic maxilla and retrognathic mandible;
- FMA is more than 28°;
- SN–MP is more than 32°;
- Small interincisal angle;
- Vertical mandibular growth.

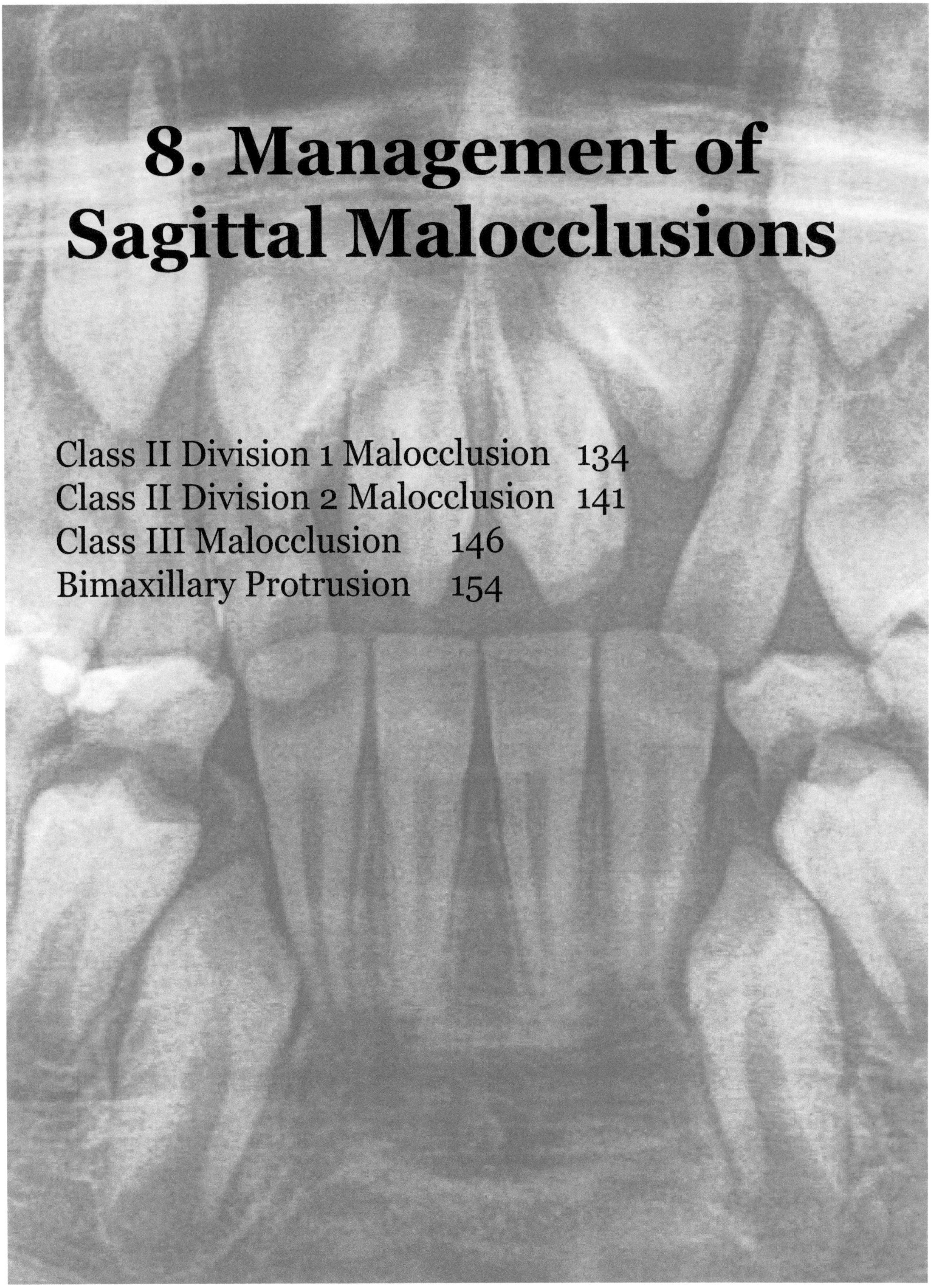

8. Management of Sagittal Malocclusions

Class II Division 1 Malocclusion

Class II malocclusion is a condition in which the lower molar is positioned distally in relation to the upper molar.

Class II malocclusion is divided into two types namely division 1 and division 2. If the molar relation is Class I on one side and Class II on the other, it is called Class II subdivision malocclusion. The incidence of Class II division 1 malocclusion is 20% (Todd and Dodd, 1975).

Etiology

- Heredity:

Heredity plays an important role as the etiology of Class II malocclusion. The inherited growth pattern of the jaw may manifest as prognathic maxilla or retrognathic mandible. Sometimes both prognathic maxilla and retrognathic mandible may be present;

- Developmental defects:

Micrognathia or small mandible may be due to congenital defects, like Pierre Robin syndrome, Treacher Collins syndrome;

- Trauma:

Birth injuries—mandible will become hypoplastic. Trauma to TMJ—causes ankylosis and retarded growth of the mandible. Intrauterine pressure may lead to asymmetry and inhibited growth of mandible;

- Habits:

Various pernicious habits like digit sucking, tongue thrusting, mouth breathing can cause Class II division 1 features;

- Posture:

Faulty body posture leads to undesirable mandibular posturing and retruded mandible;

- Diseases:

Nasopharyngeal disease will cause increased proclination and Class II malocclusion.

Clinical Features

Skeletal Features

- Prognathic maxilla;
- Retrognathic mandible;
- Combination of prognathic maxilla and retrognathic mandible (*Figure 8.1*);
- Some cases will be associated with receding chin.

Soft Tissue Features

- Convex profile;
- Posterior divergence;
- Incompetent lips or potentially incompetent lips;
- Short hypotonic upper lip;
- Due to increased overjet, there will be lip trap;
- Hyperactive lower lip/mentalis activity;

- Abnormal buccinator activity due to the posterior placement of the tongue.

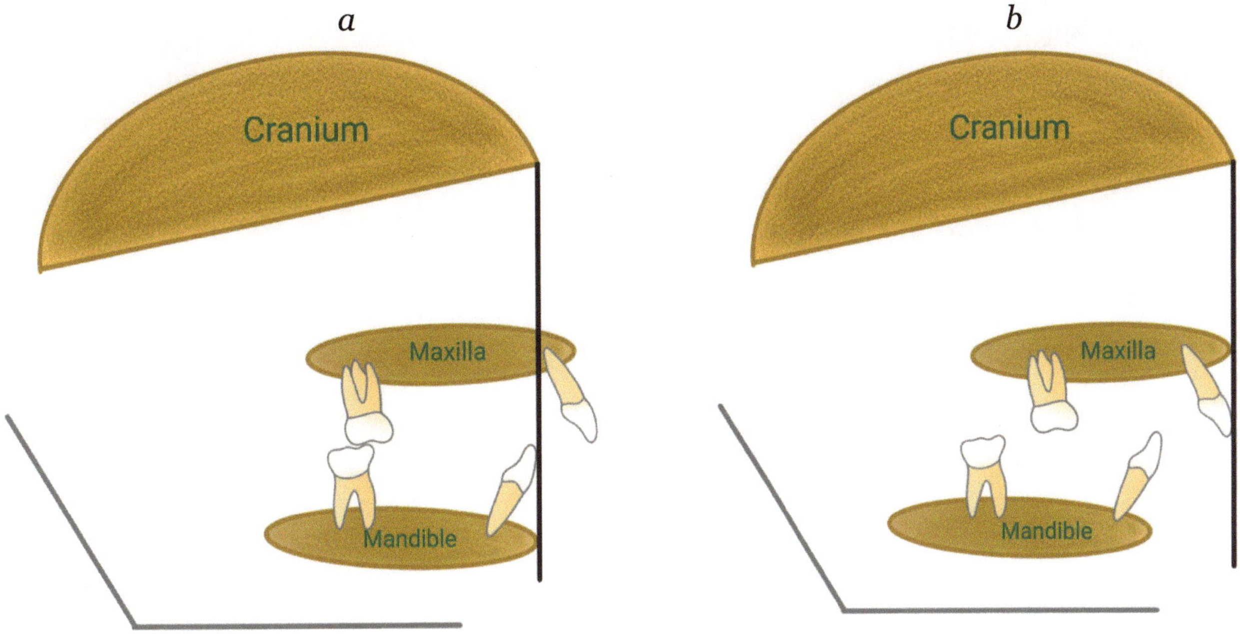

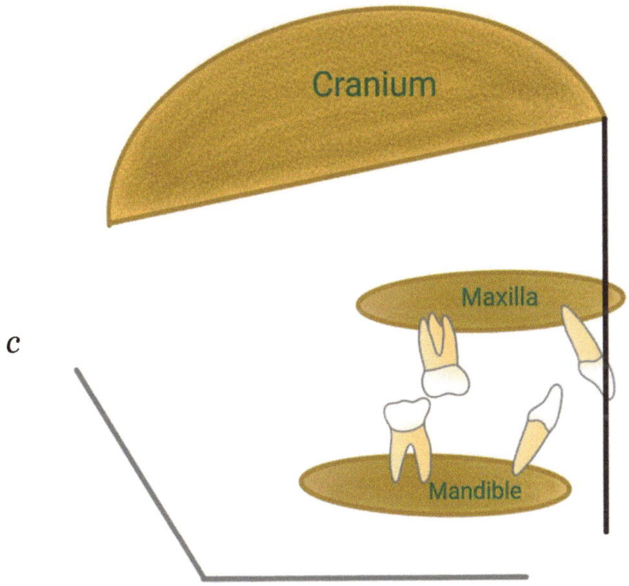

Figure 8.1 Class II due to prognathic maxilla (a), Class II due to retrognathic mandible (b), Class II due to combination of prognathic maxilla and retrognathic mandible;

Occlusal Features *(Figure 8.2)*

- Class II molar relation s Class II incisor relationship due to increased overjet;
- Overbite is frequently deep;
- If associated with thumb sucking, incomplete overbite or open bite;
- Deep curve of Spee;
- Canine relationship will be Class II;
- Crossbite and scissors bite may occasionally be present;
- Facial Growth Varying types of growth pattern are seen;
- Cases with horizontal growth pattern respond well to functional appliance therapy;
- Vertical growth patterns are difficult to treat.

Functional Features

- Abnormal swallowing pattern may be evident;

- Hyperactive mentalis;
- The path of closure will be deviated due to crossbite.

Diagnosis

Model analysis that will show arch length discrepancy;
Functional analysis will reveal aberrations in normal functions, like respiration, swallowing, and path of closure;

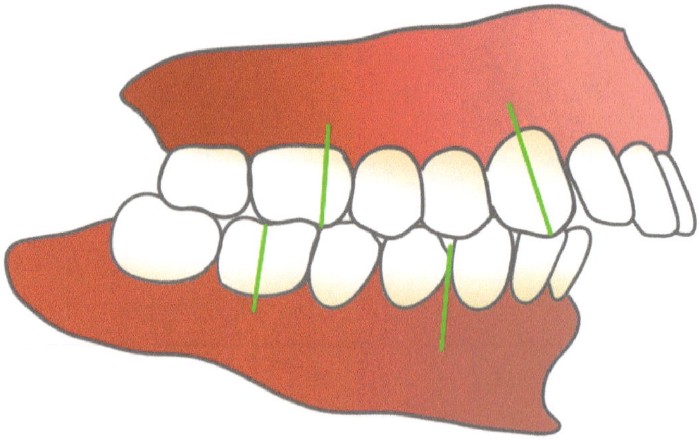

Figure 8.2 Class II division 1 Malocclusion

Cephalometric findings

Findings	Interpretation
Increased SNA > 84°	Prognathic maxilla
Decreased SNB < 78°	Retrognathic mandible
Increased ANB > 4°	Class II skeletal base
Increased upper 1 to NA angle	Proclined upper incisor
Reduced interincisal angle	Proclined upper and lower Incisor
Increased FMA > 28°	Vertical growth
Decreased FMA < 23°	Horizontal growth
Increased IMPA > 90°	Proclined lower incisors

Table 8.1 Cephalometric findings

Management

Treatment Objectives

The objectives of treatment planning in correcting a Class II division 1 malocclusion in a growing child are:
- Relieve crowding and irregularities of teeth;
- Correction or improvement of the skeletal discrepancy;
- Establish stable Class I incisor relationship;
- Establish normal overbite;
- Correction of molar and canine relation;
- Improving facial esthetics.

Management in the mixed and early permanent dentition

Treatment Plans for Class II malocclusion in growing child are listed in *Figure 8.3*.

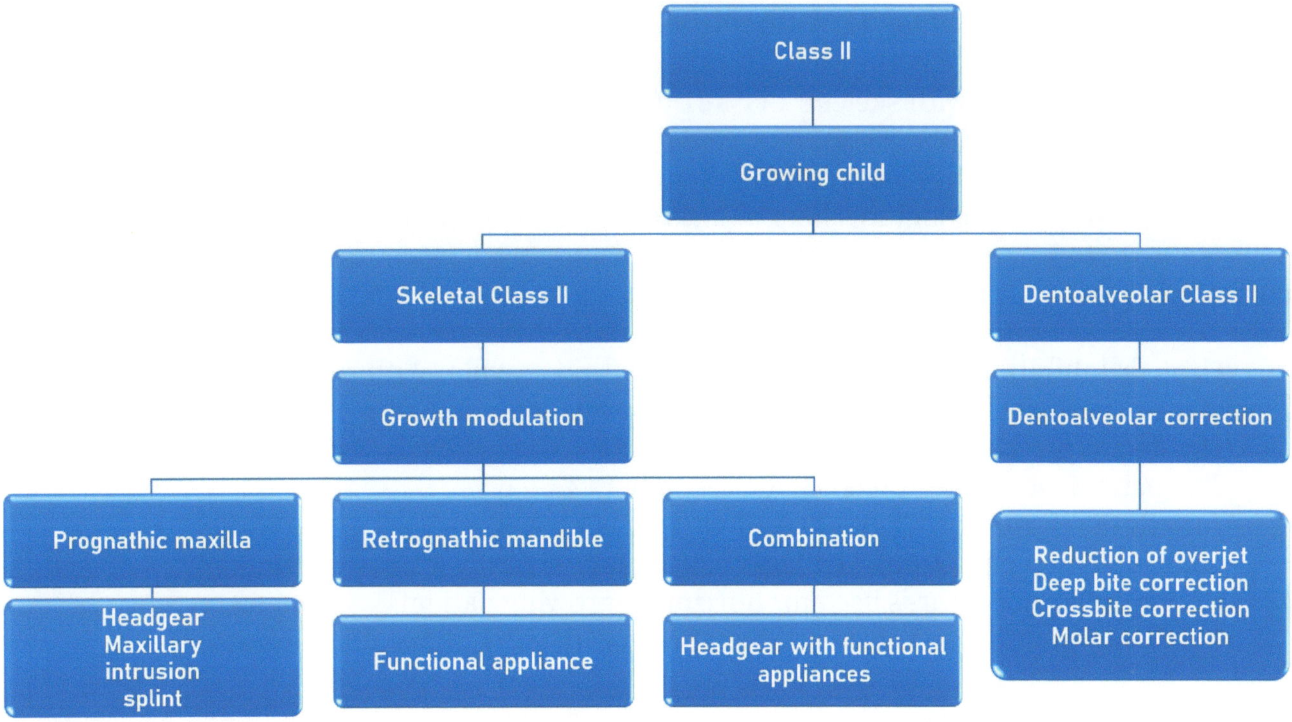

Figure 8.3 Treatment Plan for Class II Malocclusion in Growing Child

Correction of Dentoalveolar Class II with Class I Skeletal Base.

In dentoalveolar Class II, the skeletal base is normal or orthognathic. The defect lies in the dentoalveolar part (*Figure 8.4*).

- Establishment of normal incisor and molar relationship is one of the aims of early correction;
- If this is achieved, the other teeth usually settle in normal position and function;
- Correction of crowding is achieved by gaining space either by distalization of molars or extraction;
- Deep bite correction is achieved by using anterior bite planes in low angle case;
- In high angle cases, incisor intrusion is achieved using utility arches;
- Retraction of incisors is achieved by using labial bows or with fixed appliance mechanotherapy;
- Posterior crossbites are corrected using crossbite elastics;
- Any habit should be corrected simultaneously.

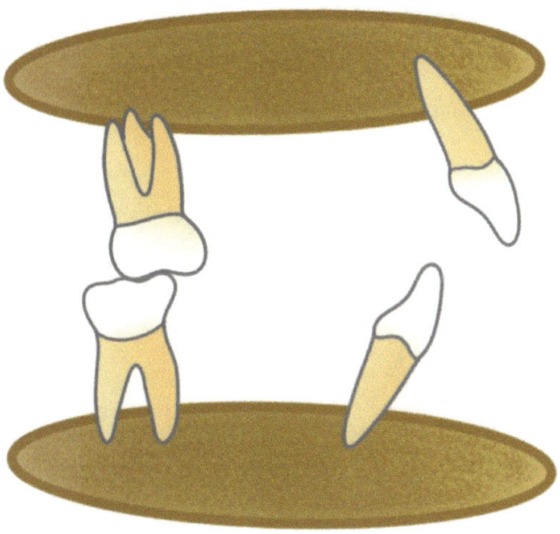

Figure 8.4 Dentoalveolar Class II.

Correction of Skeletal Class II Malocclusion:

- A growing patient with skeletal Class II malocclusion should be treated by growth modification;
  - The skeletal age and growth potential can be assessed;
  - Lateral cephalograms help to locate the skeletal problem.

Prognathic maxilla:

- Growth inhibition of the maxilla for prognathic maxilla, with distalization of upper buccal segments is achieved by using extraoral orthopedic force;
- Headgears are used for orthopedic force;
- The patient wears the appliance for 12–14 hours a day;
- An orthopedic force of 350–450 grams/side is applied;
- High-pull or occipital-pull headgear is used for vertically growing patients;
- Cervical-pull headgear is used for horizontal growing patients;
- Maxillary intrusion splint is used in patients with vertical maxillary excess.

Retrognathic mandible:

- Growth stimulation of the mandible is induced using functional appliances;
- Functional appliances act by placing the mandible in an anterior position and also by eliminating functional retrusion;
- Commonly used functional appliances for Class II correction are Activator, Frankel, Twin Block, and Bionator;
- During late mixed dentition in children with residual post-pubertal growth, fixed functional appliances, like Herbst, Jasper jumpers, are used (*Figure 8.5*).

a *b*

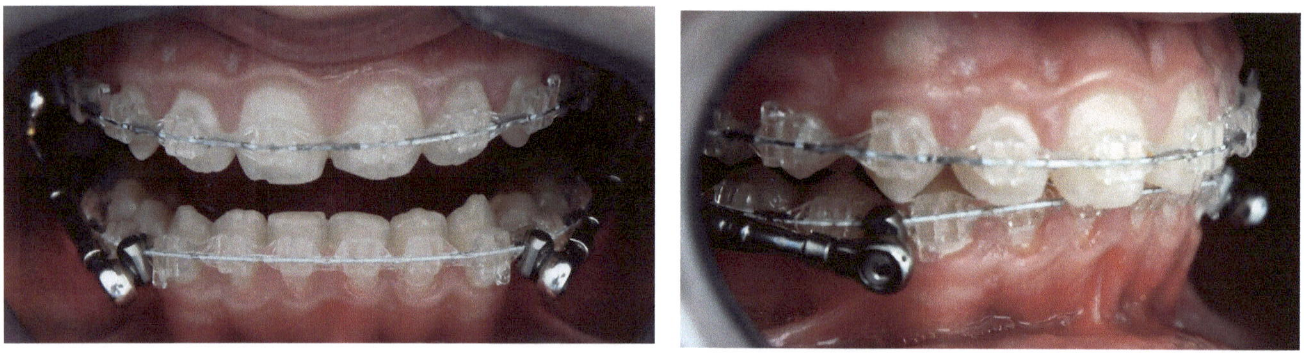

Figure 8.5 Functional treatment with PowerScope appliance

- Class II Elastics
  - Using class II elastics to correct skeletal class II in a growing adolescent is an alternative to functional appliance treatment;
  - Class II elastics are placed on the hooks of the lower first molar brackets and are stretched to a hook on the upper canine brackets (*Figure 8.6*);
  - Elastics used for class II correction should be 5/16 heavy;
  - The patient is instructed to wear the elastics full day and night and remove them for mealtimes.

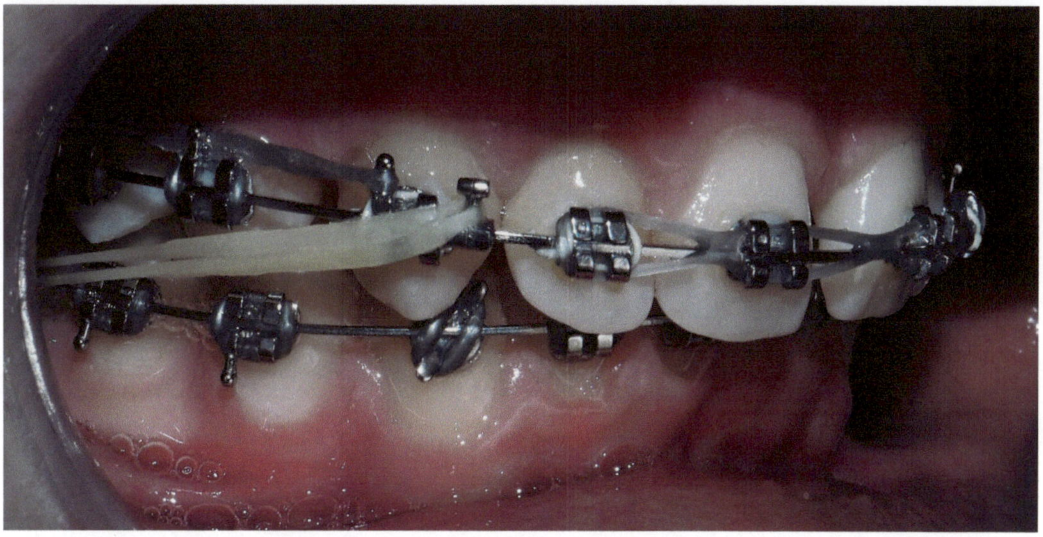

Figure 8.6 Class II elastics

Combination of prognathic maxilla and retrognathic mandible:

- Growth modification is done by a combination of headgear and functional appliances;
- Activator with headgear is commonly used.

Management of Class II Division 1 Malocclusion in an Adult

Treatment Objectives:

- Relieve crowding and irregularities of teeth;
- Correction or improvement of skeletal discrepancy either by surgery or camouflage;
- Establish stable Class I incisor relationship;
- Establish normal overbite;
- Correction of molar and canine relation;
- Improving facial esthetics.

A treatment plan for Class II correction in adult is given in the *Figure 8.7.*

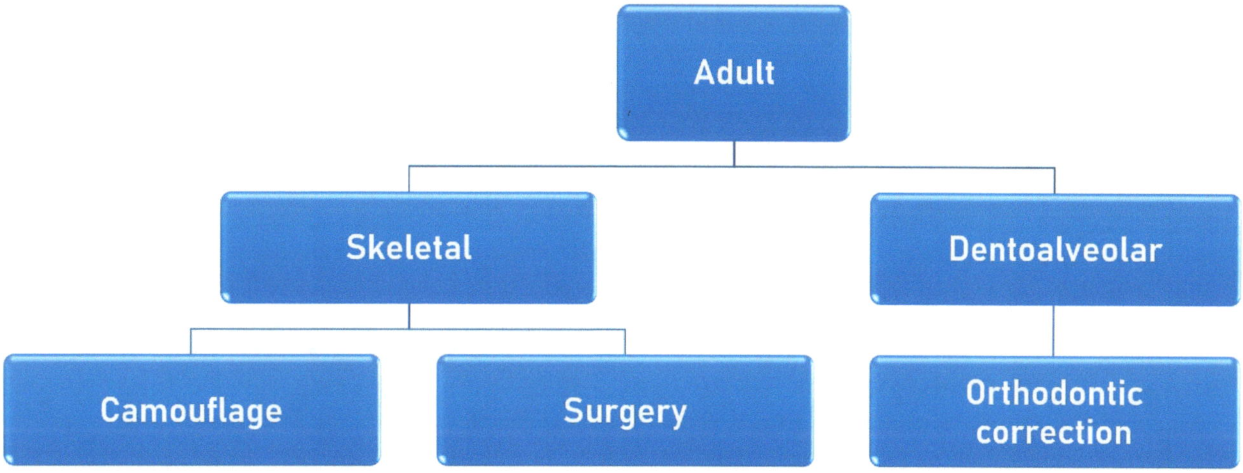

Figure 8.7 Treatment plan for Class II correction in adult

Dentoalveolar Correction

- Establishment of normal incisor and molar relationship is one of the aims of early correction;
- If this is achieved, the other teeth usually settle in normal position and function;

- Correction of crowding is achieved by gaining space either by distalization of molars or extraction;
- Deep bite correction is achieved by using anterior bite planes in low angle case;
- In high angle cases, incisor intrusion is achieved using utility arches;
- Retraction of incisors is achieved by using labial bows or with fixed appliance mechanotherapy;
- Posterior crossbites are corrected using crossbite elastics;
- Any habit should be corrected simultaneously.

Correction of skeletal deep bite

Orthodontic Camouflage:

- Orthodontic camouflage implies repositioning the teeth without correcting the skeletal problem;
- The objective of orthodontic camouflage is to correct the malocclusion which makes the underlying skeletal problem less apparent;
- Class II malocclusions often can be camouflaged.

Indications for camouflage treatment are:

- Patients too old for growth modulation;
- Mild or moderate skeletal Class II;
- Good alignment of teeth;
- Good vertical proportions.

Extractions for camouflage are done in three possible ways:

1. Extraction of upper first premolars;
2. Extraction of upper and lower first premolars;
3. Extraction of upper first and lower second premolars.

- Extraction of upper first premolars alone is done when only retraction of proclined incisors is required;
- If crowding correction or proclination correction is required in the lower arch then extraction of both upper and lower first premolars is done;
- Extraction of a lower second premolar is done for molar correction;
- Orthodontic camouflage is achieved through fixed appliance;
- Camouflage is best performed in adolescents but it is also done in adults.

Surgery

The envelope of discrepancy will act as a guideline in selecting cases for orthognathic surgery. The various surgical procedures carried out are:

- With prognathic maxilla: (a) Le Fort I osteotomy, (b) anterior maxillary osteotomy;
- Retrognathic mandible: (a) sagittal split, (b) oblique osteotomy— advancement procedure;
- Combination: Bi-jaw surgery with genioplasty, if required.

Retention

Depending on the method of correction of the malocclusion, retention protocol can differ.

- Growth modification done with a functional appliance can be retained with the night ware of the same appliance;

- In extraction cases, it is preferred to use a removable appliance as a retainer, because extraction spaces tend to reopen.

Class II Division 2 Malocclusion

Class II division 2 malocclusion is generally the result of dentoalveolar compensation for a Class II skeletal pattern by retroclination of the upper central incisors. The overbite also will be deep. The incidence of Class II division 2 malocclusion is 5% (Todd and Dodd, 1975).

Clinical Features

Skeletal Features:

- The skeletal pattern may be Class I or Class II;
- Class II skeletal pattern is usually mild when compared to division 1 pattern;
- In the vertical dimension, the lower anterior face height is smaller;
- Deep bite will be moderate to severe. Lower facial height will be reduced;
- Transversely, the maxillary arch may be broad relative to the mandibular arch.

Soft-tissue Features:

- The level of the lower lip is high relative to the upper incisor crown;
- Because the lower lip is high, it causes the upper incisors to retrocline since the skeletal pattern is not severe;
- If the skeletal pattern is severe, the upper teeth will lie outside the lower lip, and this will cause proclination as in Class II division 1 malocclusion;
- Hyperactive lower lip;
- Deep mentolabial fold;
- Because of chin prominence, the profile may be straight;
- Competent lips;
- Strong musculature will be present;
- Trauma to the palatal gingiva due to a closed bite of the lower incisor.

Occlusal Features (*Figure 8.8*)

- Class II molar relationship;
- Class II division 2 incisor relationship;

There are three types of incisor relationships.

- Retroclined upper central and lateral incisors;
- Retroclined upper central incisors and proclined lateral incisors;
- Retroclination with crowding of upper anterior teeth;

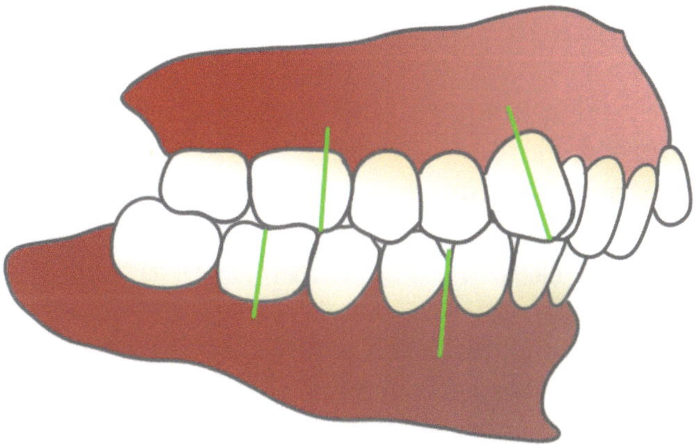

Figure 8.8 Dental features of Class II division 2 malocclusion.

Other occlusal features:

- Retroclined lower anterior teeth;
- Excessive deep overbite;
- Increased curve of Spee;

- Increased interocclusal clearance or increased freeway space;
- Class II canine relation s Lower anterior crowding;
- Anterior mandibular rotation or horizontal type of growth pattern is seen.

Functional Features

- Posterior displacement of mandible due to over closure;
- This is called functional retrusion of mandible;
- The path of the closure of mandible will be upwards and backwards;
- Usually associated with large interocclusal distance.

Management of Class II Division 2 Malocclusion

Objectives of Treatment are:

- Correction of potentially traumatic deep bite;
- Alignment of upper incisors;
- Relieving the crowding in the lower arch;
- Elimination of functional retrusion;
- Establishing Class I molar relation.

Management in the mixed and early permanent dentition

Dental—orthodontic correction

- It can be done with removable appliances;
- Removable appliances are usually used to assist in the reduction of the deep overbite;
- In mild cases, simple removable appliances alone will be enough;
- Removable appliances are not used in conditions which require premolar extraction.

Removable appliances used are:

- Hawley's appliance with anterior bite plane;
- Hawley's appliance with double cantilever springs;
- Distalization appliances like pendulum combined with a fixed appliance;
- Use of intermaxillary elastics with a fixed appliance.

Fixed Appliance in the Upper Arch

- Fixed appliance in the upper arch alone is indicated when the overbite and incisor inclination is acceptable;
- Molar distalization is done and the space gained is used to align teeth.

Upper and Lower Arch Fixed Appliance

This appliance is indicated when the following objectives are to be achieved:

- Extraction and correction of crowding;
- Overbite correction by active intrusion;
- Achieve proper interincisal angle;
- To torque the incisors;
- Skeletal malocclusion requires —functional appliances after the alignment of incisors.

Functional Appliances

- Children seeking orthodontic correction due to Class II division 2 are less when compared to Class II division 1;
- Functional appliances with modification for division 2 malocclusion are used;
- Usually, the incisors have to be aligned before giving functional appliances. (*Figure 8.9*)

Appliances used can be
- Upper inclined plane;
- Andersen Activator;
- Twin block;
- Fixed functional appliances.

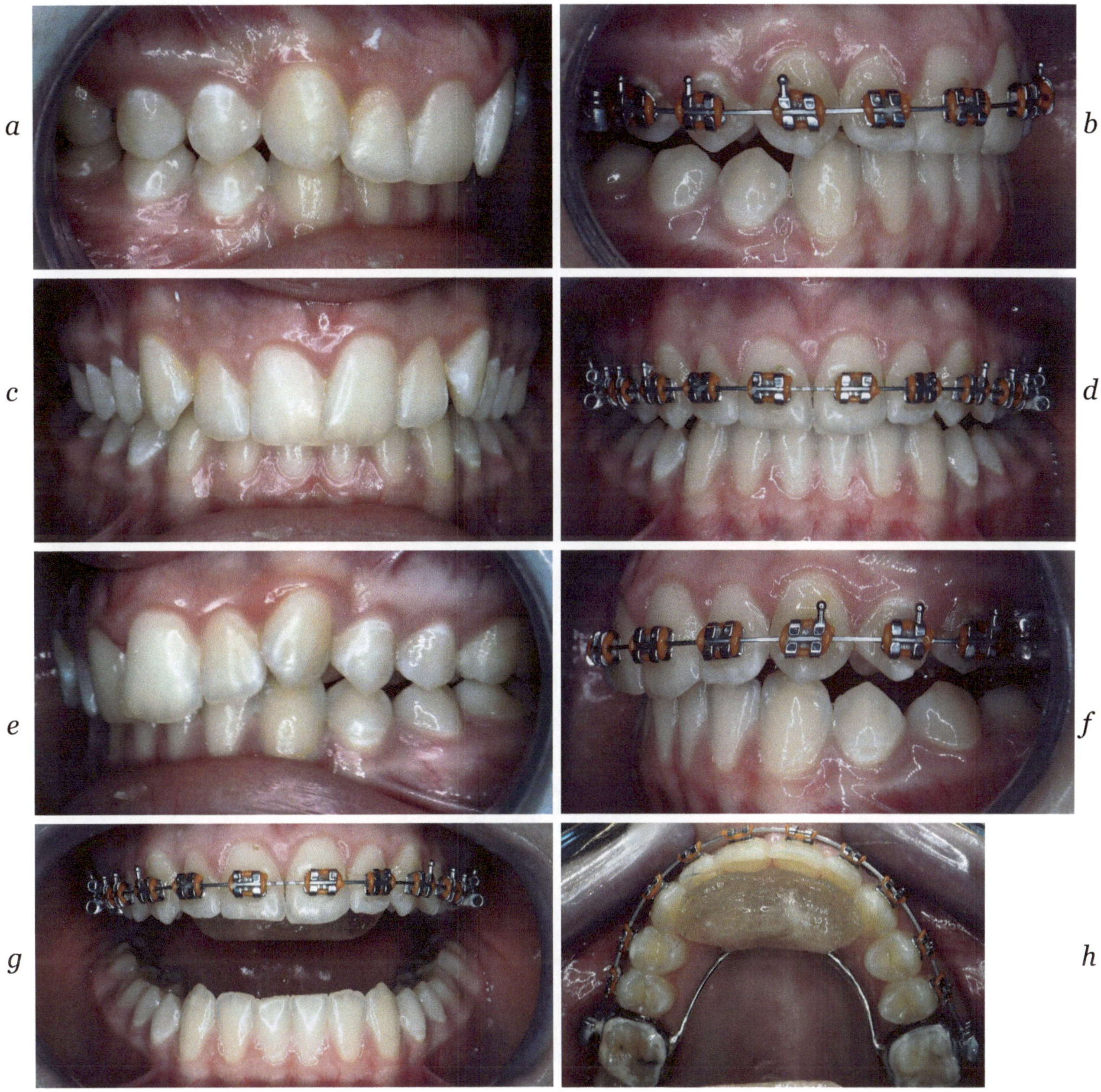

Figure 8.9 Functional treatment with an inclined plane

Management in adults

Dental malocclusion— corrected by orthodontics.

- Extraction treatment;
- Distalization treatment.

Skeletal malocclusion— corrected by:

- *Orthodontic correction;*

Camouflage treatment

- It can be performed by distalization in the upper arch if the sagittal deviation is less than ½ premolar width;
- Distalization should be done after third molar extraction;
- Distalization is a method of treatment for low angle cases because it tends to open the bite;
- Distalization can be done with a removable appliance, fixed distalizer like a pendulum, or with mini implants;
- If distalization needed is 1/3 premolar width, we can use fixed functional appliances like Forsus or Powerscope;
- If the sagittal deviation is more than ½ premolar width in an adult, we should consider extraction treatment for camouflage;
- Extraction schemes can be:
    - o Upper first premolars;
    - o Upper first premolars, lower second molars;
    - o Upper first premolars, lower incisor in a case of Bolton discrepancy.

- *Surgery;*
- *Mandibular advancement;*
- *Maxillary set back.*

Appliances used

- *Pendulum appliance (Figure 8.10)*

This appliance produces distalization with little inclination compared to other methods, and at the same time allows rotational control over the molars with minimal mesial premolar anchorage displacement.

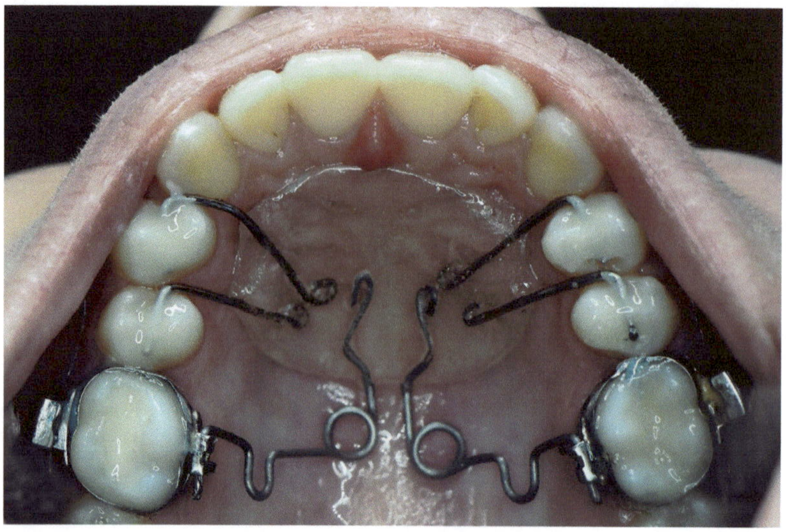

Figure 8.10 Pendulum appliance

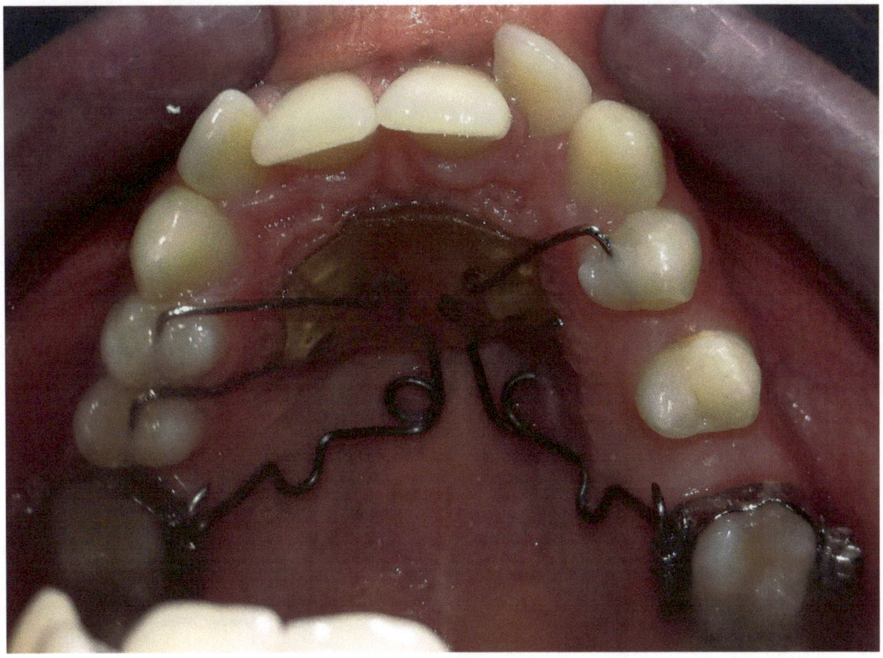

Figure 8.11 This patient needs only unilateral distalization which is easy to do with pendulum appliance because we can use the other side as an additional anchorage. After the needed amount of distalization is met, the second premolar is freed from the appliance and left to distalize with the force of the supracrestal interdental fibers

This distalizer has 3 sections:

1. An ample Nance button that leans on the palatine vault behind the incisor teeth for anchorage;
2. A pair of TMA 0.032" wires. When we cement the Pendulum, the arms will be parallel to each other, then they are inserted in the molar band sheaths. Posterior adjustments are done pressing the center of the adjustment loop;

- Depending upon the amount of degrees of activation of the arms, will be the amount of force produced;
- If they are activated to 90°, the distalizing force will be 350 g, if they are activated 60°, the force will be 250 g; if they are activated 40°, the force will be 125 g. These activations must be done before we cement the Pendulum;

3. One or two pairs of rests that are cemented or banded on the premolars;
4. An expansion screw to correct transversal problems. This appliance is called "Pendex' (*Figure 8.12*);

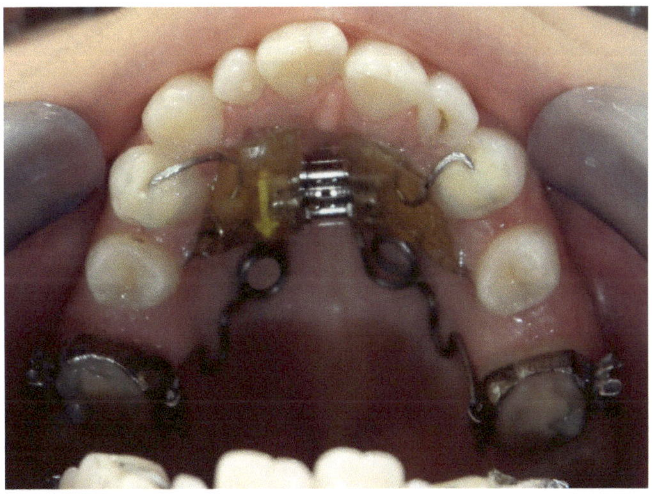

Figure 8.12 Pendex appliance

Retention

- Prolonged retention should be planned;
- Precision is done for the incisors;
- In cases treated after growth, fixed permanent retention is advisable.

Class III Malocclusion

Class III malocclusion is found in about 3% of the population. Class III malocclusion is a condition in which the lower molar is positioned mesial to the upper molar.

Etiology

Environmental factors play a small role in the genesis of Class III malocclusion.

Functional Factors

- Unfavorable anterior incisal guidance promotes Class III relationship;
- If functional cases are not treated, they can become a true Class III malocclusion;
- Premature loss of deciduous molars also may cause mandibular displacement;
- Loss of posterior teeth results in loss of posterior proprioceptive support in habitual occlusion.

Soft-tissue Factors

- A flat anterior positioned tongue that lies low in the mouth is said to cause Class III malocclusion;
- Lack of eruption of posterior teeth due to lateral tongue thrust results in overclosure of the mandible. This causes autorotation which leads to Class III development.

Heredity

Heredity plays an important role in skeletal or true Class III malocclusion.

Clinical Features

Occlusal Features *(Figure 8.13)*

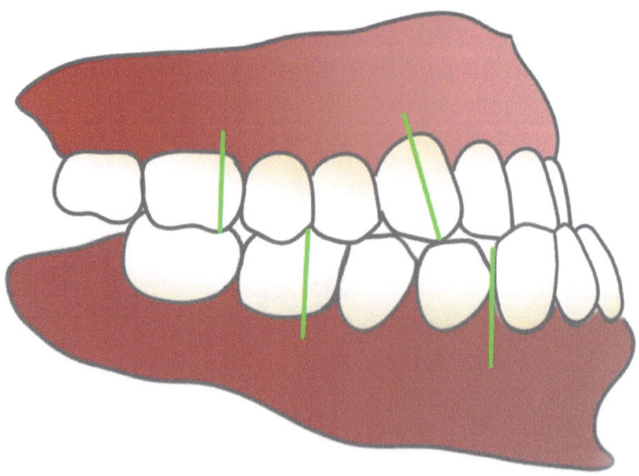

Figure 8.13 Dental features of Class III malocclusion

- Class III molar relation. The lower dental arch is in anterior relation to the maxillary arch. Mesiobuccal cusp of the upper first permanent molar occludes with the interdental space between the lower first and second permanent molars;
- Class III canine relation. Upper canine occludes with the interdental space between lower first and second premolars;
- The severity of the incisor malrelationship varies greatly;
- It could be edge-to-edge or reverse overjet;
- Frequently, the lower incisors are retroclined;
- The overbite also varies between cases;
- Deep bite or open bite will be seen;
- Crowding will be present in some cases;
- The upper arch is narrow and the lower arch is broad. This could lead to a crossbite.

Skeletal Features

- Usually, Class III skeletal pattern exists (Guyer et al, 1986): Retrognathic maxilla, prognathic mandible, or combination *(Figure 8.14)*;
- Sometimes the skeletal pattern will be Class I with dentoalveolar Class III *(Figure 8.15)*;
- Class III malocclusion is associated with both increased and reduced facial height or average facial height. Accordingly, the Frankfort mandibular angles are high, low or average;
- In the transverse plane in many cases maxilla is narrow and the mandibular base is wide.

Soft Tissue Features *(Figure 8.16)*

- Profile is concave;
- There is anterior divergence;
- Lips are frequently incompetent;
- The upper lip may be short;
- The tongue is more anteriorly placed.

Functional Features

- There is a forward displacement of mandible;
- Lateral mandibular displacement is also found when there is unilateral crossbite;
- In pseudo-Class III, patients will have Class I skeletal pattern, the abnormality is due to tilting of the tooth;
- The path of closure is upwards forwards and forwards;
- Facial growth is unfavorable in most of the Class III cases;
- Vertical facial growth increases the tendency to open the bite;
- Excessive horizontal growth causes the reverse overjet to become worse.

Diagnosis

- The model analysis will show arch length discrepancy;
- Functional analysis will reveal aberrations in normal function, like respiration, swallowing, and path of closure;
- Cephalometric Findings (*Table 8.2).*

a *b*

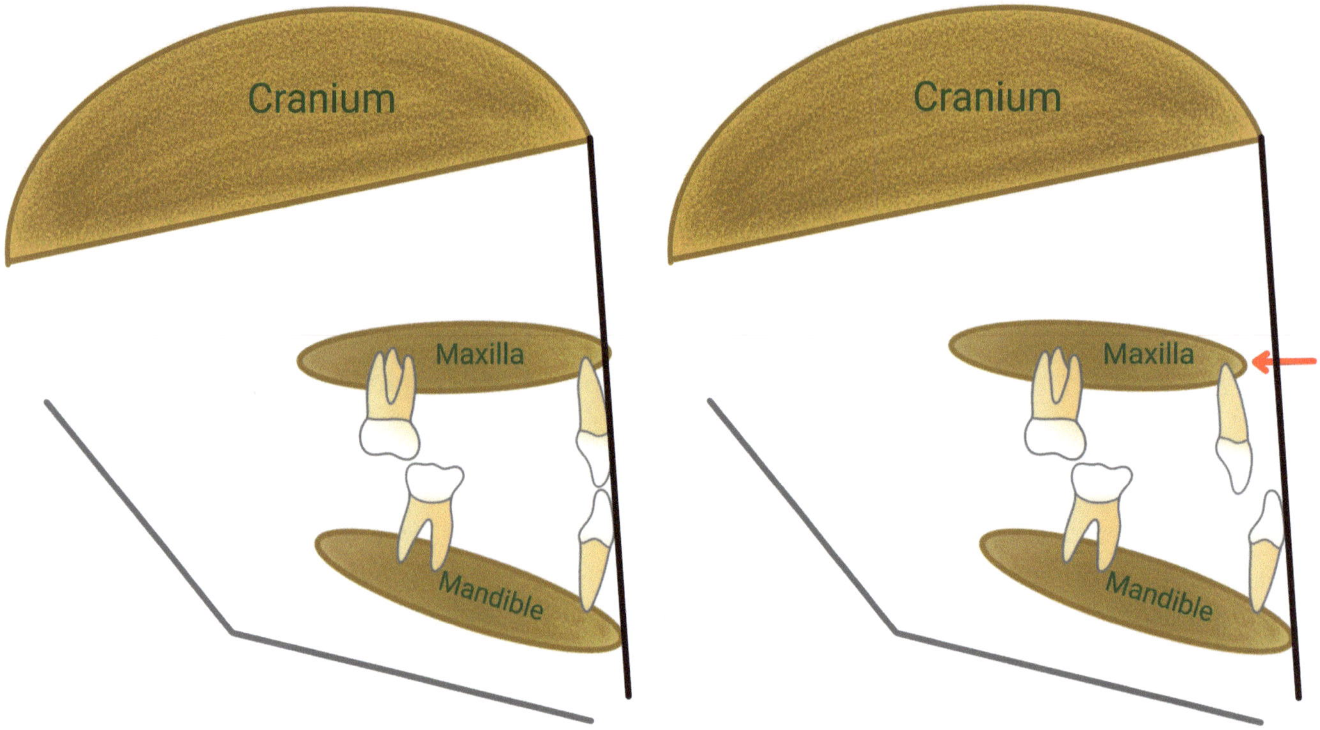

c

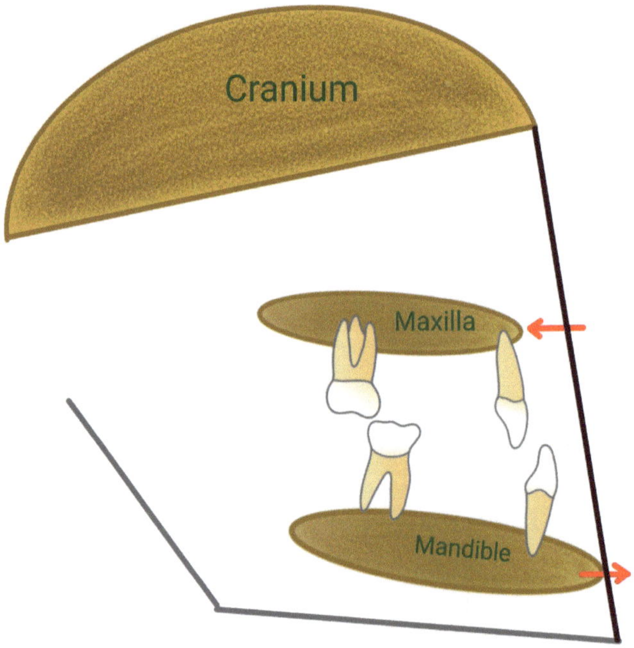

Figure 8.14 Prognathic mandible(a) Retrognathic maxilla (b) and combination of a prognathic mandible and retrognathic maxilla (c).

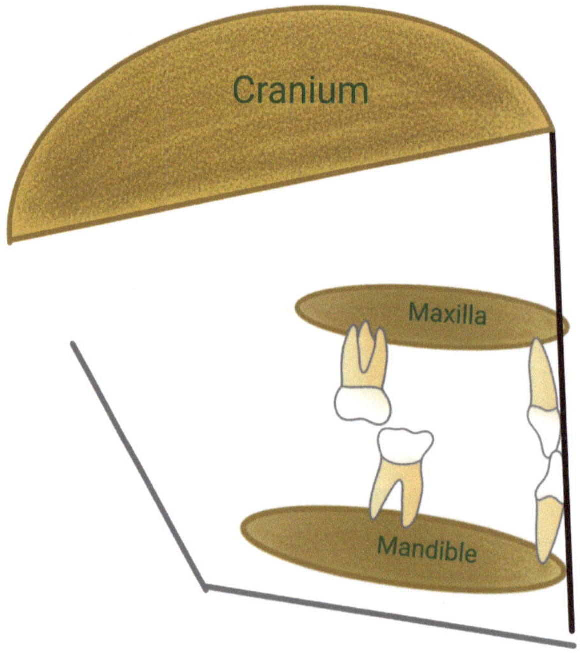

Figure 8.15 Dentoalveolar Class III on Class I skeletal basis

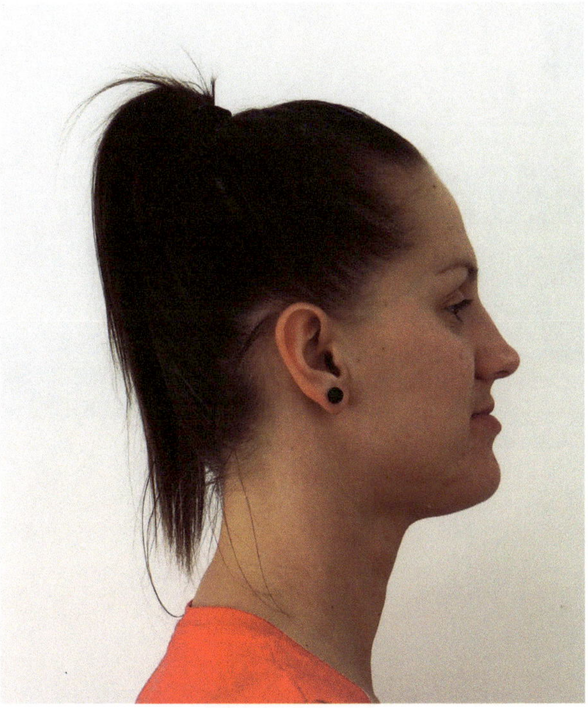

Figure 8.16 Soft tissue features of Class III patient.

Findings	Interpretation
Decreased SNA < 78°	Retrognathic maxilla
Increased SNB > 82°	Prognathic mandible
Decreased ANB < 1° or negative	Class III skeletal base
Increased upper 1 to NA	Proclined upper incisors
Reduced interincisal angle	Proclined upper and lower Incisors
Increased FMA > 28°	Vertical growth
Decreased FMA < 23°	Horizontal growth
Increased IMPA > 90°	Proclined lower incisors
Decreased IMPA < 90°	Retroclined lower incisors

Table 8.2 Cephalometric findings in Class III malocclusion

Management for Class III malocclusion is shown in *Figure 8.17.*

Treatment Objectives are

- To achieve growth modulation in a skeletal case;
- To relieve crowding and produce alignment of teeth;
- To correct incisor relationship to obtain normal overjet and overbite;
- To eliminate anteroposterior and unilateral lateral crossbite;
- Stable molar relationship.

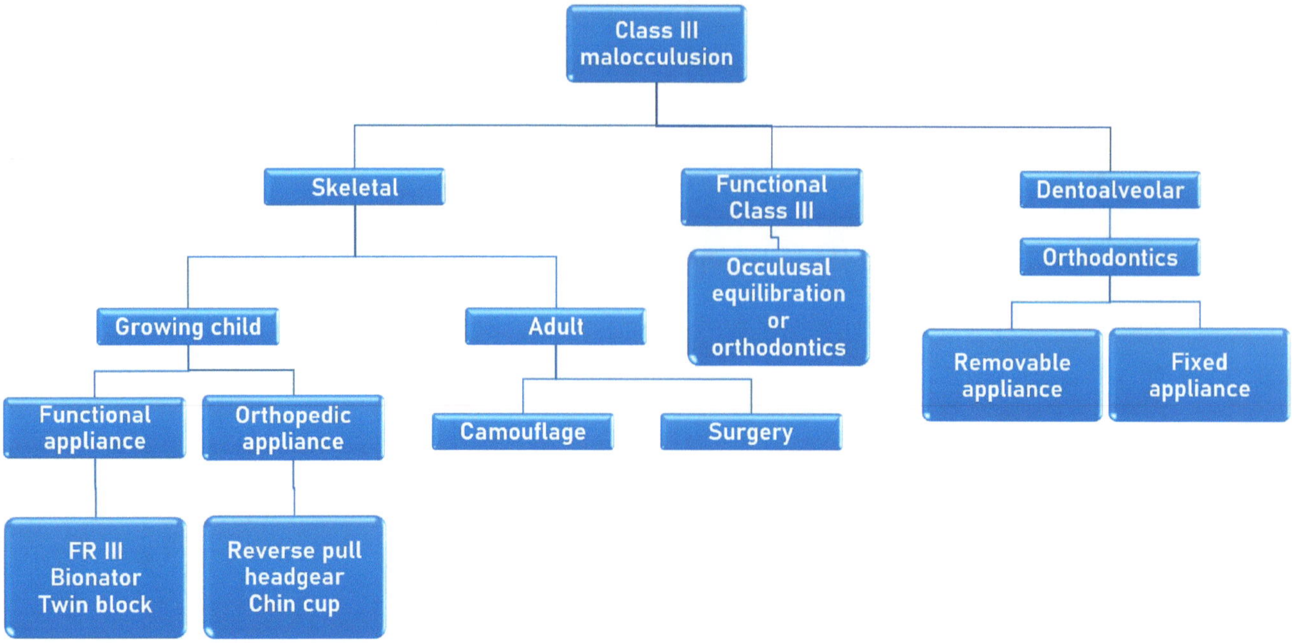

Figure 8.17 Treatment plan for Class III malocclusion

Management in the mixed and early permanent dentition

Treatment depends on the causing facial structure.

Retrognathic maxilla

- When midface deficiency is diagnosed, functional appliances are indicated in primary dentition or early mixed dentition;
- FR III is used. Other functional appliances that can be used are reverse Activator, reverse Bionator and Twin block for Class III;
- Reverse-pull headgears are also used in cases with maxillary deficiency.

Mandibular prognathism

- Extraoral appliance, like chin cap, is used as an early form of treatment.

Combination of factors

- Devices which combine midface protraction and chin cap are ideal for the cases;
- Reverse-pull headgear can be used;
- FR III with a chin cap can be used.

Management in adults

Camouflage

- This can be used in mild skeletal Class III problems;
- Usually, camouflage is less successful in Class III when compared to Class II problems;
- Lower premolars are extracted and combined with Class III elastics to produce good dental occlusion;
- The drawback with camouflage is the retraction of lower incisors make the chin more

prominent;

- The other extraction pattern for Class III camouflage is the extraction of upper second premolars and lower first premolars (*Figure 8.18*);
- This is followed by Class III intermaxillary elastics which aids in lower incisor retraction and molar correction.

a b c d e f

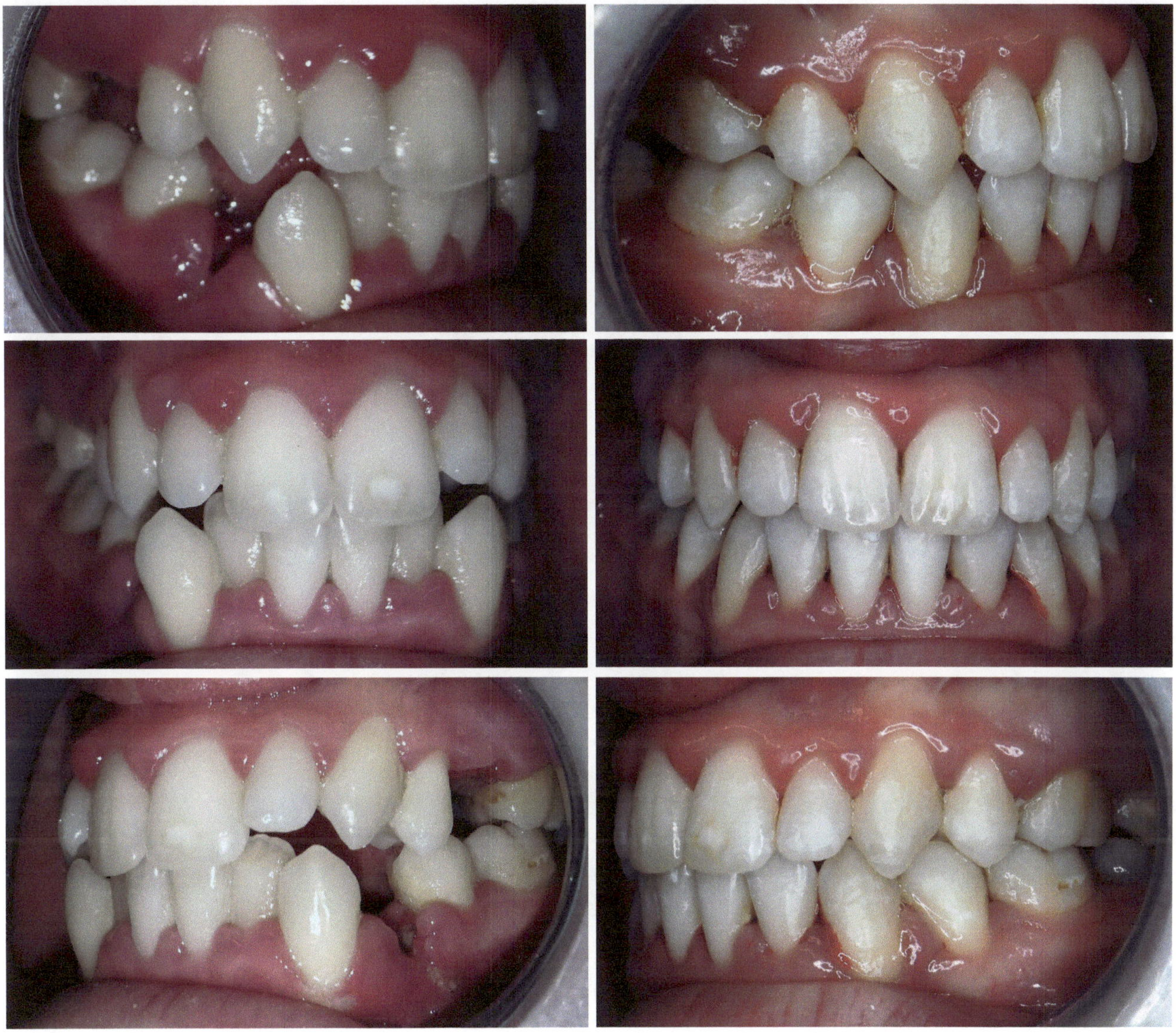

Figure 8.18 Treatment of mild Class III with upper second and lower first premolar extraction.

Surgical management

The maxilla may be advanced or mandible pushed back as the condition demands. Sometimes a combination of upper and lower jaw surgery is performed with reduction genioplasty.

Functional Class III or Pseudo-Class III

This is a postural malrelationship due to reflex functional mandibular protrusion.

- There is a shift from Class I to Class III as the mandible closes;
- Early treatment consists of occlusal equilibration;
- Late treatment consists of correcting the anterior crossbite or functional interference.

Dentoalveolar Correction can be done with:

- Removable appliances: Removable appliances are effective when one or two incisors are in crossbite associated with functional displacement;
    - Effective during mixed dentition period;
    - Adequate overbite is essential.
- Appliances, like anterior expansion plates and Z springs, are used to achieve labial movement of palatally placed incisors;
- Fixed appliances: In a suitable case, fixed appliance gives excellent result;
    - Case selection is critical;
    - Cases are treated either by extraction or by nonextraction (Figure 8.19).

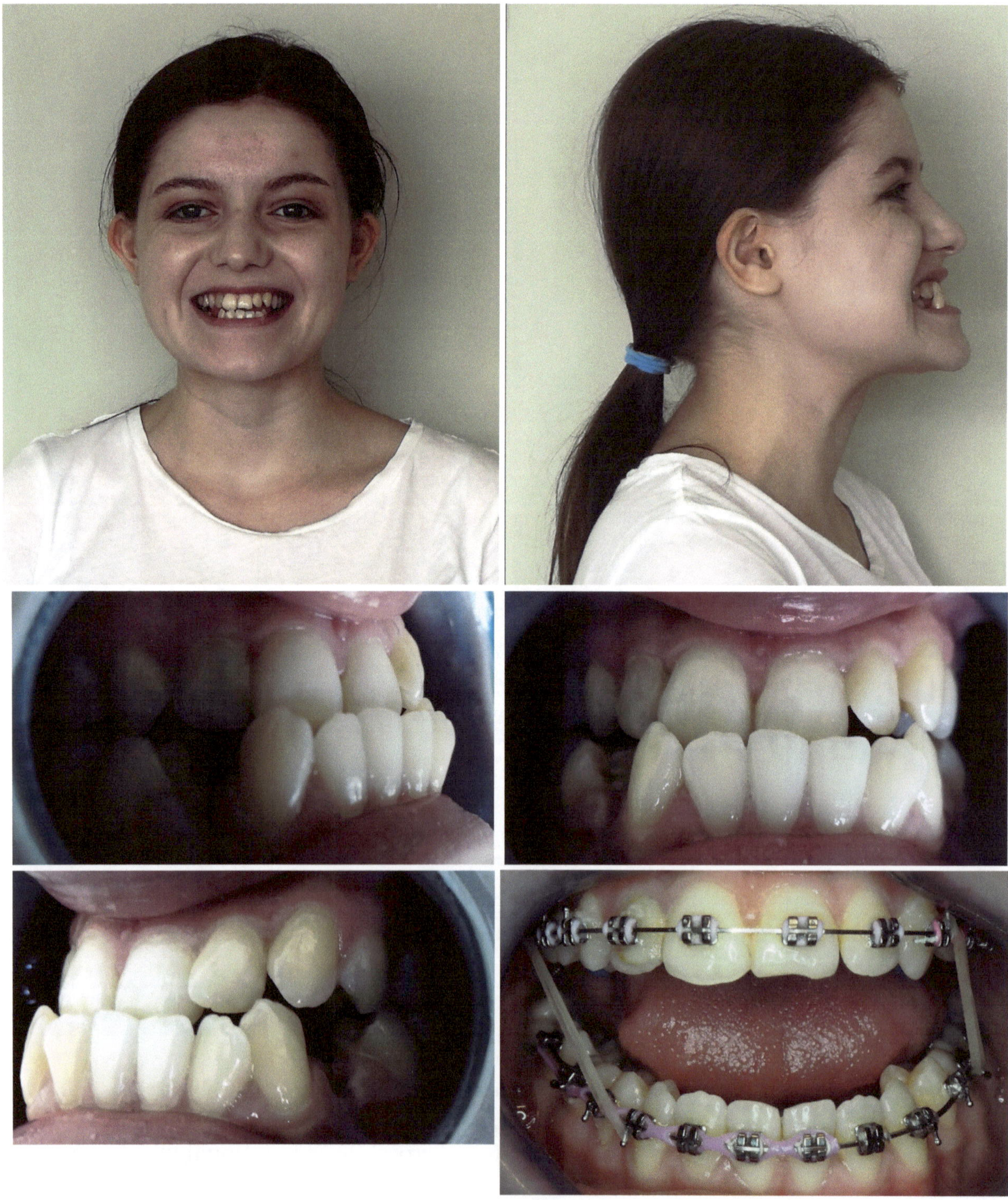

a *b* *c* *d* *e* *f*

g

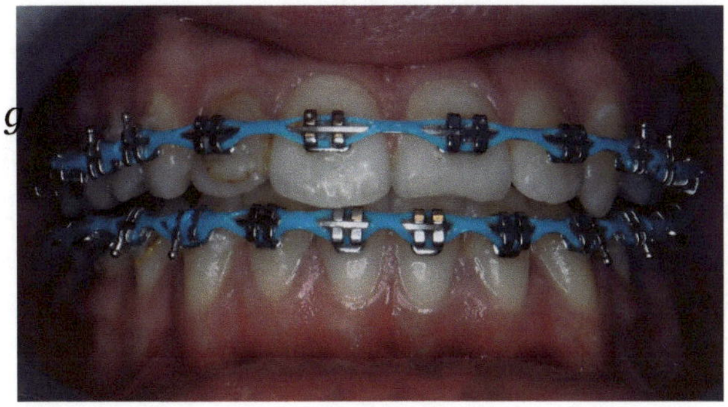

Figure 8.19 Treatment of functional Class III with upper and lower premolar extraction. Start of treatment after extraction of premolars (a,b,c,d,e). Correction of midline with intermaxillary elastics (f). Finishing the case (g).

Clinical features or differences between pseudo- and true-Class III malocclusion are depicted in *Table 8.3*.

Pseudo-Class III	True-Class III
This has a normal Class I skeletal base	Has a Class III skeletal base
Class I molar relationship in rest position	Class III molar relationship in rest position
Associated with functional interference when mandible moves from rest position to occlusion	May not be associated with functional interferences. Not a rule
There is shift from Class I to Class III molar relationship as the mandible closes in centric occlusion	Class III in centric occlusion
Patient can move mandible backwards to edge-to-edge or normal overbite	Patient cannot move mandible backward to edge-to-edge
Path of closure is upwards and forwards up to initial contact and then forwards	Path of closure is upwards and forwards
Usually associated with deep bite	Varying overbite present
There is overclosure of mandible	May or may not be associated with overclosure
Associated with large freeway space	May not be associated with large freeway space
Maxillary arch may be constricted	Well-developed maxillary arch
This is a postural malrelationship due to reflex mandibular protraction	It is a skeletal dysplasia involving mandibular hypertrophy
Profile of the patient improves as the mandible drops from centric to rest position	No improvement in profile

Table 8.3 Pseudo- and true-Class III malocclusion differences.

Management of Pseudo-class III

- Occlusal equilibration: In the early stages, patients can be treated by equilibration alone;
- Inclined plane: Inclined planes act as an extension of the lower incisal edges by contacting the palatal surfaces of maxillary incisors. On closing, the mandible is forced to be retruded. Maxillary teeth are tipped labially;
- If the bite is shallow, then posterior bite blocks with Z springs to move the palatally placed maxillary incisors can be given.

Retention

- Retention after pseudo-Class III correction is not needed. The occlusal contacts support the bite;
- A removable functional appliance is the best retainer after correcting class III dentoalveolar or skeletal bite.

Bimaxillary Protrusion

Classification

They are: 1. Bimaxillary prognathism, and
2. Bimaxillary dental protrusion.

Bimaxillary Prognathism

- Bimaxillary prognathism is a skeletal problem in which both maxilla and mandible are placed forward than normal in relation to cranium;
- Because bimaxillary prognathism is a problem in the basic morphology and growth pattern of the bony skeleton, interception does not produce very satisfactory results;
- Bimaxillary prognathism is seen as an ethnic type of malocclusion;
- Bimaxillary prognathism may exist alone or in combination with bimaxillary dental protrusion (*Figure 8.20*).

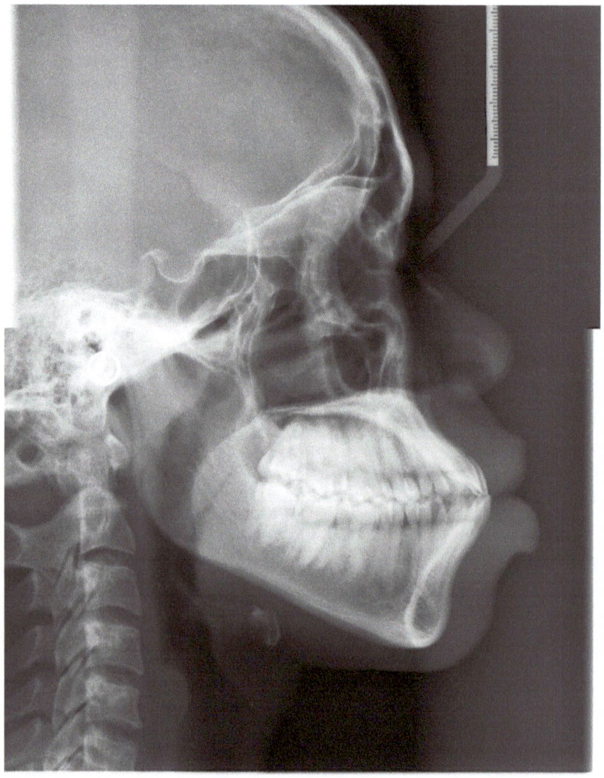

Figure 8.20 Bimaxillary prognathism
In this case, the patient presents with excessive spacing, and the treatment plan does not need to involve extraction.

Management

- Treatment consists of camouflage or combined orthodontics and surgery;
- Camouflage treatment consists of symmetric extraction of premolars (mostly first premolar) and retraction of incisors;
- More severe cases are treated by combined orthodontics and surgery.

Bimaxillary Dental Protrusion

Bimaxillary dental protrusion is a proclination of both upper and lower dentitions on a normal bony base.
The diagnosis is confirmed by measuring the interincisal angle.

Management

- Treatment consists of symmetric extraction of four first premolars and treatment with fixed appliance mechanotherapy. Results are more satisfactory than the treatment of bimaxillary prognathism.

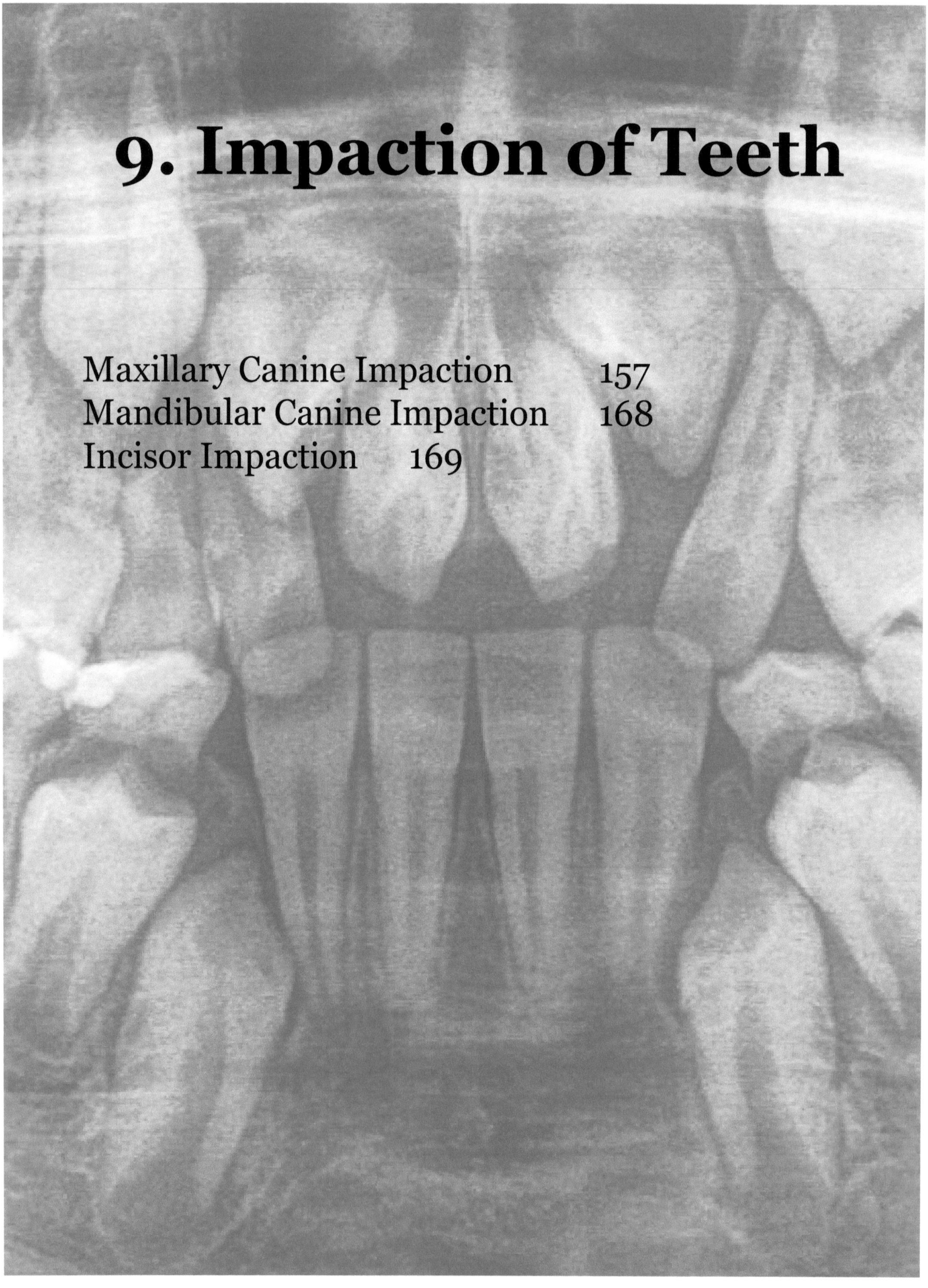

9. Impaction of Teeth

Tooth impaction is an intraosseously displaced position of the teeth and an abnormal eruption pathway that results in a prognosis of a delayed or failed eruption.
Impacted teeth are commonly found anomaly in dental practice.

Any tooth can be impacted, but the following are the most frequently impacted teeth:
• Mandibular third molars;
• Maxillary canines;
• Maxillary third molars;
• Maxillary and mandibular second premolars;
• Maxillary central incisors.

Maxillary Canine Impaction

Canines are prone to ectopic eruption and impaction because of their high and deep position in alveolar bone, their extended developmental period, and their long and tortuous eruption route. Adjacent teeth or other local factors may also narrow the eruption path of the canine because of its late appearance in the eruption sequence.

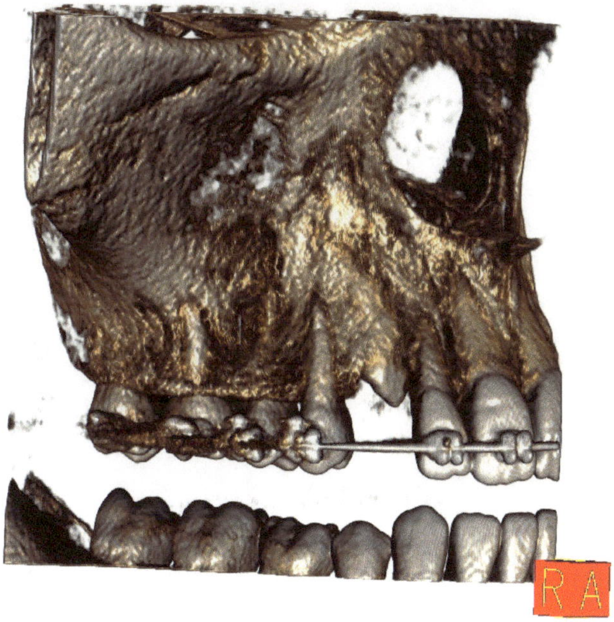

Figure 9.1 Impacted maxillary canine in an adult patient.

Prevalence

- In the maxilla is more than three times that in the mandible;
- maxillary canine impaction ranges between 1% and 3% of patients;
- For the mandibular canine, the incidence of impaction is about 0.35%;
- This anomaly is twice as common in females as it is in males;
- Most affected patients have unilaterally impacted maxillary canines, and only 8% have bilateral impactions;
- Canine impaction has a high family association and is five times more common in Europeans than in Asians;
- Buccal canine impactions are mostly associated with inadequate space and are positioned more vertically;
- Palatally impacted canines are positioned more horizontally.

Etiology

Guidance theory

Guidance theory contends that this anomaly develops because of the presence of local predisposing causes.

- Arch length deficiency;
- When there is arch length discrepancy or space loss in the maxillary canine area, the canine becomes impacted buccally;
- When the maxillary lateral incisor is missing, the canine becomes impacted palatally.

The following are the most common local factors that can cause canine impaction:

- Missing lateral incisor *(Figure 9.2)*;

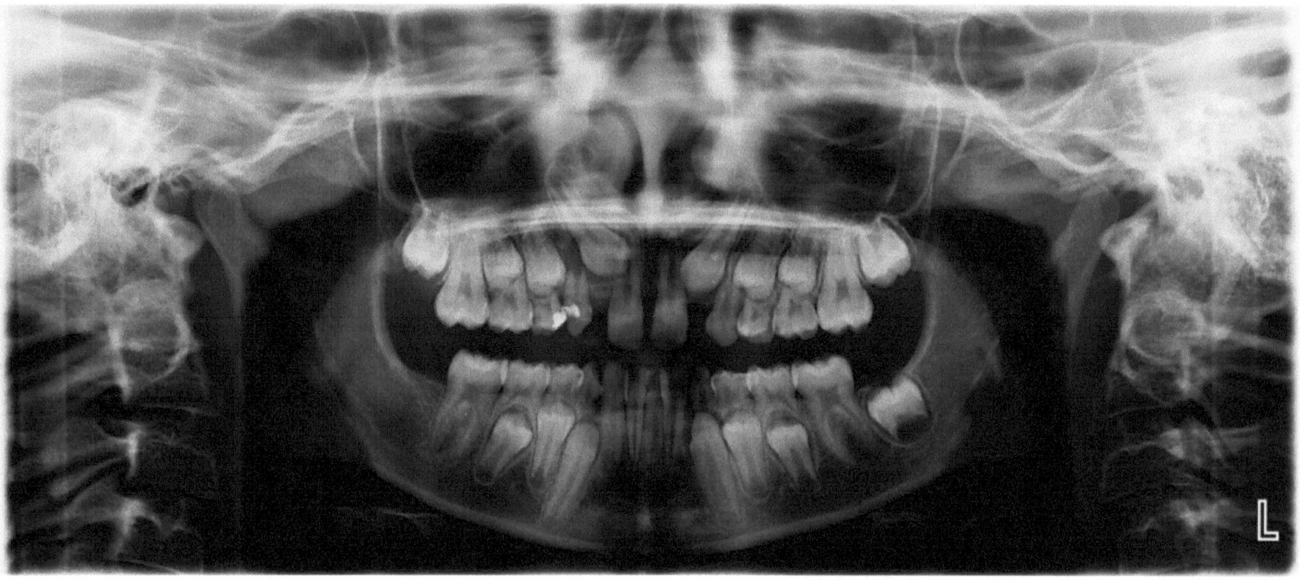

Figure 9.2 Impaction of an upper canine tooth with missing lateral incisor

- Peg-shaped lateral incisor;
- Supernumerary tooth or odontoma;
- Space deficiency;
- Dysplasia in the maxillary-premaxillary suture;
- Some Class II division 2 malocclusions.

Genetic theory

- According to genetic theory, disturbance of maxillary permanent canine eruption is due to an abnormal developmental condition of the dental lamina.

Factors associated with palatal impaction

- Space deficiency;
- Trauma;
- Overretention of the primary canine;
- Premature loss of the primary canine;
- Failure of the primary canine root to resorb, creating a potential mechanical obstacle for canine eruption;
- Abnormal position of the tooth bud;

- Disturbances in tooth eruption;
- Localized pathologic lesions such as cysts and odontomas;
- Abnormal sequence of eruption;
- Missing lateral incisors;
- Anomalous abnormal size of the lateral incisor or abnormal form of the lateral incisor roots (dilacerations of the root);
- Variation in the timing of lateral incisor root formation;
- Ankylosis of the permanent canine;
- Presence of a supernumerary tooth;
- Presence of an alveolar cleft.

Factors associated with labial canine impaction

- Space deficiency during the transitional dentition;
- Premature loss of the primary canine followed by a midline shift;
- Anterior dental crossbite that decreases the anterior arch circumferences;
- Deflecting the canine buccally;
- Ectopic migration of the permanent canine over the adjacent teeth;
- Overretention of the primary canine.

Consequences of impacted maxillary canines

- Migration of the adjacent teeth and loss of arch length;
- Development of cystic lesions and infection;
- Root resorption of the nearby lateral incisors;
- Overretention of primary canines.
- Loss of arch length;
- Transposition;
- Periodontal defects.

Diagnosis

Clinical examination

- Digital palpation of the buccal bulge of the canine in the sulcus above the primary canine root, Impaction of the permanent canine is indicated if the buccal canine bulge is not palpable in children older than 10 years and the primary canine is retained and shows no signs of mobility;
- Distobuccal inclination of the lateral incisors.

Clinical signs of canine impaction

- Delayed eruption of the permanent canine;
- Prolonged retention of the primary canine, especially asymmetric exfoliation of the primary canine;
- Absence of a normal labial canine bulge;
- Presence of a palatal bulge *(Figure 9.3)*;
- Distal tipping of the lateral incisor crown *(Figure 9.4)*;
- Retroclined position of the lateral incisor (if its root is forced buccally and its crown palatally by the palatally impacted canine).

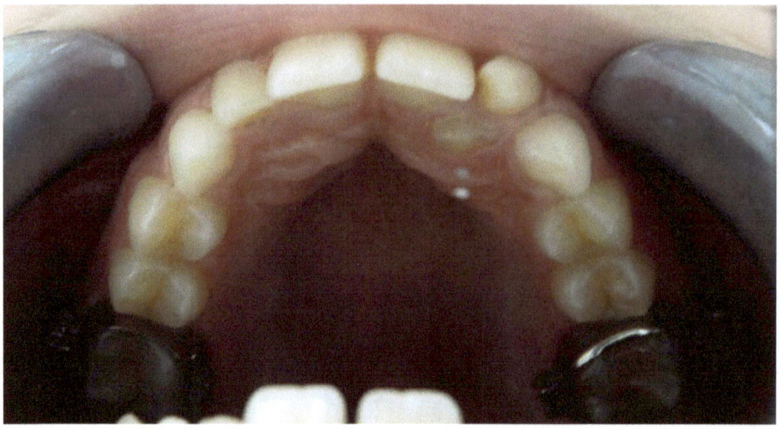

Figure 9.3 Palatal bulge of impacted canines

a b

c d

e f

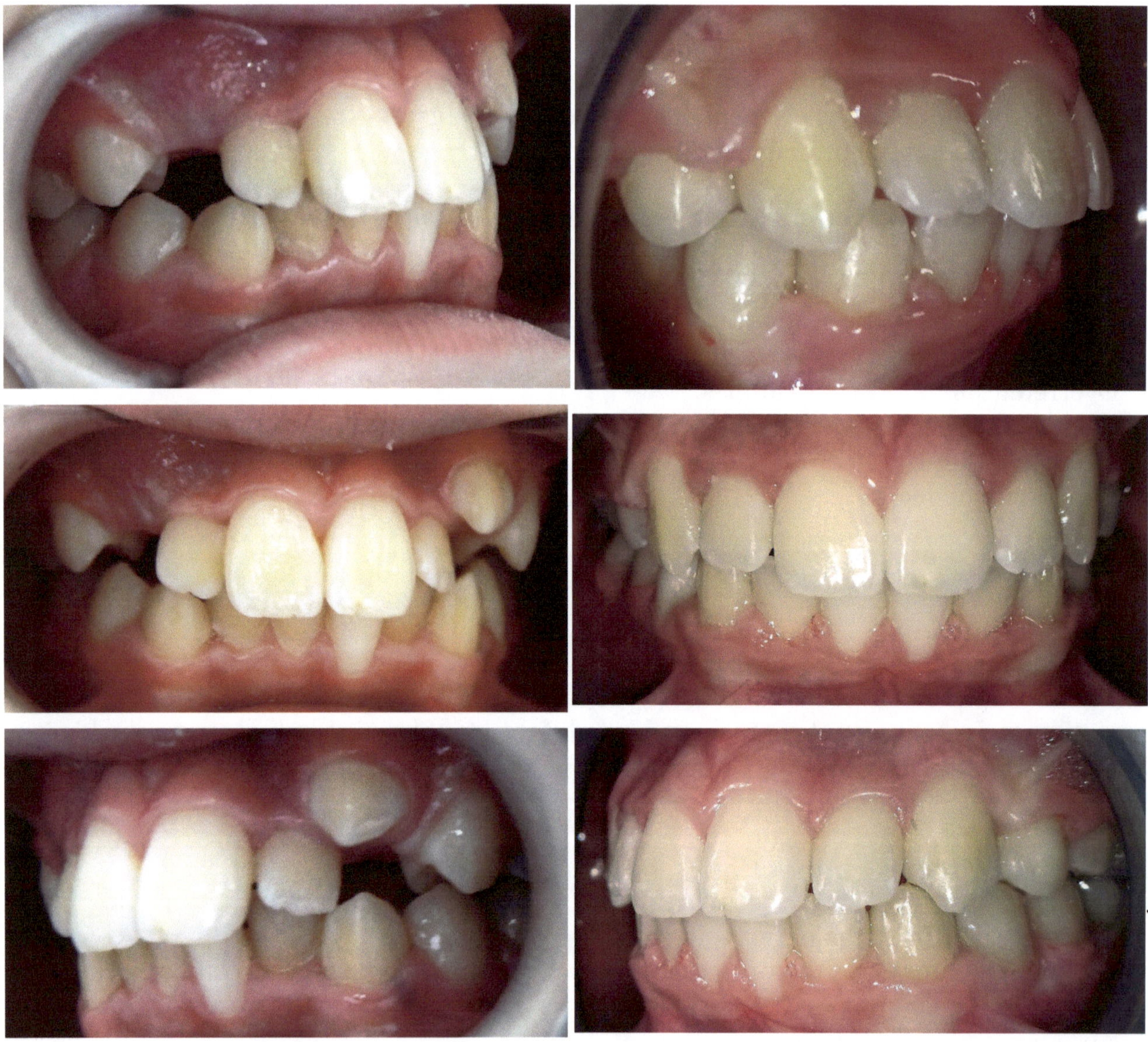

Figure 9.4 Distal tipping of lateral incisor under the pressure of impacted canine. Before treatment (a,b,c) and after treatment (d,e,f)

Radiographic evaluation

1. Periapical radiographs.
- Clark's rule technique - two different angulations are taken in the same horizontal plane. If the object moves to the same side of the angulation, the subject (in this case, the canine) is located more lingually (palatally); if it moves to the opposite direction, the object is more buccally positioned.

2. Occlusal radiographs.
- Determine the position of the involved tooth in the buccolingual and mesiodistal directions.

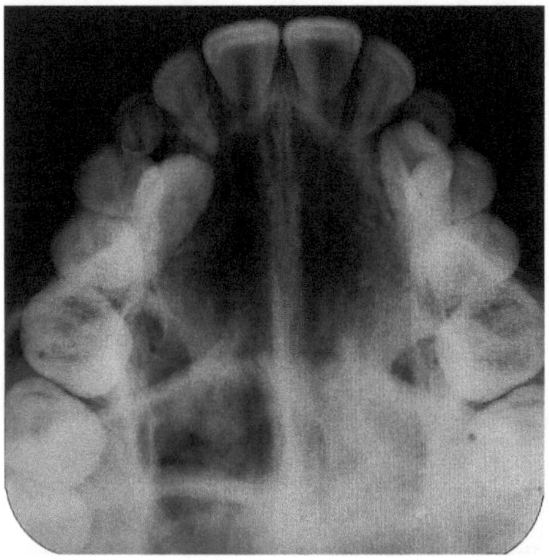

Figure 9.5 Impacted upper canine occlusal view.

3. Lateral and frontal cephalometric radiographs.
- Lateral cephalometric radiographs can show the anteroposterior position of the canine relative to the incisors;
- Frontal radiographs can show the vertical and lateral positions of the canines relative to the incisors.

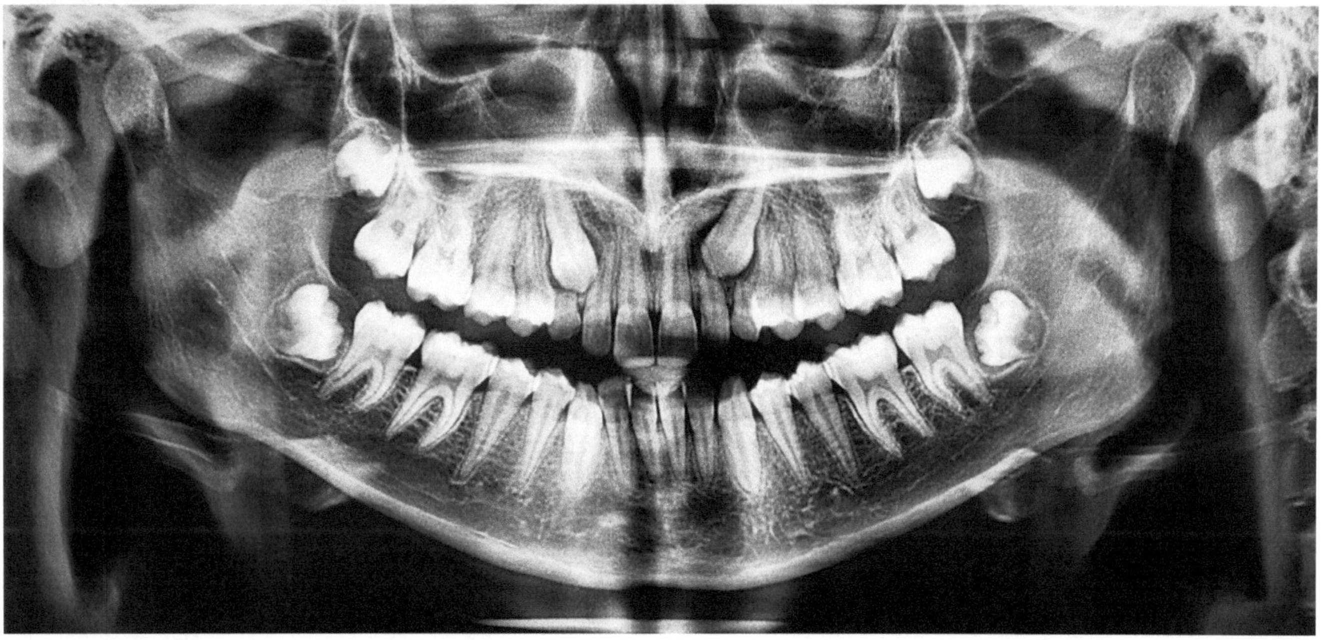

Figure 9.6 Panoramic radiograph of patient with impacted canines. Computed tomography scans of the same patient.

4. Computed tomography scans.

5. Panoramic radiographs.

- Show other developmental anomalies, such as supernumerary teeth, missing teeth, odontomas, other pathologic conditions, the conditions of the primary roots and their successors, and the conditions of permanent root development (*Figure 9.7*);

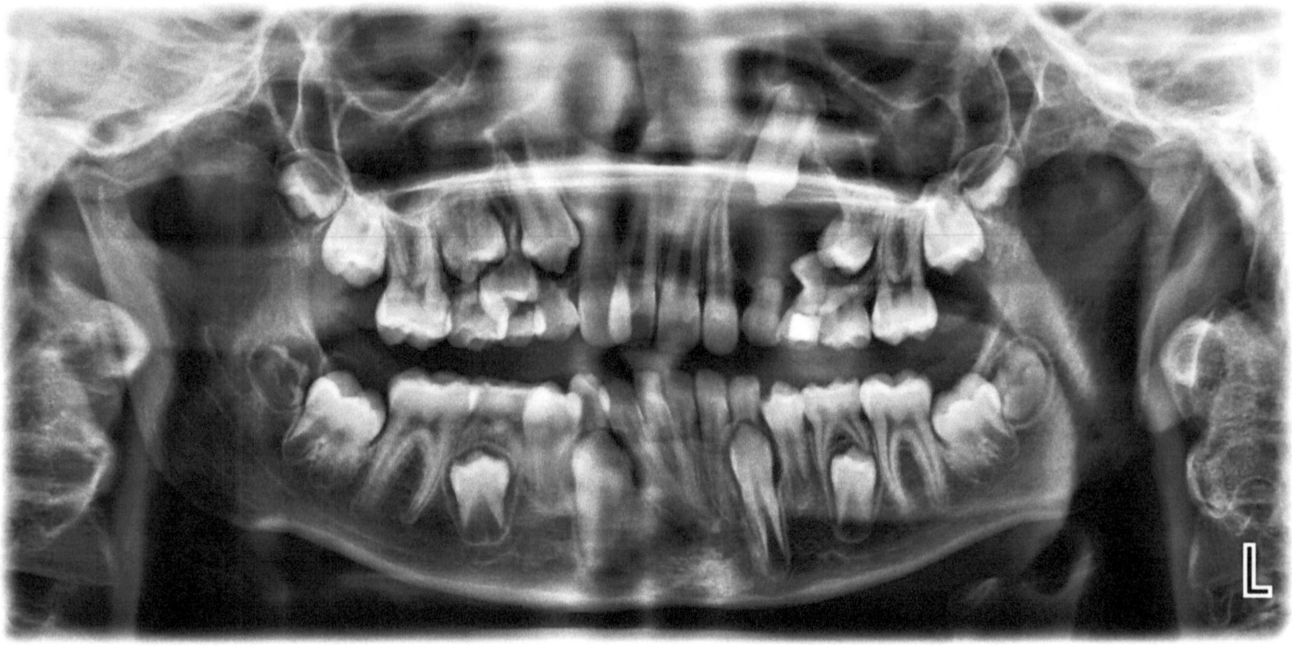

Figure 9.7 Cystic formation associated with impacted upper canine

- The film or the screen that captures the image is located palatally of two objects, the canine, and incisors;
- If the area of superimposition of the two images is dominated by the opacity representing the shape of the lateral incisor, it means that the lateral incisor is closer to the film, indicating that the canine is located more buccally;
- If the area is dominated by the opaque contours of the canine, it means that the canine is closer to the film, indicative of a more palatally positioned canine;
- If the tooth is angled more than 31 degrees relative to the midline, its chances of eruption after primary extraction are decreased.

Management

Treatment options for impacted maxillary canines are:

- Observation during the mixed dentition;
- Interceptive treatment;
- Surgical exposure of the canine and orthodontic treatment;
- Autotransplantation of the canine;
- Extraction of the impacted canine and space closure;
- Extraction of the impacted canine and prosthetic or implant replacement;
- Periodic radiograph observation (in adults when the impacted canine is located very high or horizontally and because of either high risk or the patient's desire for no treatment).

Observation should be done during the early mixed dentition stage

- If the canine does not show any change in position after 10 to 12 months and the possibility of lateral incisor root resorption is evident, exposure of the canine and bonding attachment for orthodontic traction is indicated;
- Age 8 years is the best time to begin observation of the maxillary canines and that the posi-

tional changes over the next 2 years require careful observation.

Treatment in the mixed and early permanent dentition

Interceptive treatment

Interceptive treatment, or guidance of eruption, for canine impaction is a series of procedures that should begin when the canine starts its long intrabony movement toward its final position. Interceptive options are:

- Removal of the obstacle causing deflection of the canine, such as a supernumerary tooth, odontoma, cyst, or ankylosed primary tooth;
- Creation of space, if space deficiency is the cause of this anomaly. Depending on the occlusion and age of the patient, different tactics can be applied for providing the necessary space:
  - Distalization of the buccal segment in some Class II mixed dentition treatment;
  - Correction of maxillary anterior dental crossbite if retroclination of the maxillary incisors has resulted in space deficiency for maxillary canines or if correction of crossbite increases the arch circumference in the anterior segment;
  - Closure of the space that sometimes remains between the incisors, even after the complete eruption of the lateral incisors.
- Extraction of the primary canine at the right time is advocated by many investigators in the following conditions:
  - The permanent canine is mesially displaced and does not follow the guidance of the lateral incisor root;
  - The permanent lateral incisor crown is somewhat distally inclined, indicating the presence of permanent canine crown force;
  - The buccal canine bulge cannot be palpated;
  - An over-retained primary canine is present and shows no signs of mobility.
- The next step in any case of canine guidance would be 2 × 4 bonding, slow alignment of the maxillary incisors, and closure of any diastema or dental spacing present between incisors to facilitate the eruption of the permanent canine;
- Surgical exposure of the canine and orthodontic treatment is the next step (*Figure 9.8*).

If impacted canines are in their final stage of development in the permanent dentition, the clinician must consider orthodontic treatment combined with surgical exposure of the canine to bring it into occlusion.

Pretreatment considerations.

An impacted canine can be located palatally or buccally, can be ectopic or nonectopic, and can be unilateral or bilateral; each of these situations requires different surgical techniques and different orthodontic approaches. Among the factors that must be considered are:

- The inclination of the impacted tooth;
- The position of the impacted crown and its proximity to adjacent teeth;
- The cause of impaction;
- The age of the patient and the amount of root development.

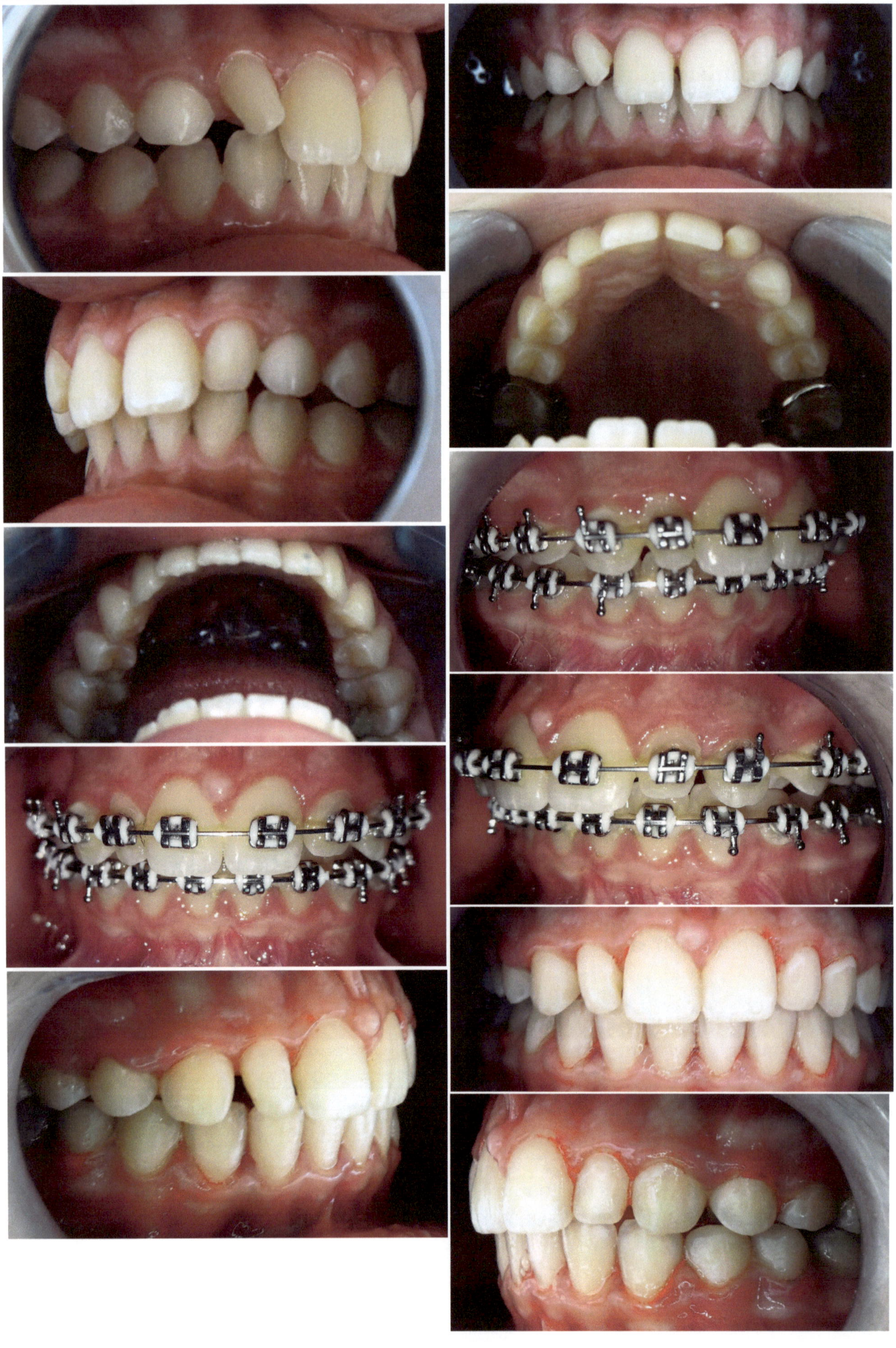

a *b* *c* *d* *e* *f* *g* *h* *i* *j* *k*

l 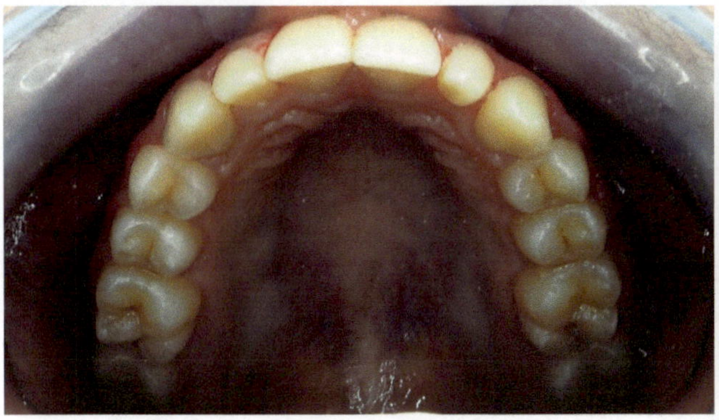 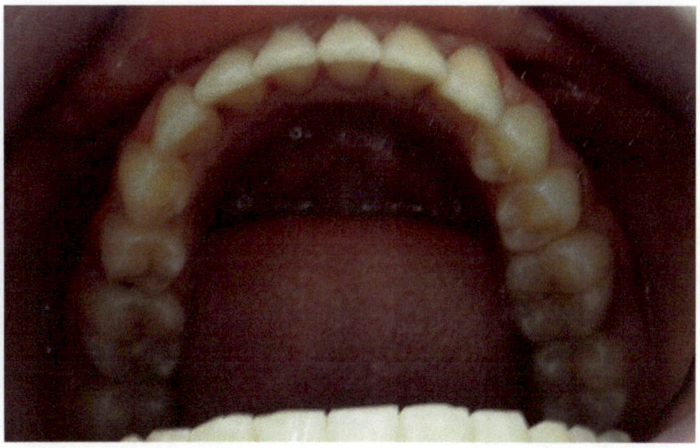 m

Figure 9.8 Before (a,b,c,d,e), during (f,g,h) and after (i,j,k,l,m) treatment of impacted canines in the upper arch.

Surgical approach

Basic orthodontic procedures for correction of canine impaction include:

1. Prepare complete records, including clinical and paraclinical examinations, to enable clear identification of the problem and design accurate surgical and orthodontic techniques;
2. Accomplish orthodontic preparation prior to surgical intervention; this can include leveling, correction of rotation, elimination of crowding, and creation of space for the impacted tooth if tipping of adjacent teeth has resulted in insufficient space (*Figure 9.9 a,b,c,d,e*);
3. After all orthodontic movement is completed, refer the case for surgical intervention. The surgical approach should be based on the buccal or palatal inclination and vertical position of the impacted tooth and its proximity to adjacent teeth (*Figure 9.9 f,g*);
4. After a week or more of post-surgical healing, initiate orthodontic movement of the crown toward the edentulous site (*Figure 9.9 h,i,j*);
5. Design the direction and the amount of force delivered for traction of the impacted tooth to smooth the eruption path and prevent any damage to the impacted tooth and its supporting structure as well as the adjacent teeth.

a 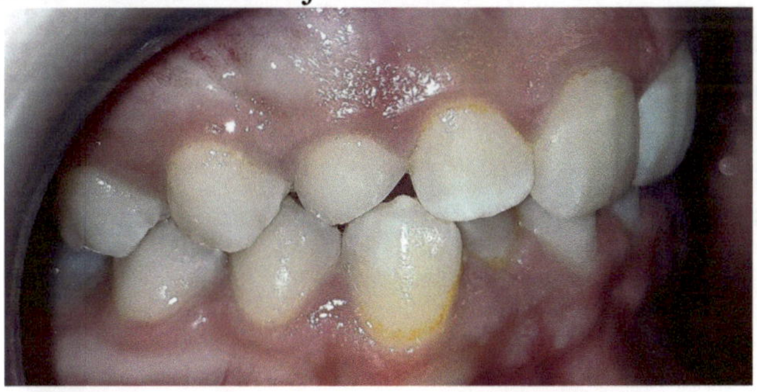 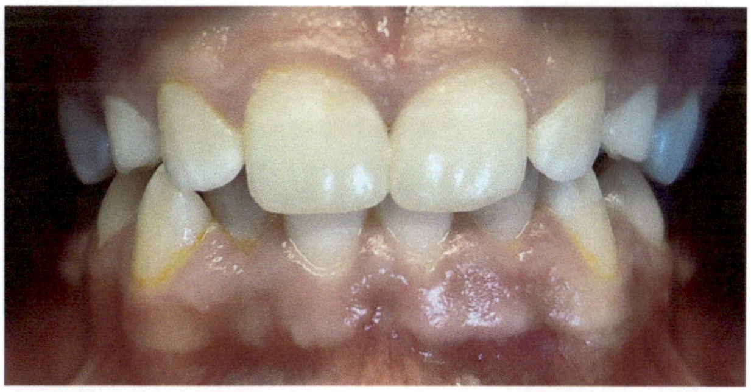 b

c 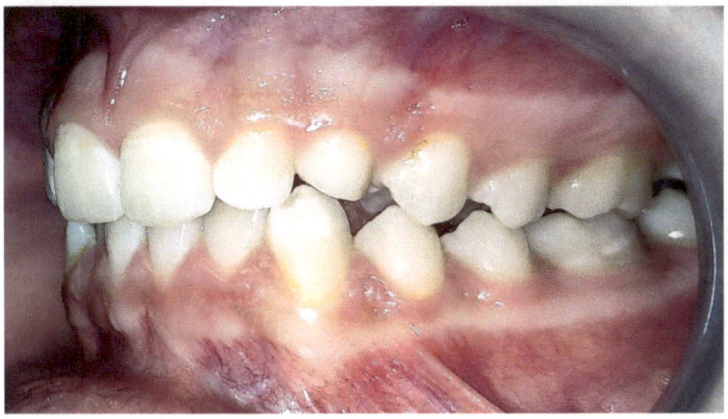 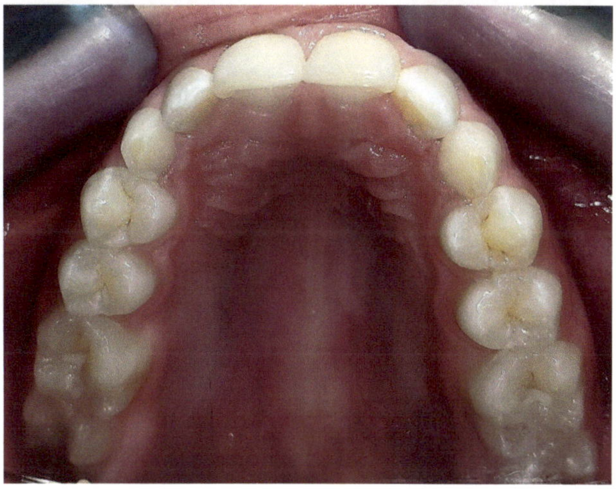 d

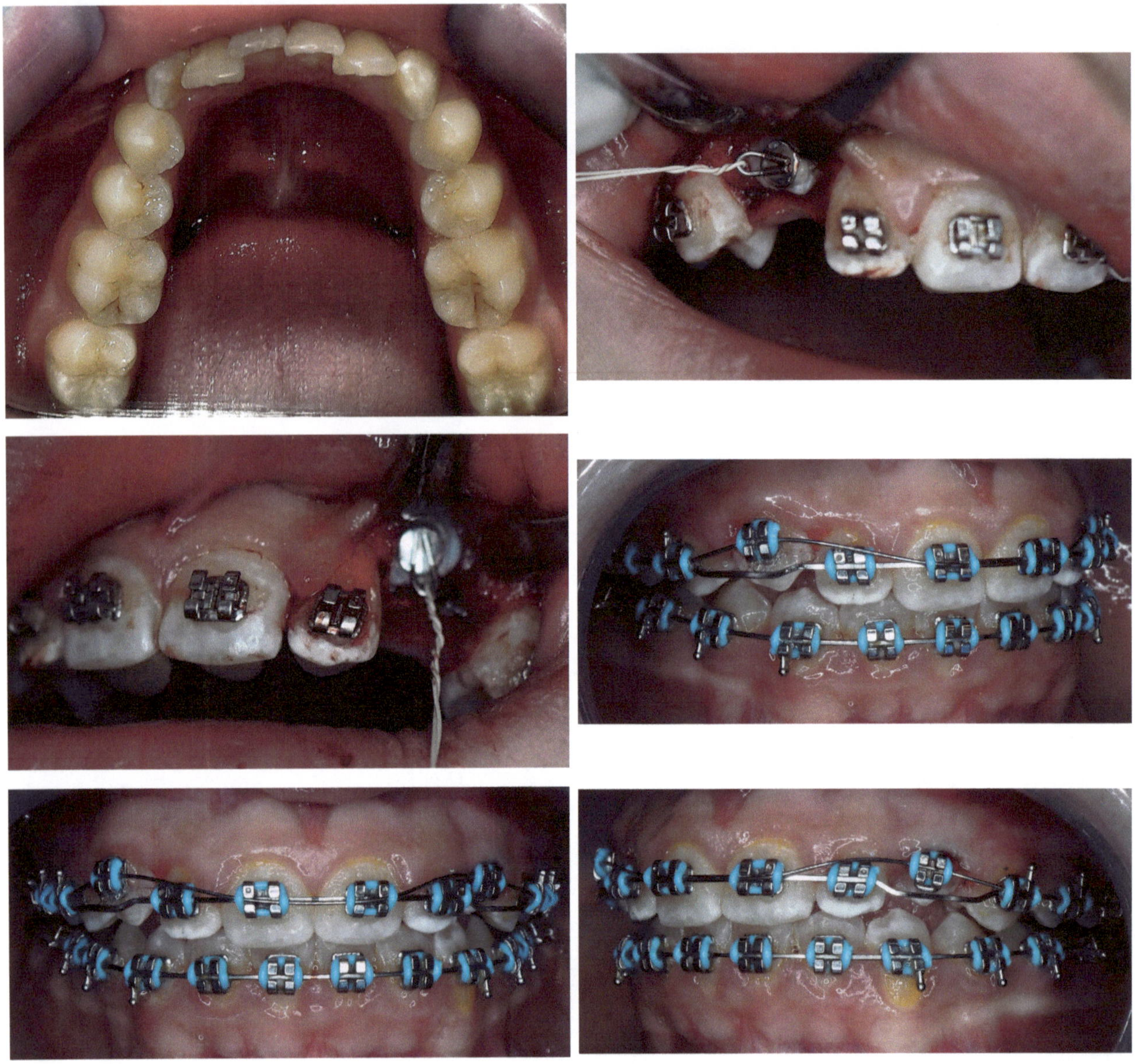

e f g h i j

Figure 9.9 Patient with two impacted upper canines before treatment (a,b,c,d,e). Surgical exposure (f,g). Orthodontic alignment of the canines (h,i,j).

Anchorage preparation. Use:

1. Modified transpalatal arch;
2. Mini-implant or vertical and horizontal loop;
3. Auxiliary labial archwire, spring or chain;
4. Elastic traction.

If tooth movement is not detectable after the application of reasonable orthodontic force for 2 to 3 weeks, ankylosis of the impacted tooth is confirmed. The best option in this situation is the extraction of the ankylosed canine and substitution with the first premolar in that quadrant.

Autotransplantation of the canine

- When the impacted tooth is ankylosed;
- If the patient desires to minimize or eliminate orthodontic treatment;
- When the patient has a physical or mental disability and may benefit from limitation or elimination of orthodontic treatment;

Complications associated with autotransplantation include
- Root resorption;
- Devitalization;
- Pulpal obliteration;
- Ankylosis of the transplanted tooth.

Extraction of the impacted canine and space closure or prosthetic replacement

Indications for extraction
- When the tooth is impacted very deeply and severely inclined;
- When the tooth's position and proximity to incisor roots contraindicate any tooth movement;
- When the impacted tooth is ankylosed and patient compliance is not sufficient for transplantation.

Management in the permanent dentition

In some situations, impacted canines may go undetected by the patient or patient refused early treatment. Most often primary canine has not been exfoliated and plays an esthetic role in the smile.
Reasons for adults to seek treatment for impacted canine
- Loss of primary canine;
- Esthetic concerns with the small primary canine;
- Esthetic concerns with missing tooth and space in the arch if a primary tooth is lost;
- Sometimes impacted canines can erupt at a later age.

Treatment options

Orthodontic treatment with surgical exposure and traction of the canine

- The first stage is to align the arches using fixed appliance therapy;
- When we have the space needed for the canine, the patient undergoes surgical exposure and bonding of the impacted tooth;
- If the impacted canine crown is with close contact with incisor root we can perform surgery before bonding of the other teeth;
- The impacted tooth is moved away from the root before incisor movement is initiated;
- For anchorage we can use a TPA with loops for hooking elastics from impacted canine;
- The orthodontic eruption of the canine is done with auxiliary wires like ballista spring (made of 0.018-inch Stainless steel or 0.016 x 0.022 inch SS wire) *(Figure 9.10);*

a *b*

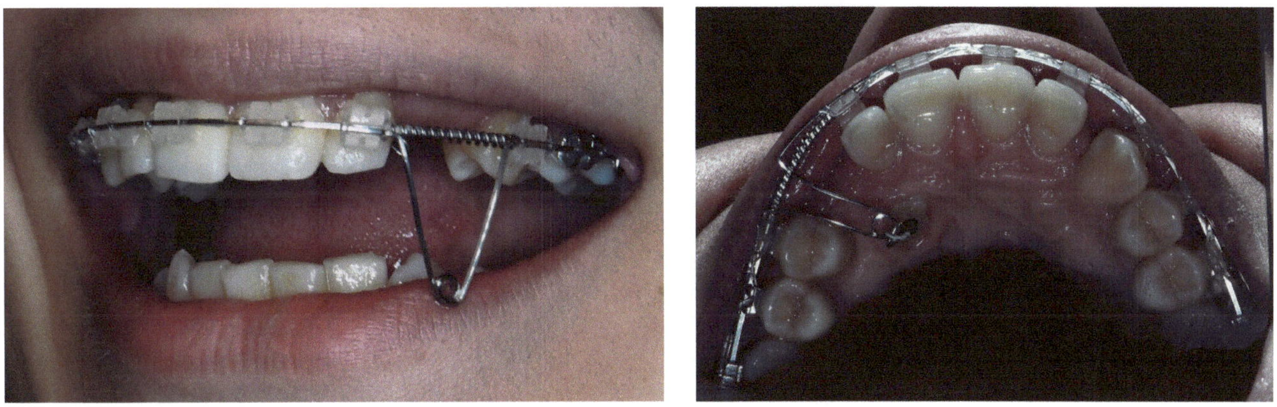

Figure 9.10 Ballista spring before activation (a), activated (b).

- After the eruption of the canine, we perform traction with elastics or soft piggy back wire;
- Canine brought to the arch is ligated and aligned;
- Additional torqueing bends or springs may be used for torque control.

Extraction of the impacted tooth and space closure

- Space closure is indicated when we have Class II malocclusion with protruding upper front teeth;
- In open bite cases extraction can aid to bite correction;
- If the canine is anchylosed.

Extraction and implant replacement

- Ankylosed canine;
- The patient does not want orthodontic treatment.

Mandibular Canine Impaction

Mandibular canine impaction is rare compared with maxillary canine impaction (*Figure 9.12*).

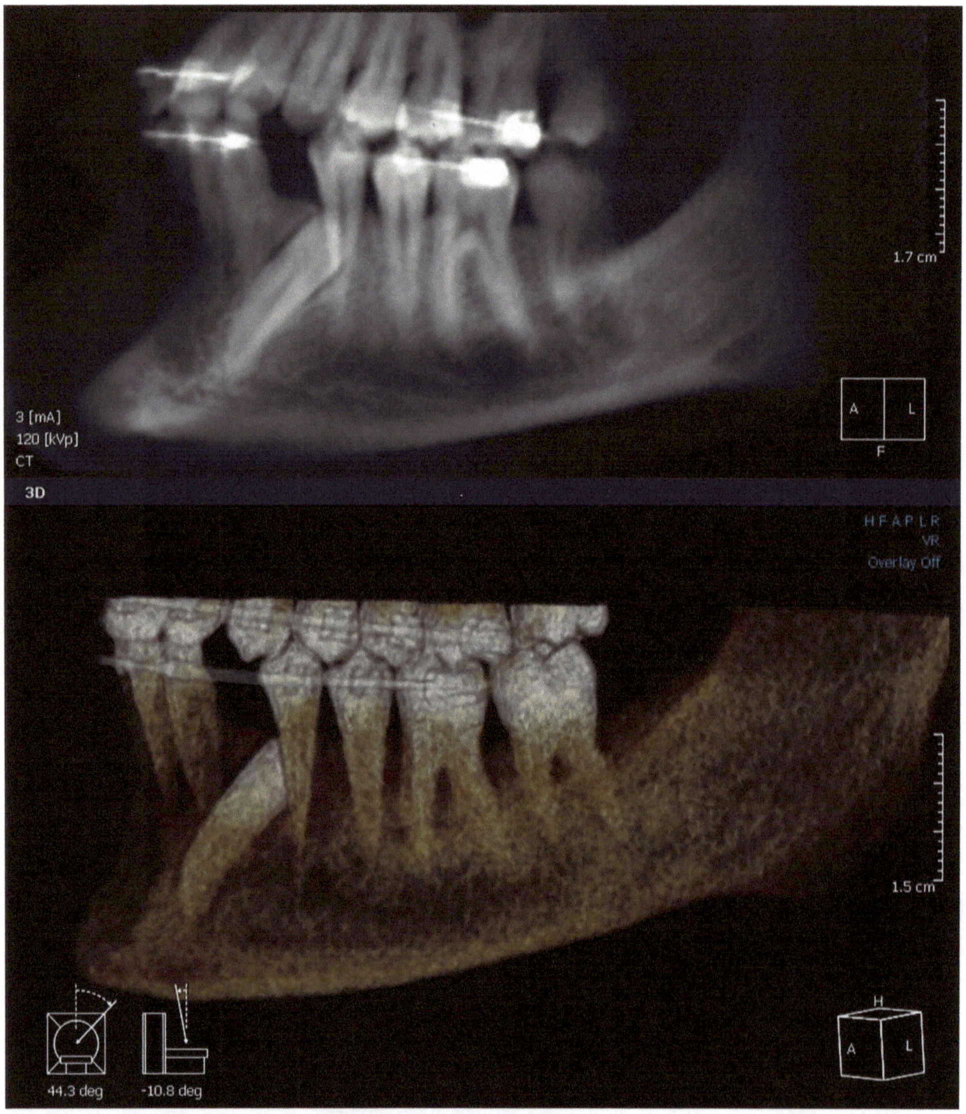

Figure 9.11 Impacted mandibular canine

Factors for impaction of mandibular canines

- Inadequate space;
- The presence of a supernumerary tooth or odontoma;
- Premature loss of the primary canine;
- Hereditary factors;
- Functional disturbances of the endocrine glands, tumors, cysts, and trauma.

Management options for mandibular impaction

- Interceptive treatment
  - If we detect on radiograph lower canine with an inclination of 30° to the midline, we should extract primary canine and if indicated, extract primary first molar on the problem side.
- Observation
  - Indicated if the canine is deeply impacted and asymptomatic and no associated pathosis is evident. Periodic radiographic follow-up is necessary;
  - In this situation, if the primary canine is in good condition and has a good root length, it can be maintained in the arch.
- Exposure and orthodontic traction;
- Autotransplantation;
- Extraction.

Incisor Impaction

Impaction of the anterior teeth creates occlusal problems and can have serious dental, esthetic, and psychological consequences for patients.

Etiology of incisor impaction

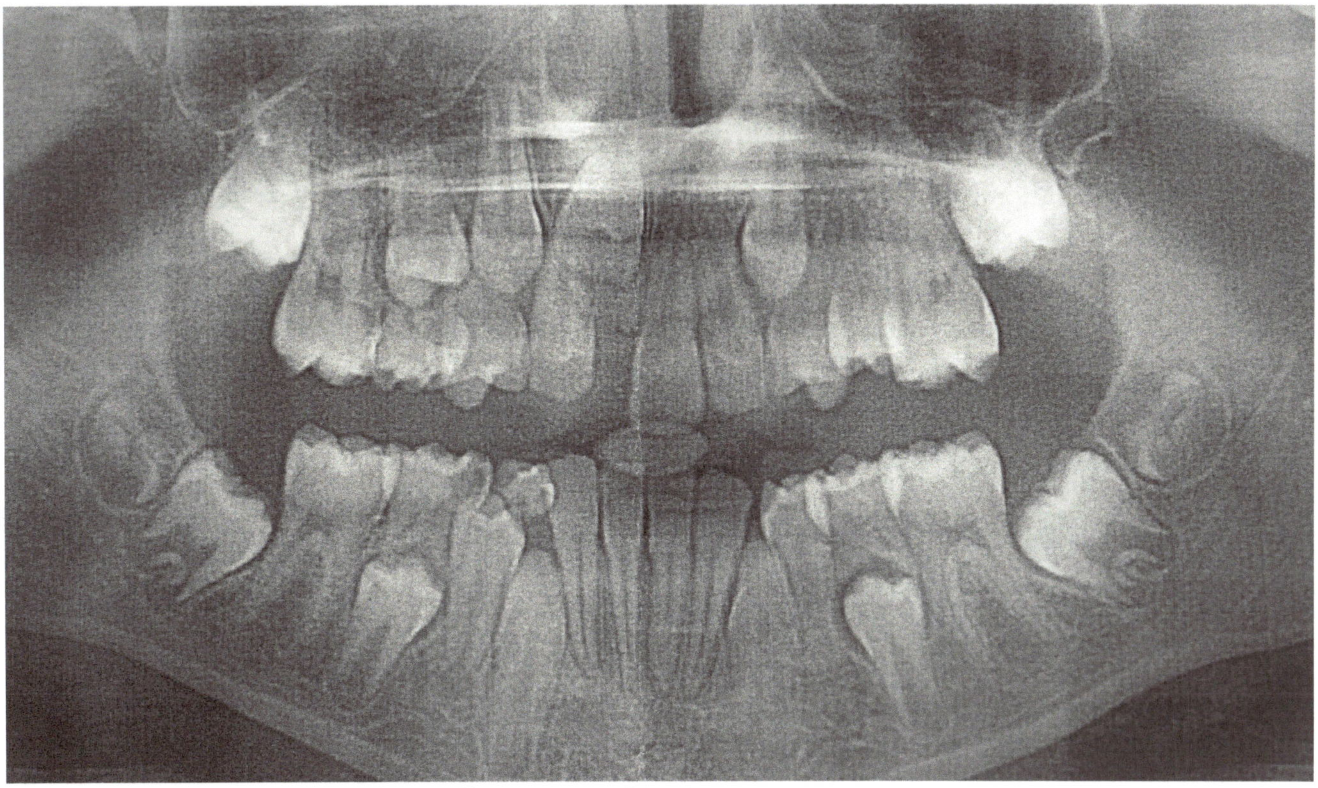

Figure 9.12 Dilaceration of maxillary central incisor

Trauma

- Trauma to the maxillary primary anterior teeth can be the reason for permanent tooth bud displacement, root dilaceration, complete arrest of root formation, enamel dysplasia, retarded eruption, failure of eruption, impaction, and transposition;
- Radiographic follow-up for children who suffered dental trauma at an early age is important to monitor possible sequelae in the permanent successors even before their eruption.

Supernumerary teeth or odontomas

- The best management is early detection and extraction of any supernumerary and primary teeth, if present, and maintaining the space for permanent tooth eruption;
- After removal of the supernumerary tooth and space maintenance, spontaneous eruption of the permanent incisors occurs.

Hypodontia or peg-shaped lateral incisors

- Congenital absence or abnormal shape of the lateral incisors also disrupts anterior tooth eruption, resulting in problems such as diastema and canine impaction.

Bone barriers or fibrotic tissue

Sclerotic tissue or dense bone that covers incisors, which is common following the premature loss of primary incisors, can interfere with the normal eruption pattern of incisors.

This can result in:
- Delayed eruption;
- Space loss and consequently crowding of the incisors;
- An abnormal sequence of eruption;
- Impaction of the incisors.

Space loss can result in:
- Crowding of the permanent incisors;
- Delayed eruption;
- Failed eruption;
- Impaction of the incisors.

Diagnosis

- Delayed exfoliation of primary incisors;
- Delayed eruption of permanent incisors;
- Asymmetric eruption of permanent incisors;
- Severe diastemata;
- Abnormal sequence of eruption (eg, eruption of maxillary lateral incisors before central incisors).

Interceptive treatment for incisor impaction

- Recognition of the cause: radiographic examination;
- Elimination of the cause, such as extraction of a supernumerary tooth or an odontoma, maintenance or regaining of necessary space for the permanent incisors, or removal of bone

barriers or fibrotic tissue that is preventing eruption;

- After removal of the obstacle, maintenance of the space for permanent eruption and prevention of a midline shift;
- If there is no significant progress of permanent tooth eruption after the elimination of the cause and maintenance of the necessary space for 6 to 12 months, surgical exposure and orthodontic traction of the impacted incisor to the normal position is the only option.

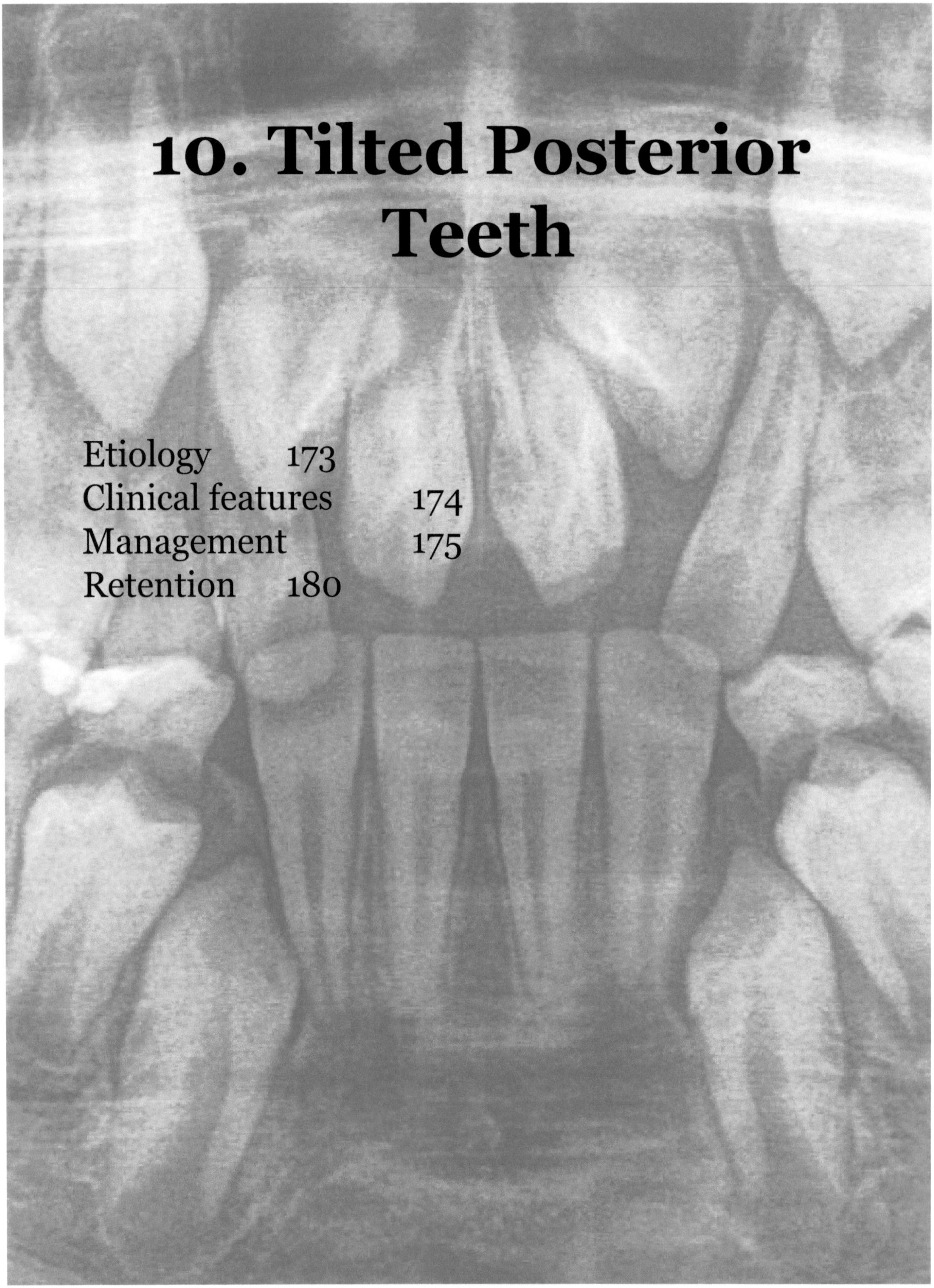

10. Tilted Posterior Teeth

The most common tilted tooth is the lower second molar. Although always mesially inclined, the degree of tilt is variable and often has a lingual component.

Etiology

The tilted molar results from loss of arch integrity at a site immediately mesial to it.

- Missing teeth *(Figure 10.1)* ;
  - The first mandibular molar is probably the most common tooth to be lost, thus rendering the second molar the most commonly tilted tooth.

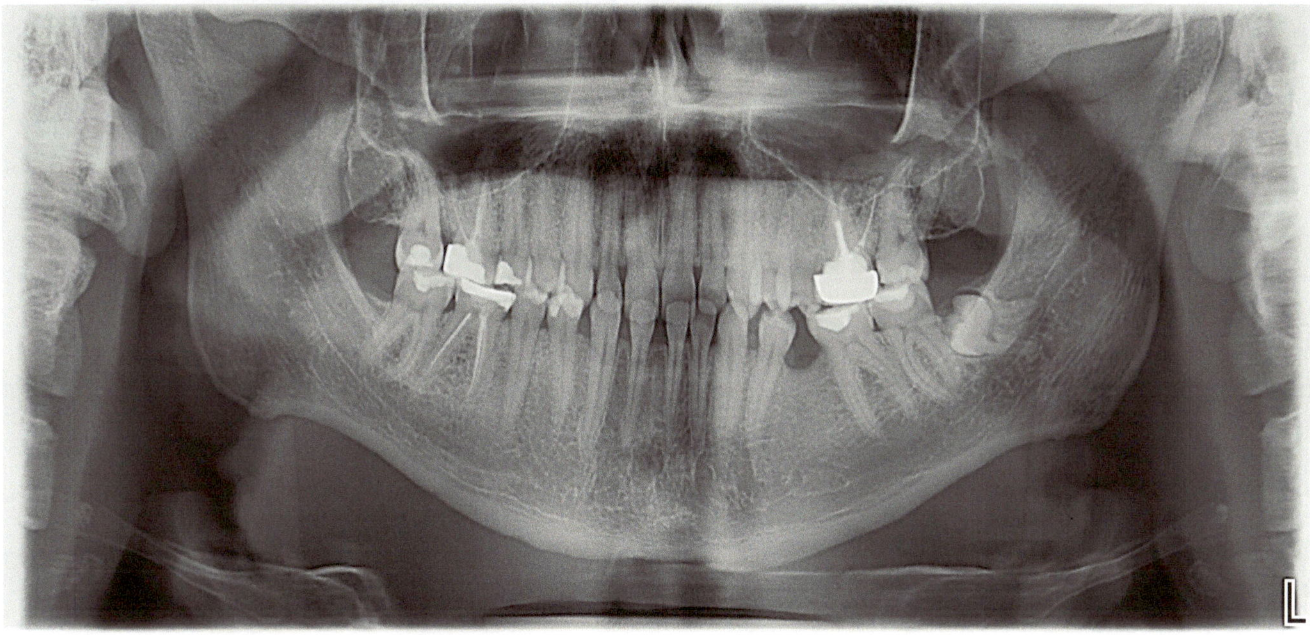

Figure 10.1 Tilted first mandibular molars because of agenesis of second premolars

- Loss of tooth tissue *(Figure 10.2)*;
  - Proximal caries - mesial movement of the posterior tooth into the carious cavity will occur as the unchecked response to the anterior component of force.

a *b*

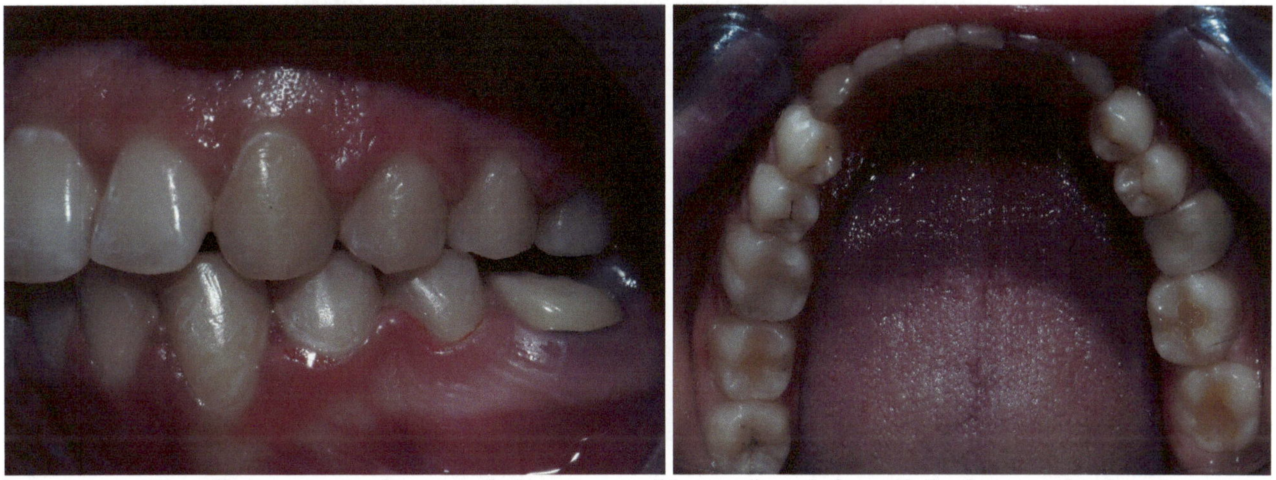

Figure 10.2 Smaller restoration made because of loss of arch length before orthodontic treatment. Space gained after treatment (a, b)

- Ectopic eruption *(Figure 10.3)*;
  - Ectopic eruption of a second premolar is usually due to the early loss of its deciduous predecessor;

- The first permanent molar tilts mesially before the second premolar erupts into the arch;
- The premolar then has insufficient space in the arch and erupts ectopically, usually on the lingual.

a *b*

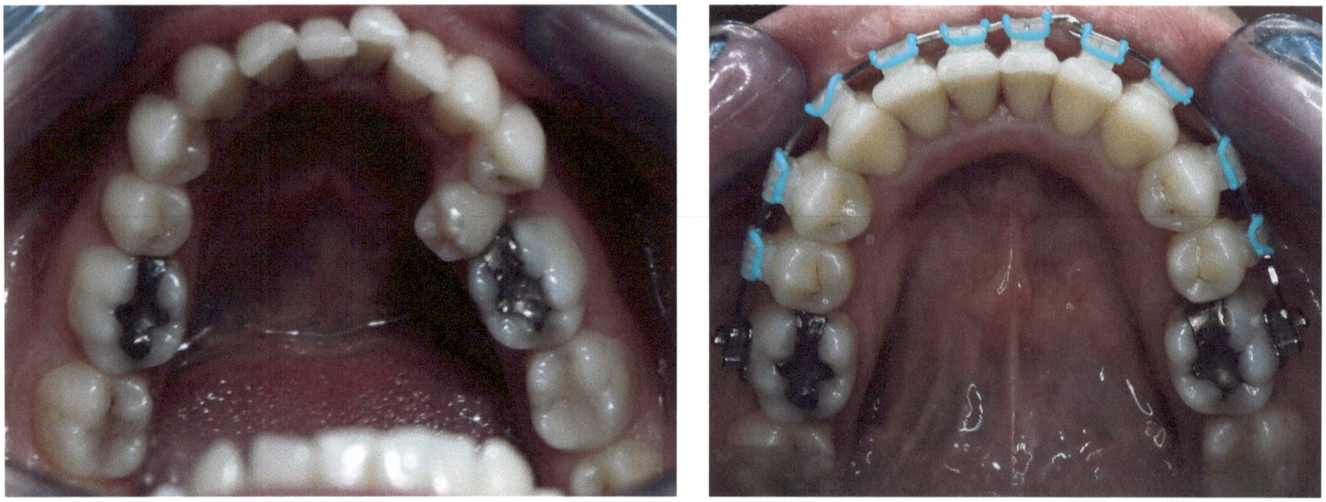

Figure 10.3 Lingual position of the second mandibular premolar because of loss of arch length. Before treatment (a), during treatment(b).

Clinical features

Tilting of the molar

- If teeth which normally occlude with a tilted molar be missing, supraversion of the tilted tooth will also occur.

Tilting of the premolar

- The premolar usually tilts distally,
- Distal tilting does not occur in the following circumstances:

1. In a Class II malocclusion where the contact exists between upper and lower canines;
2. When the tongue may be inserted into an extraction space where more than one tooth has been removed. This has the effect of limiting the distal movement.

Space loss.

- Tilting of a molar and premolar toward each other reduces the space previously occupied by the extracted tooth;
- It is impossible to restore the space with a pontic of normal size.

Transfer of forces

A tilted tooth cannot withstand vertical occlusal forces in an efficient way, since occlusal forces are not transferred through the vertical axis of the tooth *(Figure 10.4)*.

Changes in the occlusal plane are caused by premature contacts

- Infrabony pocket is formed;
- Alveolar crest height is reduced;
- Supraversion of the opposing tooth.

Prevention

- The missing tooth should be replaced as soon as possible by a fixed or removable partial denture;
- A space maintainer should be placed until permanent restoration can be made *(Figure 10.5)*.

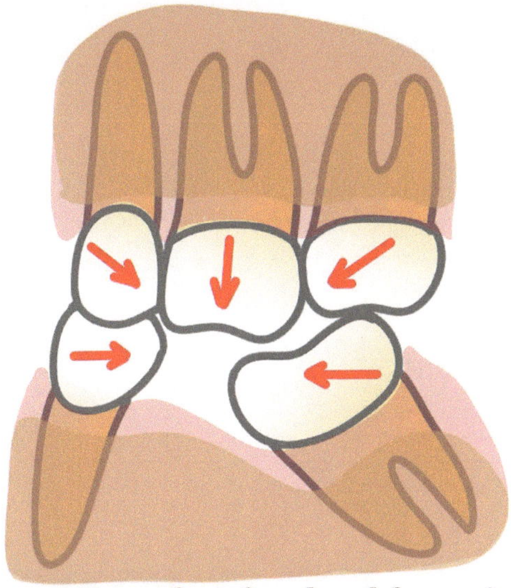

Figure 10.4 Transfer of occlusal forces in the circumstances of a missing tooth.

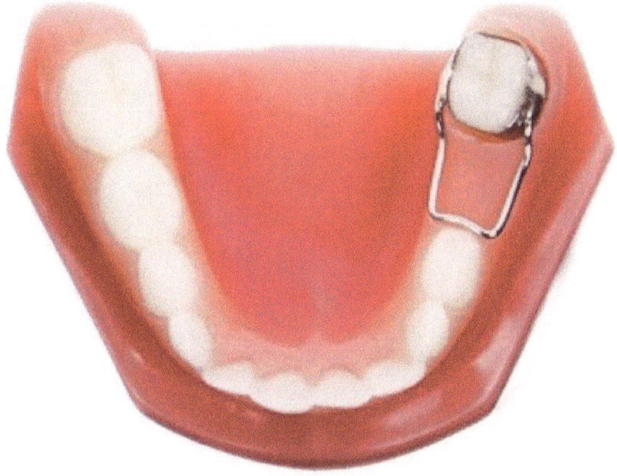

Figure 10.5 Band and loop space maintainer

Management

Possible tooth movements include:
- Mesial or distal movement of crown or root or both;
- Correction of axial inclination of the teeth adjacent to the area of tooth loss;
- Correction of the buccolingual position of crown and root;
- Correction of rotation and occlusal movement of individual teeth if required.

Other considerations:
- Space available for tooth movement;
- The absence or presence and position of antagonist teeth;
- The number of teeth to be moved.

In most cases, the tooth position can be corrected in 10-14 weeks.

Treatment in the mixed dentition

Appliances

- Removable appliances can be used;
  - Hawley appliance with screw positioned mesial to the tilted tooth is a good option if space is lost and needs to be reopened *(Figure 10.6)*;
  - Removable devices are easier to construct;
  - They may be used to tip individual teeth mesially, distally, buccally, and palatally with great efficiency;
  - They cannot move teeth bodily, nor can they produce root movement;
  - They can be used to temporarily increase the occlusal vertical dimension, clearing the teeth to be moved from occlusal interference;

- The insertion of a Hawley-type device with a bite plane has the effect of separating the teeth.

- 2 x 4 bonding can be used

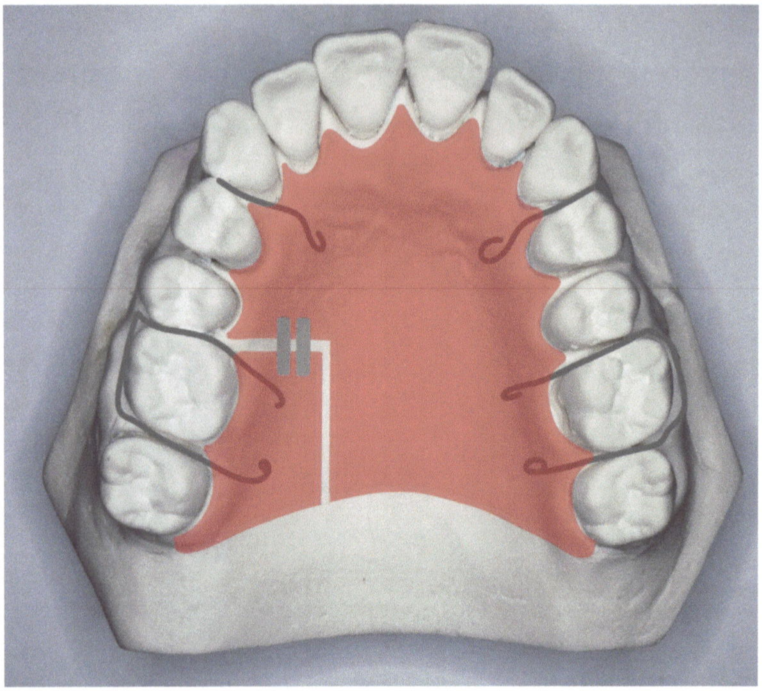

Figure 10.6 Hawley type space regainer

Management in the permanent dentition

Both removable and fixed orthodontic devices are suitable for the movement of teeth in the adult. The fixed appliance technique provides us with more options. When treating tilted teeth there will be an anchor unit and an active unit.

Anchor unit

- To provide a resistance, all the teeth as far forward as the canine in the treatment quadrant should be bonded;
- The canine on the contralateral side of the arch should also be bonded and linked to the anchor unit by a bonded canine-to canine lingual arch;
- This is mandatory in the mandibular arch and may be advisable in the maxillary arch;
- The teeth in the anchor unit should be ligated together securely;
- Lingual attachments on bicuspids may be useful for correcting minor rotations.

Active unit

- The molars to be uprighted should also be banded and carry brackets or tubes;
- Lingual attachments should be placed to help correct or prevent unwanted rotations.

Plain archwire with compressed coil spring (Figure 10.7)

- If a straight wire of suitable dimensions can be placed, a coil spring between the tipped molar and distal bicuspid will upright the molar by distal crown movement;
- The reciprocal forces will move the anchor teeth mesially;
- Light forces should be employed, and occlusal interferences, if any, should be removed at regular intervals;

- It is recommended that a wire of sufficient stiffness 0·018 or 0·017 x 0·022 inch, should be used.

Helical uprighting spring (Figure 10.8)

- Fabricated from a medium-size rectangular wire;
- May be used to upright a single tipped terminal molar;
- The spring causes considerable occlusal as well as distal crown movement;
- This appliance should only be used when the terminal molar has an occlusal antagonist;
- Frequent occlusal adjustments are necessary to reduce developing interferences.

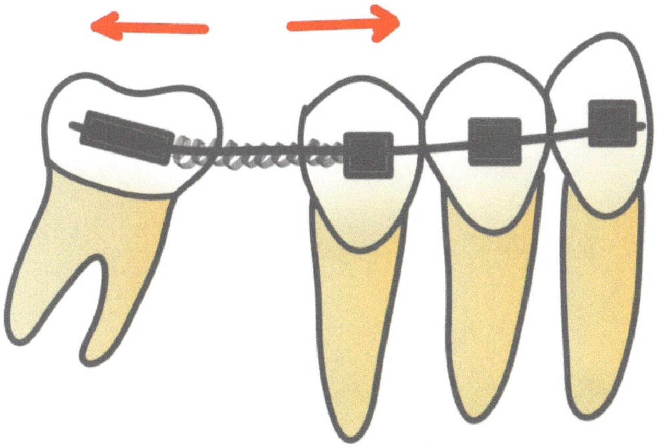

Figure 10.7 Plain archwire with compressed coil spring.

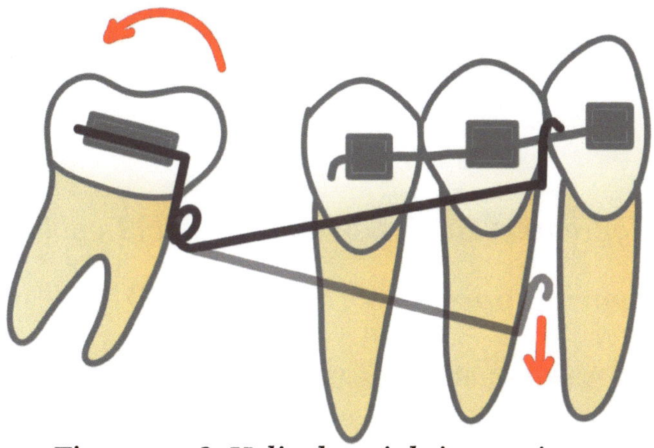

Figure 10.8 Helical uprighting spring.

Single T-loop appliance (Figure 10.9)

- Fabricated from a light rectangular wire;
- This spring may be used to upright a single terminal molar with or without an antagonist;
- The wire may be adjusted to control the teeth in all three planes;
- The molar is uprighted by distal crown movement, or if the T-loop is activated in an antero-posterior direction, by mesial root movement (Figure 10.10).

a

b

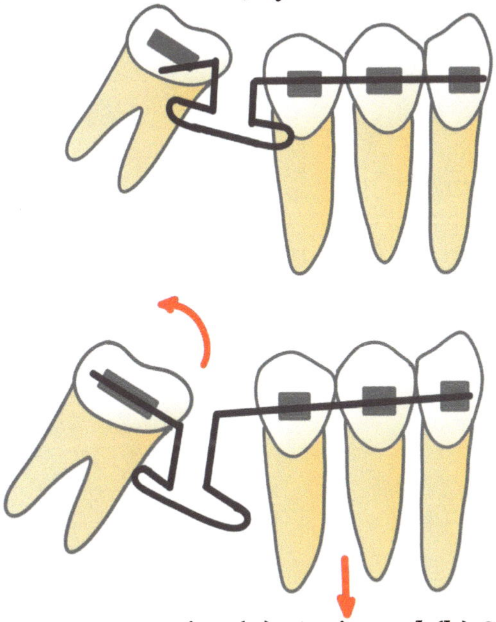

Figure 10.9 Passive (a), Activated (b) Single T-loop appliance.

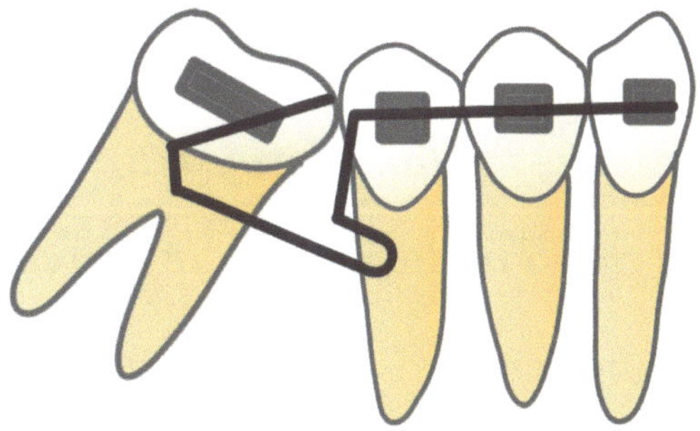

Figure 10.10 Distal T-loop uprighting spring.

Double T-loop appliance (Figure 10.11)

- Fabricated from a light rectangular wire and used to upright two tipped molars, either by distal crown movement or mesial root movement;
- Careful attention must be paid to the available anchorage.

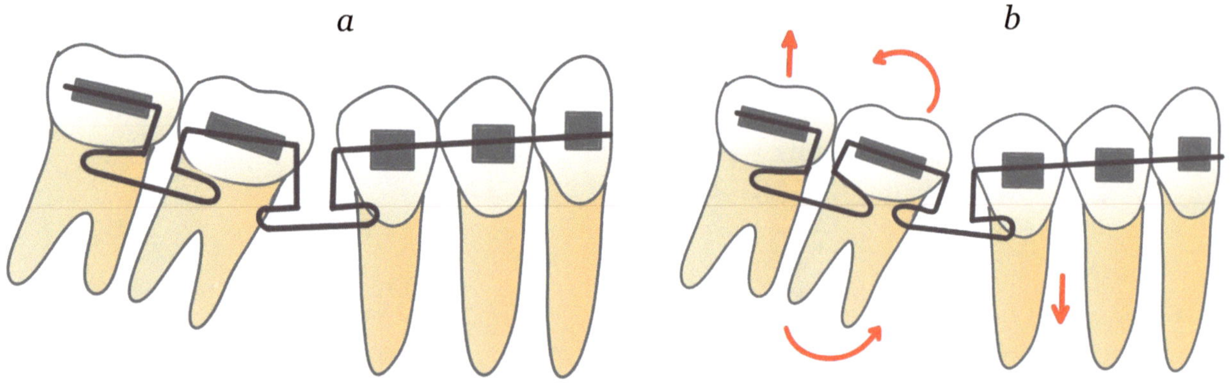

Figure 10.11 Passive (a), Activated (b) Double T-loop appliance.

Box spring appliance (Figure 10.12)

- An alternative design to the double T-loop and may be used when the vestibular depth is shallow. The most frequent problems encountered with these appliances are soft tissue irritations from the loops;
- Unwanted movement of anchor teeth is minimized by using light forces and incorporating an across-arch stabilizing splint.

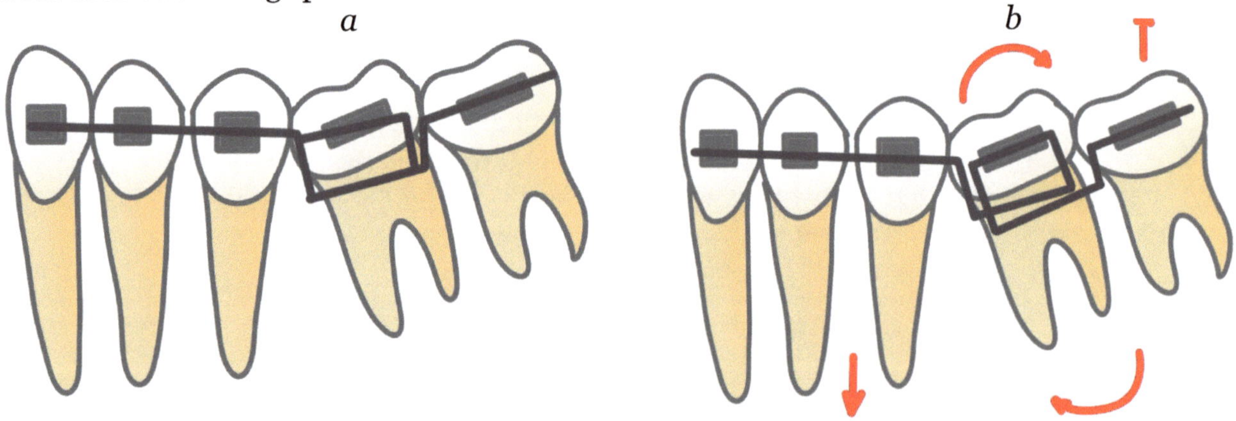

Figure 10.12 Passive (a), Activated (b) Box spring appliance.

Uprighting tilted molars using inverted piggy back wire (Figure 10.13)

- The main archwire is used to anchorage all other teeth except the tilted molar;
- Another light round NiTi wire is ligated to all the brackets and passes the buccal tube of the molar and is inserted from the distal end.

Uprighting molars using miniscrew anchorage

1. *Direct anchorage:*

- In direct anchorage the force is applied directly from the miniscrew to the molar to be uprighted;

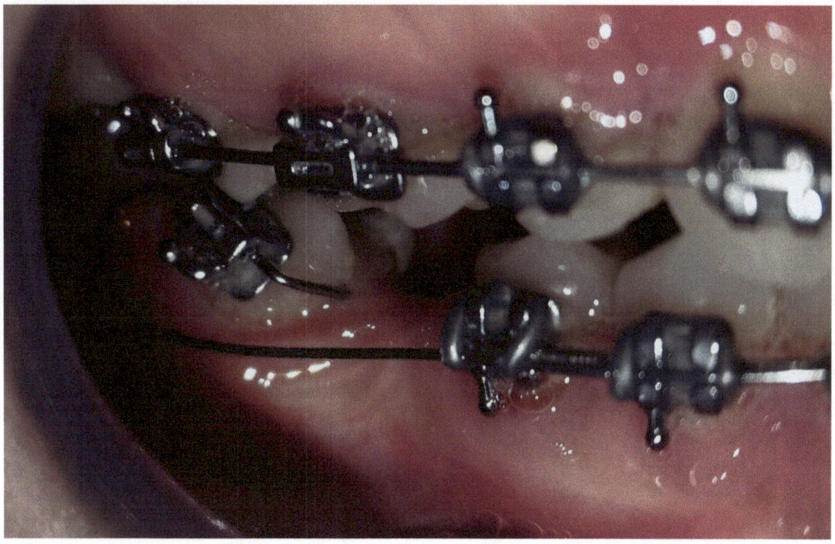

Figure 10.13 Inverted accessory wire inserted from the distal end of the molar tube

Uprighting with intrusion.

- Two miniscrews are vertically positioned on the alveolar crest area and a bracket is bonded on a resin uniting the two miniscrews (*Figure 10.14*);

a b c

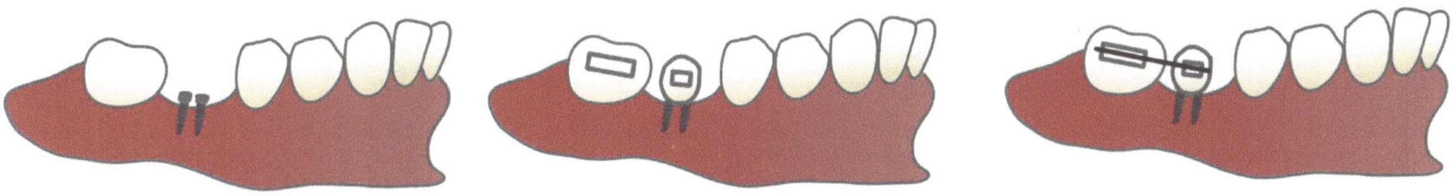

Figure 10.14 Direct anchorage with two miniscrews. Two miniscrews inserted on the alveolar crest (a), Bracket bonded on miniscrews (b), 0.017 x 0.025 –inch TMA wire activated (c)

- A segment of .017 x .025" TMA wire from this bracket to the molar tube is activated in order to result in uprighting spring or a .017 x .025" stainless steel segment of wire with an uprighting spring;
- Another option of direct anchorage includes the use of a cantilever direct activated on the miniscrew (*Figure 10.15*);
- The cantilever consists of a piece of wire with one end inserted into the tube of the molar and the other end is tied to the miniscrew;
- Wire used is TMA .017 x .025".

a b

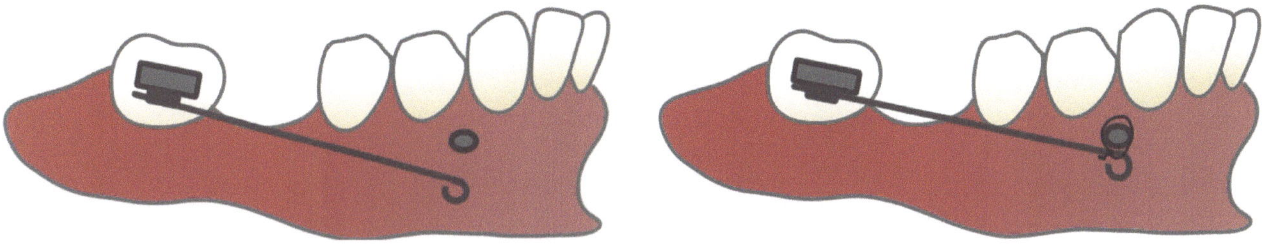

Figure 10.15 Direct anchorage using cantilever. Passive (a), Active (b).

2. *Indirect anchorage*

- The miniscrews used can be conical in shape with 7, 9 or 11 mm in length, 1.3 or 1.6 mm in diameter;

- Immediate loading is employed;
- In cases in which one molar is uprighted, a moment of force of 800g.mm is used;
- For two-molar uprighting, the force used is 1200g.mm;
- Treatment time can vary from 3 to 10 months.

- For indirect anchorage, a segment of .019 x .025" stainless steel wire is positioned on the miniscrew neck and inserted into brackets bonded at the cuspid and the premolars *(Figure 10.16)*;
- The uprighting force is obtained using a cantilever (TMA .017 x .025"). Consisting of a piece of wire with one end inserted into the tube of the molar; the other end of the wire is applied to the reactive unit at a single point of contact;
- In situations in which both intrusion and uprighting of the molar are necessary, a two-cantilever mechanic can be applied (*Figure 10.17*);
- In this case, there is a second cantilever inserted on a criss-cross tube inserted between the first and second premolars and tied to the molar tube activated to exert an intrusion force.

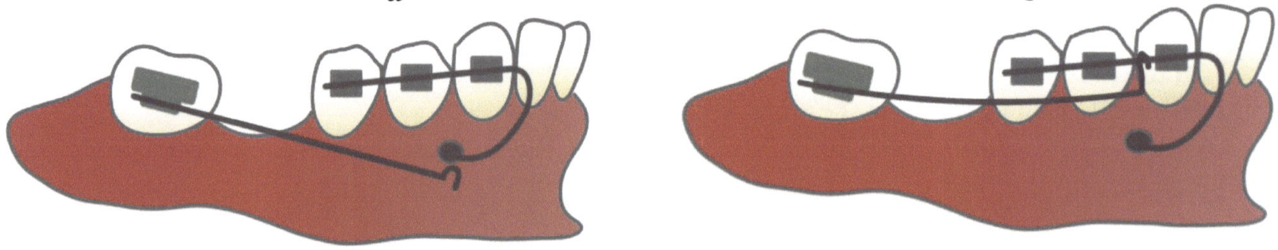

Figure 10.16 Indirect anchorage with cantilever spring. Passive (a), Active (b).

Retention

Once the teeth have been repositioned they must be retained. If a fixed or removable prosthesis is placed on the teeth that have been uprighted then this will provide the long-term retention. There are two methods of intermediate splinting:

1. Extracoronal splinting *(Figure 10.18)*;
- An 0·019 x 0·025 inch wire designed to fit the brackets passively, prevent any tooth movement, and be free of occlusal forces may be used;
- This type of retention should not be used for prolonged periods because orthodontic appliances make effective oral hygiene maintenance difficult.

2. Intracoronal splinting (*Figure 10.19*);
- Shallow cavities are prepared in the abutment teeth and a splint of 0·019 x 0·025 in. wire is secured intracoronally with composite;
- It causes very little gingival irritation and may be left in place for a considerable time.

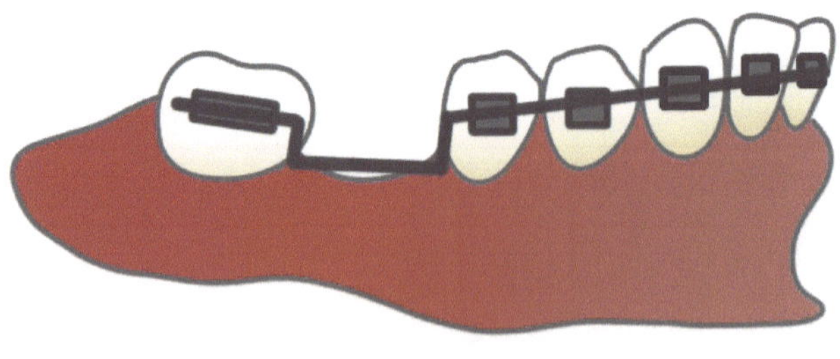

Figure 10.18 Extracoronal splinting

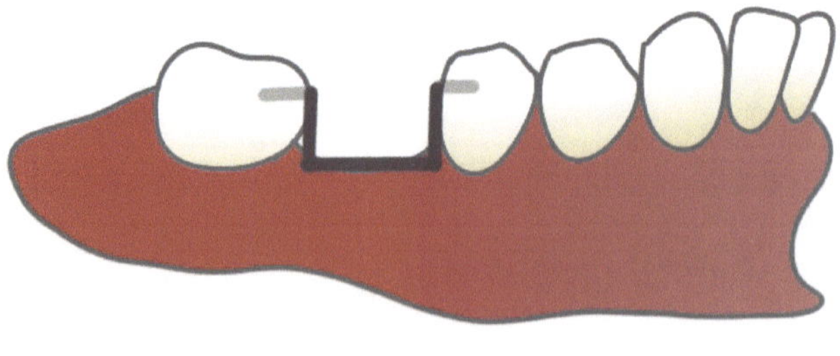

Figure 10.19

References

Adair SM. Pacifier use in children: A review of recent literature. Pediatr Dent 2003;25:449–458.
Ahmad S, Bister D, Cobourne MT. The clinical features and etiological basis of primary eruption failure. Eur J Orthod 2006;28:535–540.
Alqerban A, Jacobs R, Fieuws S, Willems G. Comparison of two cone beam computed tomographic systems versus panoramic imaging for localization of impacted maxillary canines and detection of root resorption. Eur J Orthod 2011;33:93–102.
Bahreman A. Early-Age Orthodontic Treatment. Quintessence Publishing, 2013.
Balshi TJ. Osseointegration and orthodontics: modern treatment for congenitally missing teeth. Int J Periodontics Restorative Dent 1993;13(6),494–505.
Becker A. In defense of the guidance theory of palatal canine displacement. Angle Orthod 1995;65:95–98.
Berkovitz BK. How teeth erupt. Dent Update 1990;17:206– 210.
Bernard JP, Schatz JP, Christou P, Belser U and Kiliaridis S. Longterm vertical changes of the anterior maxillary teeth adjacent to single implants in young and mature adults. A retrospective study. J Clin Periodontal 2004; 31(11), 1024–1028.
Bhat MA, Laway BA, Mantoo S, Choudry K, Kotwal S, Mir SA. Cleidocranial dysplasia: A rare cause of disproportionate severe short stature. Oman Med J 2012;27:408–410.
Biagi R, Butti AC, Salvato A. Premature loss of maxillary primary incisor and delayed eruption of its successor: Report of a case. Eur J Paediatr Dent 2011;12:194–197.
Birte Melsen. Adult Orthodontics. Wiley-Blackwell 2012.
Bishara SE. Impacted maxillary canines: A review. Am J Orthod Dentofacial Orthop 1992;101:159–171.
Bosshardt DD, Schroeder HE. Cementogenesis reviewed: A comparison between human premolars and rodent molars. Anat Rec 1996;245:267–292.
Bruun RA, Hertzberg JL, Tayer BH. Oral habits: Non-nutritive sucking and tongue thrusting. Am Assoc Orthod Orthod Dialogue 1991;4:2–3.
Bryant P, Gale E, Rugh J. Oral Motor Behavior Workshop, 16–17 May 1979 [Report NIH 79-1845]. Bethesda, MD: National Institutes of Health, 1979.
Cinar DN. The advantages and disadvantages of pacifier use. Contemp Nurse 2004;17:109–112.
Da Silva Assunção LR, Ferelle A, Iwakura ML, Cunha RF. Effects on permanent teeth after luxation injuries to the primary predecessors: A study in children assisted at an emergency service. Dent Traumatol 2009;25:165–170.
Dean JA, Avery DR, McDonald RE. Dentistry for the Child and Adolescent, ed 9. St Louis: Mosby, 2010:111.
Dietschi D and Schatz JP. Current restorative modalities for young patients with missing anterior teeth. Quintessence Int 1997; 28(4), 231–240.
Ely NJ, Sherriff M, Cobourne MT. Dental transposition as a disorder of genetic origin. Eur J Orthod 2006;28:145–151.
Frank CA, Long M. Periodontal concerns associated with the orthodontic treatment of impacted teeth. Am J Orthod Dentofacial Orthop 2002;121:639–649.
Frazier-Bowers SA, Simmons D, Koehler K, Zhou J. Genetic analysis of familial non-syndromic primary failure of eruption. Orthod Craniofac Res 2009;12:74–81.
Freilich MA, Niekrash CE, Katz RV and Simonsen RJ. The effects of resin-bonded and conventional

fixed partial dentures on the periodontium: restoration type evaluated. J Am Dent Assoc 1990; 121, 265–269.
Garib DG, Peck S, Gomes SC. Increased occurrence of dental anomalies, associated with second premolar agenesis. Angle Orthod 2009;79:436–441.
Góis EG, Ribeiro-Júnior HC, Vale MP, et al. Influence of nonnutritive sucking habits, breathing pattern and adenoid size on the development of malocclusion. Angle Orthod 2008;78:647–654.
Graber TM, Rakosi T, Petrovic AG. Dentofacial Orthopedics with Functional Appliances, ed 2. St Louis: Mosby, 1997.
Gupta N, Gupta SD, Varshney S, Singh R, Bist SS, Barthwala J. Orthodontic treatment after adenoidectomy patients: Effect on jaw relations in saggital plane. Indian J Otolaryngol Head Neck Surg 2009;61:153–156.
Haas R, Mensdorff-Pouilly N, Mailath G and Watzek G. Branemark single tooth implants: a preliminary report of 76 implants. J Prosthet Dent 1995; 73(3), 247–279.
Hartsfield JK Jr. Premature exfoliation of teeth in childhood and adolescence. Adv Pediatr 1994;41:453–470.
Haselden K, Hobkirk JA, Goodman JR, Jones SP, Hemmings KW. Root resorption in retained deciduous canine and molar teeth without permanent successors in patients with severe hypodontia. Int J Paediatr Dent
Hepper PG, Wells DL, Lynch C. Prenatal thumb sucking is related to postnatal handedness. Neuropsychologia 2005;43:313–315.
Hitchcock S. Endorsing safe infant sleep: A call to action. Nurs Womens Health 2012;16:386–396.
Huber KL, Suri L, Taneja P. Eruption disturbances of the maxillary incisors: A literature review. J Clin Pediatr Dent 2008;32:221–230.
Jacobs SG. The impacted maxillary canine. Further observations on aetiology, radiographic localization, prevention/interception of impaction, and when to suspect impaction. Aust Dent J 1996;41:310–316.
Jeryl D English; Sercan Akyalcin; Timo Peltomaki, Kate Litschel. Mosby's Orthodontic Review. Mosby 2014.
Kinzer GA, Kokich VO Jr. Managing congenitally missing lateral incisors. 3. Single-tooth implants. J Esthet Restor Dent 2005;17:202–210.
Kokich VG and Spear FM. Guidelines for managing the orthodonticrestorative patient. Semin Orthod 1997; 3(1), 3–20.
Kokich VG. Surgical and orthodontic management of impacted maxillary canines. Am J Orthod Dentofacial Or-thop 1980;126:278–283.
Kosowicz J, Rzymski K. Abnormalities of tooth development in pituitary dwarfism. Oral Surg Oral Med Oral Pathol 1977;44:853–863.
Kurol J, Olson L. Ankylosis of primary molars—A future periodontal threat to first permanent molars? Eur J Orthod 1991;13:404–409.
Kurol J,Thilander B. Infraocclusion of primary molars with aplasia of the permanent successor: A longitudinal study. Angle Orthod 1984;54:283–294.
Levy SM, Slager SL, Warren JJ, Levy BT, Nowak AJ. Associations of pacifier use, digit sucking, and child care attendance with cessation of breast feeding. J Fam Pract 2002;51:465.
Linden G. Periodontal destruction and loss of the remaining natural teeth. Commun Dent Oral Epidemiol 1988; 16, 19–21.
Liu JF. Characteristics of premaxillary supernumerary teeth: A survey of 112 cases. ASDC J Dent Child 1995;62: 262–265.
Lygidakis NA, Bafis S, Vidaki E. Case report: Surgical luxation and elevation as treatment approach for secondary eruption failure of permanent molars. Eur Arch Paediatr Dent 2009;10(suppl 1):46–

48.
Lynham A. Panoramic radiographic survey of hypodontia in Australian Defence Force recruits. Aust Dent J 1990;35:19–22.
Maruko E, Hayes C, Evans CA, Padwa B, Mulliken JB. Hypodontia in hemifacial microsomia. Cleft Palate Craniofac J 2001;38:15–19.
Matsumoto MA, Itikawa CE, Valera FC, Faria G, Anselmo-Lima WT. Long-term effects of rapid maxillary expansion on nasal area and nasal airway. Am J Rhinol Allergy 2010;24:161–165.
Mc Cafferty J, Al Awadi E, O'Connell AC. Case report: Management of severe posterior open bite due to primary failure of eruption. Eur Arch Paediatr Dent 2010;11:155–158.
Meiers JC and Freilich MA. Chairside prefabricated fiber-reinforced resin composite fixed partial dentures. Quintessence Int 1999; 32(2), 99–104.
Millar BJ and Taylor NG. Lateral thinking: the management of missing upper lateral incisors. Br Dent J 1995; 179(3), 99–106.
Moimaz SA, Zina LG, Saliba NA, Saliba O. Association between breast-feeding practices and sucking habits: A cross-sectional study of children in their first year of life. J Indian Soc Pedod Prev Dent 2008;26:102–106.
Mostowska A, Kobielak A, Trzeciak WH. Molecular basis of non-syndromic tooth agenesis: Mutations of MSX1 and PAX9 reflect their role in patterning human dentition. Eur J Oral Sci 2003;111:365–370.
Oesterle LJ and Cronin RJ Jr. Adult growth, aging, and the singletooth implant. Int J Oral Maxillofac Implants 2000; 15(2), 252–260.
Olive RJ. Factors influencing the non-surgical eruption of palatally impacted canines. Aust Orthod J 2005;21:95–101.
Ovsenik M. Incorrect orofacial functions until 5 years of age and their association with posterior crossbite. Am J Orthod Dentofacial Orthop 2009;136:375–381.
Pavoni C, Mucedero M, Laganà G, Paoloni V, Cozza P. Impacted maxillary incisors: Diagnosis and predictive measurements. Ann Stomatol (Roma) 2012;3:100–105.
Peck S, Peck L, Kataja M. Concomitant occurrence of canine malposition and tooth agenesis: Evidence of orofacial genetic fields. Am J Orthod Dentofacial Orthop 2002;122:657–660.
Peng CL, Jost-Brinkmann PG, Yoshida N, Miethke RR, Lin CT. Differential diagnosis between infantile and mature swallowing with ultrasonography. Eur J Orthod 2003;25:451–456.
Peterka M, Peterková R, Likovský Z. Timing of exchange of the maxillary deciduous and permanent teeth in boys with three types of orofacial clefts. Cleft Palate Craniofac J 1996;33:318–323.
Peterka M, Tvrdek M, Müllerová Z. Tooth eruption in patients with cleft lip and palate. Acta Chir Plast 1993;35:154– 158.
Peterson JE, Schneider PE. Oral habits: A behavioral approach. Pediatr Clin North Am 1991;38:1289–1307.
Priest GF. Single tooth implants and their role in preserving remaining teeth: a 10-year survival study. Int J Oral Maxillofac Implants 1999; 14(2), 181–188.
Proffit WR, Frazier-Bowers SA. Mechanism and control of tooth eruption: Overview and clinical implications. Orthod Craniofac Res 2009;12:59–66.
Quirynen M, Mongardini C, Lambrechts P, De Geyseleer C, Vanherle G and Van Steenberghe D. A long-term evaluation of compositebonded natural/resin teeth as replacement of lower incisors with terminal periodontitis. J Periodontol 1999; 2, 205–212.
Rada RE (1999) Mechanical stabilization in the mandibular anterior segment. Quintessence Int 30, 243–248.
Richardson G and Russell KA. Congenitally missing maxillary lateral incisor and orthodontic treatment considerations for the singletooth implant. J Can Dent Assoc 2001; 67(1), 25–28.
Robertsson S and Mohlin B. The congenitally missing upper lateral incisor. A retrospective study of

orthodontic space closure versus restorative treatment. Eur J Orthod 2000; 22(6), 697–710.
Romberg E, Wood M, Thompson VP, Morisson GV and Suzuki JB. 10-year periodontal response to resin-bonded bridges. J Periodontol 1995; 66, 973–977.
Salama H and Salama M. The role of orthodontic extrusive remodeling in the enhancement of soft and hard tissue profiles prior to implant placement: a systematic approach to the management of extraction site defects. Int J Periodontics Restorative Dent 1993; 13(4), 312–33.
Samama Y, Lboukili L and Purer R. Predictability of resin-bonded splints in the treatment of pa tients periodontitis: a retrospective study. Perio 2004; 1(3), 227–235.
Samama Y. Fixed bonded prosthodontics: a 10-year follow-up report. Part II: Clinical assessment. Int J Periodontics Restorative Dent 1996; 16(1), 52–59.
Sattur A, Naikmasur VG, Shrivastava R, Babshet M. Familial hypophosphatemic rickets. J Indian Soc Pedod Prev Dent 2010;28:302–306.
Sexton S, Natale R. Risks and benefits of pacifiers. Am Fam Physician 2009;79:681–685.
Shah R, Boyd M. Studies of permanent tooth anomalies in 1,886 Canadian individuals. J Can Dent Assoc 1978;6:265– 268.
Shapira J, Chaushu S, Becker A. Prevalence of tooth transposition, third molar agenesis, and maxillary canine impaction in individuals with Down syndrome. Angle Orthod 2000;70:290–296.
Shapira Y, Kuftinec MM. Early diagnosis and interception of potential maxillary canine impaction. J Am Dent Assoc 1998;129:1450–1454.
Shumaker DB. A comparison of chronologic age and physiologic age as predictors of tooth eruption. Am J Orthod 1974;66:50–57.
Souki BQ, Pimenta GB, Souki MQ, Franco LP, Becker HM, Pinto JA. Prevalence of malocclusion among mouth breathing children: Do expectations meet reality? Int J Pediatr Otorhinolaryngol 2009;73:767–773.
Spear FM, Mathews DM and Kokich VG. Interdisciplinary management of single-tooth implants. Semin Orthod 1997; 3(1), 45–72.
Sridhar Premkumar. Textbook of orthodontics. ELSEVIER 2015.
Stellzig-Eisenhauer A, Decker E, Meyer-Marcotty P, et al. Primary failure of eruption (PFE)—Clinical and molecular genetics analysis. J Orofac Orthop 2010;71:6–16.
Suri L, Gagari E, Vastardis H. Delayed tooth eruption: Pathogenesis, diagnosis, and treatment. A literature review. Am J Orthod Dentofacial Orthop 2004;126:432–445.
Tejasvi MLA, Babu BB. Erupted compound odontomas: A case report. J Dent Res Dent Clin Dent Prospects 2011;5:33–36.
Ten Cate AR. Oral Histology: Development, Structure, and Function, ed 8. St Louis: Mosby-Year Book, 2012.
Thilander B, Odman J, Grondahl K and Friberg B. Osseointegrated implants in adolescents. An alternative in replacing missing teeth? Eur J Orthod 1994; 16(2), 84–95.
Thompson GW, Popovich F. Probability of congenitally missing teeth: Results in 1,191 children in the Burlington Growth centre in Toronto. Community Dent Oral Epidemiol 1974;2:26–32.
Vadiati Saberi B, Shakoorpour A. Apert syndrome: Report of a case with emphasis on oral manifestations. J Dent (Tehran) 2011;8:90–95.
Walker L, Enciso R, Mah J. Three-dimensional localization of maxillary canines with cone-beam computed tomography. Am J Orthod Dentofacial Orthop 2005;128:418–423.
Warford JH Jr, Grandhi RK, Tira DE. Prediction of maxillary canine impaction using sectors and angular measurement. Am J Orthod Dentofacial Orthop 2003;124:651–655.
Weinberger SJ. Correction of bilateral ectopic eruption of first permanent molars using a fixed appliance. Pediatr Dent 1992;14:382–383.
Wise GE. Cellular and molecular basis of tooth eruption. Orthod Craniofac Res 2009;12:67–73.

www.ingramcontent.com/pod-product-compliance
Lightning Source LLC
Chambersburg PA
CBHW041321210926
51847CB00002B/13
9786199164006